Integrated M
Treatment for
Borderline Personality
Disorder

A Practical Guide to Combining Effective Treatment Methods

W. John Livesley
Department of Psychiatry, University of British Columbia

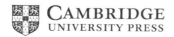
CAMBRIDGE
UNIVERSITY PRESS

CAMBRIDGE
UNIVERSITY PRESS

University Printing House, Cambridge CB2 8BS, United Kingdom

Cambridge University Press is part of the University of Cambridge.

It furthers the University's mission by disseminating knowledge in the pursuit of education, learning and research at the highest international levels of excellence.

www.cambridge.org
Information on this title: www.cambridge.org/9781107679740

© W. John Livesley 2017

First published 2017

Printed in the United Kingdom by Clays, St Ives plc

A catalogue record for this publication is available from the British Library

ISBN 978-1-107-67974-0 Paperback

To my wife Ann, with love

Contents

Preface

This book describes an integrated, evidence-based approach to the treatment of border-line personality disorder. My intention is to state as simply as possible the basic principles needed for comprehensive treatment by trying to strip the treatment of borderline personality disorder to its essentials and describe these essentials in straight-forward, common-sense language that is as free as possible from jargon and unnecessary theoretical speculation. The volume is intended to be read by anyone with an interest in treating borderline personality disorder. Although designed primarily for mental health professionals from all disciplines ranging from those with modest training to seasoned therapists, the volume may also be of interest to informed family members, significant others, and those with the disorder.

For some time now, I have been convinced of the need to radically rethink how borderline personality disorder is treated. The development of effective treatments for this disorder is one of the unheralded successes of contemporary mental health. It is easy to forget that less than a generation ago, it was widely assumed that personality disorder was untreatable. We now know that this is not the case – patients can be helped with appropriate treatment and some improve without. However, we still do not know the optimal way to treat borderline personality disorder, and even after successful treatment, many patients continue to have substantial residual difficulties.

Until the early 1990s, treatment was largely dominated by psychoanalytic therapies, and few empirical studies were available to guide psychotherapists who wanted to pursue evidence-based treatment. The situation has changed dramatically over that last two decades, with the publication of more than half-a-dozen manualized treatments and the emergence of randomized controlled trials testifying to their efficacy. These achievements encouraged the idea that treatment should be based on one of the specialized therapies shown to be effective. I have never found this idea convincing. None of these therapies offers comprehensive coverage of the diverse problems of most patients. Each therapy is based on a theory of the disorder that shapes the treatment methods used. The problem is that most theories focus on a limited aspect of borderline problems and hence current treatments are not comprehensive. Also, each treatment contains effective interventions. Reliance on a single therapy means that many effective methods are not used simply because they are part of a different model. Under these circumstances, it seems more sensible to adopt an eclectic and integrated approach that combines the effective ingredients of all treatments rather than selecting one of them.

Another reason why I find integration appealing is that it makes it easier to tailor treatment to the problems and needs of individual patients. I am struck by the sheer diversity, hetero-geneity, and individuality of the patients I have treated. Although all would have met diagnostic criteria for borderline personality disorder, they differed widely in severity, in how the disorder was manifested, and in other personality characteristics that contributed to the clinical picture. These differences usually had a big effect on treatment. This led me to question the merits of the one-approach-fits-all strategy of manualized and specialized treatments. These considerations led to an interest in how to integrate effective interventions to create a more comprehensive treatment that could be tailored to the differing problems and personalities of my patients.

Although my interest in integration was initially based on the nature of borderline pathology and the conceptual limitations of current therapies, empirical research began to support the idea. Current evidence suggests that the different specialized therapies produce similar results and that they were not substantially better than either good clinical care or supportive therapy. This added new impetus to the idea of a unified trans-theoretical approach and the development of a trans-diagnostic model that could be used to treat all forms of personality disorder. There seems little point in pursuing expensive and highly specialized treatments that do not differ in effectiveness or produce better outcomes than good clinical care or less-expensive supportive therapy. A more effective, and certainly less expensive, strategy would be to integrate interventions that work from all treatments regardless of their theoretical origins.

The framework provided for understanding and treating borderline personality disorder is intended to be used by clinicians with differing degrees of training and experience, including support staff, nurses, social workers, occupational therapists, psychotherapists, clinical and forensic psychologists, and psychiatrists. The framework is also applicable to most treatment settings, including community mental health services, private office practice, hospital inpatient and outpatient services, and the full range of forensic mental health services. Important components of the framework can be implemented by mental health support staff with relatively little professional training given modest instruction and ongoing support. This is important because borderline personality disorder is a relatively common condition and our health care systems cannot afford expensive specialized care delivered by highly trained professionals.

The book is designed to be read in two ways. First, it provides a narrative about how to treat borderline personality disorder using an integrated approach. The narrative begins by describing the nature of the disorder because a nuanced understanding is needed for effective treatment. It then offers a step-by-step description of the treatment process organized around interventions based on mechanisms of change common to all effective treatments. More specific interventions drawn from all effective therapies are then added to this core to address specific problems and impairments. Second, the book is also intended to be a workbook that therapists can dip into and re-read when dealing with a given problem or impairment in their patients. To make the book easier to use in this way, chapters are relatively short, and each deals with a relatively specific issue.

One of the central problems that I have grappled with in writing this book is the very term "borderline personality disorder." I do not like the term and would be happy to see it replaced by something more descriptive. My concerns are three-fold. First, the term "borderline" is commonly used as a pejorative and a stigmatizing label. Second, the term is not descriptive of these patients' problems. Originally, it was used to describe patients who showed features at the borders of psychosis and neurosis. However, this meaning was lost long ago and became meaningless when psychiatric nosology abandoned the concept of neurosis. Third, the term is invariably used to refer to patients who meet the DSM criteria for the diagnosis. However, I find the DSM criteria set inadequate. Since they were originally designed to ensure reliable diagnosis, they tend to focus on the more superficial aspects of the disorder and neglect many of the subtleties and complexities of the condition including the conflicted nature of most patients' experience. Nevertheless, although I do not like the term, I have no doubts about the importance of the problem. There are clearly a large number of patients who show high levels of lability and instability that is disabling and profoundly affects their emotional and interpersonal lives and their sense of self and identity. The question is what term would best capture this constellation of features. Since an alternative is not readily available, I decided regretfully to stick with the traditional term but with the understanding that I am defining it slightly differently from the DSM criteria set, although the two definitions are highly overlapping.

I have many debts and obligations to acknowledge. My overriding debt of gratitude is to the many patients that I have worked with over the years. Borderline personality disorder is not something readily learned from books. We know so little about it that there is little substitute for talking with patients about their experiences, problems, and concerns. I have learned much from such talks and from my patients' remarkable insights into their problems. My patients more than anything or anyone have structured my understanding of borderline personality disorder and its treatment and at different times in the last forty years; the things they have told me have radically changed my thinking.

Since the frameworks described for understanding and treating borderline personality disorder are intended to offer an eclectic and integrated perspective, there is nothing new to the integrated modular approach described. Rather I have drawn extensively on the writings of many authors both on the treatment of personality disorder and on normal and disordered personality, and I need to recognize their contributions. However, in the interests of having a readable text that can be easily referred to when treating specific patients, I decided against have extensive citations in the text and opted instead for endnotes to document my sources with more detailed citations in a references section.

I am also very grateful to the late Richard Marley and his colleagues at Cambridge University Press. I greatly appreciated Richard's support, his patience, and his remarkable tolerance of my somewhat idiosyncratic approach to writing this book. Sadly, Richard died before the project was completed. My children Dawn and Adrian also provided helpful comments on how readable the manuscript was. Finally, but not least, I am enormously grateful to my wife, Ann, who is a wonderful and constant source of support. She has tolerated my obsession with trying to understand personality disorder for many decades and her attentiveness and caring helped ensure the completion of this volume.

Introduction

This book describes a different way to treat borderline personality disorder (BPD). Rather than using one of the manualized treatments developed in recent years, a trans-theoretical approach is proposed that combines principles, strategies, and interventions from all effective treatments. Reluctantly, I decided that a name was needed for this approach and decided on integrated modular treatment (IMT). However, my intention is not to develop yet another therapy described by a three-letter acronym but rather to show how therapists can make use of effective methods from all therapies without adopting either the total treatment package or the underlying theory.

This is not how BPD is currently treated. Treatment is usually based on one or more of the following specialized treatments shown to be effective in randomized controlled trials: dialectical behaviour therapy (DBT), transference-focused therapy (TFT), schema-focused therapy (SFT), mentalizing-based therapy (MBT), cognitive-behavioural therapy (CBT), cognitive-analytic therapy (CAT), and systems training for emotional predictability and problem-solving (STEPPS).[1] Since these treatments do not differ in effectiveness, however, there are no scientific grounds for selecting one approach over another. Nor do they produce better outcomes than good clinical care or supportive therapy. Hence, it may be more effective to combine the effective ingredients of all therapies rather than choose among them.

There are other reasons to pursue integration. Current treatments are not comprehensive: most are based on theories that explain BPD largely in terms of a single impairment, which then becomes the main focus of therapy with other impairments receiving less attention. Thus, DBT considers emotional dysregulation to be the primary problem. MBT assumes that it is impaired mentalizing (difficulty understanding the mental states of self and others). SFT focuses primarily on early maladaptive schemas – beliefs that originated in dysfunctional relationships with significant others during early development. Finally, TFT assumes that problems are largely due to disturbances in the structure of personality. Each explanation has merit: BPD does indeed involve emotional dysregulation, dysfunctional cognitions, impaired mentalizing, and structural problems with personality, but patients do not have just one of these impairments, they have all of them. Hence, a trans-theoretical approach makes more sense.

Current therapies are also limited by the use of "one method fits all patients" approach that neglects the enormous heterogeneity of BPD: patients differ substantially in severity, co-occurring disorders, and coexisting personality characteristics, and these differences impact treatment. This suggests the need for a more patient-focused approach with treatment tailored to needs and psychopathology of individual patients.

This chapter provides a broad overview of an integrated approach. It begins by describing briefly the main features of BPD followed by a discussion of the implications of treatment outcome studies. Finally, it provides an overview of IMT to orientate the reader to the approach.

1.1 Borderline Personality Disorder

BPD occurs in 0.5 to 3.9 per cent (median 1.4 per cent) of the population.[2] Estimates vary because of differences in samples and in definition and assessment methods. Also diagnostic thresholds – the DSM-5 requires the presence of five out of nine criteria – are arbitrary and a different threshold (four or six criteria) would lead to different prevalence rates. Nevertheless, it is obviously a common disorder.

Individuals with BPD tend to have significant health and social problems leading to heavy demands on social and health care services. Interestingly, health problems are not confined to mental health difficulties: BPD is associated with a higher incidence of medical conditions that do not appear to be directly related to the disorder. The condition is also associated with increased mortality. Some of this increase is due to suicide – approximately 9 per cent complete suicide.[3] However, suicide does not totally explain increased mortality – other factors contribute as well, including alcohol and substance misuse.

1.1.1 Major Characteristics

Throughout this book, BPD is conceptualized as a pervasive pattern of instability and dysregulation involving unstable emotions, unstable and conflicted relationships, unstable sense of self or identity, unstable cognitive processes, and behavioural instability that is assumed to result from the interaction of genetic predispositions and multiple environmental influences. The instability is so pervasive and consistent that patients with the disorder have been described as "stably unstable."[4] However, instability is not the only pervasive feature. The disorder is also characterized by intense conflict and equally intense rigidity. The conflict is both external in the form of conflicted relationships and internal in the sense that these patients are often at war with themselves as they struggle with inconsistent feelings and to suppress painful feelings and memories and deny important aspects of their personality and experience. They are also rigid in thought and action. Events are interpreted in relatively fixed ways and it is difficult to change perspective and see things from alternative viewpoints. Their modes of action are also rigid: they persistently respond to situations in the same way despite these responses being unproductive. The features of BPD are described in detail in Chapter 3. It should be noted, however, that the disorder is described a little differently here than in DSM-5 largely because the DSM description is based primarily on committee decisions whereas here greater emphasis is given to research findings.[5]

Emotional dysregulation is a central impairment that influences how other features are expressed. Life for people with BPD is a roller coaster of unstable, intense, and chaotic emotions. Crises are common and typically involve a collage of anxiety, fearfulness, threat, despair, sadness, anger, rage, and shame. Interpersonal problems largely revolve around conflict between strong attachment and dependency needs and fear of abandonment and rejection. This creates unstable relationships because intense neediness leads to an urgent need for contact with significant others when stressed, which then activates fear of rejection. Instability in self or identity is shown by a poorly developed and an unstable sense of self. Many individuals also show a tendency for their thinking to become disorganized when stressed, which may progress to suspiciousness and brief stress-related psychotic episodes. Behavioural instability typically occurs in the context of emotional crises and usually involves deliberate self-harm, suicidality, and sometimes regressive and dissociative behaviours.

1.1.2 Heterogeneity

Although diagnostic systems such as DSM-5 treat all individuals who meet diagnostic guidelines as the same, patients differ extensively in ways that affect outcome and treatment planning. Differences in severity of personality pathology, for example, are more important than the type of disorder in predicting outcome.[6] Severity also influences treatment planning: in general, increasing severity suggests less intense treatment, more modest goals, and greater reliance on supportive methods.

The features of BPD do not occur in isolation but rather in the context of a variety of other personality dispositions that influence treatment both positively and negatively. The co-occurrence of compulsivity, for example, is usually beneficial because it leads to greater diligence in pursuing treatment goals. Traits such as sensation seeking and recklessness, on the other hand, hinder treatment because they involve intolerance of boredom and a craving for excitement that may contribute to interpersonal crises and various maladaptive behaviours. In contrast, social apprehensiveness may hinder the formation of an effective treatment relationship. This suggests that although contemporary therapies neglect heterogeneity, it has important consequences that need to be taken into account when planning and implementing treatment.

1.2 Treatment Outcome

A major achievement in the study of BPD in recent years is the accumulation of evidence that treatment is effective and that the magnitude of outcome change compares favourably with that for other mental disorders. This is a remarkable achievement given the therapeutic nihilism that existed previously.

1.2.1 Results of Outcome Studies

Evidence of the effectiveness of specific therapies is generally taken to imply that evidence-based treatment should use one or more of these therapies. Initially, the idea seemed reasonable because these treatments are more effective than treatment as usual. However, recent research points to a different conclusion for three reasons. First, these therapies do not differ significantly in outcome.[7] One study suggested that SFT is more effective than TFT. However, differences in outcome were small and largely offset by concerns that the quality of therapy was not comparable for the two treatments.[8]

Second, the specialized therapies do not produce better outcomes than good clinical care designed specifically for BPD. Thus far, only DBT, MBT, and CAT[9] have been compared to general care but there is no reason to assume the other specialized therapies would fare better. Also, the fact that these studies involved different therapies and were conducted by different investigators in different countries (Canada, England, and Australia) lends confidence to the robustness of the findings.

Third, the specialized therapies are not better than supportive therapy. One study compared short-term CBT with short-term Rogerian supportive therapy.[10] Although the authors interpreted their findings as indicating that cognitive therapy was more effective, differences were small and unlikely to be clinically significant. More importantly, outcome was poor for both therapies, suggesting that short-term therapy lasting a dozen or so sessions may be unhelpful in treating this disorder. A longer-term study comparing nearly two years of MBT with psychodynamic supportive therapy found few differences[11] despite that fact that the supportive therapy group received only about one-third the amount to therapy as the MBT group. The results are consistent with an earlier study showing that the long-term supportive therapy was as effective as more intensive TFT and DBT.[12]

1.2.2 Implications of Outcome Studies

Outcome studies clearly show that BPD can be treated effectively without using a specialized therapy. They also support an integrated approach: since all effective therapies incorporate treatment methods that work, a more rational strategy is to combine the effective components of all therapies rather than use a single therapy and thereby fail to use effective components of other methods. Integration is particularly pertinent given the limited focus of most specialized therapies: although individually none of the specialized therapies address all features of BPD, when taken together they cover most impairments. This has prompted suggestions that combinations of these therapies should be used – common suggestions are DBT and MBT, and DBT and TFT. However, this is a cumbersome and expensive option. It would be simpler and less confusing to select interventions that work from all approaches without trying to combine the different theories and concepts on which these therapies are based.[13]

The rationale for trans-theoretical treatment is further strengthened by evidence that similar outcome across treatments arises from change mechanisms common to all effective therapies. Evaluations of these mechanisms[14] point to the importance of such factors as a structured approach, a collaborative therapeutic relationship, an empathic and validating stance, and a consistent treatment process that facilitates motivation for change and encourages self-reflection. These are the kinds of factors emphasized in treatments based on good clinical care that were used to evaluate the effectiveness of the specialized therapies. Since these general factors account for most of outcome change, it seems most appropriate to organize evidence-based treatment around generic mechanisms.

Nevertheless, each specialized therapy contains interventions specific to that approach that probably contribute to their effectiveness. We cannot be sure because current studies do not provide information on the mechanisms responsible for positive outcomes. However, the need to use a comprehensive set of interventions that address all components of BPD suggests that IMT should also include an eclectic array of specific treatment methods.

1.3 What Is Integrated Modular Treatment?

IMT is a patient-focused, evidence-based approach to treating BPD (and other personality disorders) that uses a broad array of treatment principles and methods selected to meet the needs and problems of the individual. The term "integration" is widely used: proponents of most therapies commonly claim that their approach is integrated even though it relies on a limited conceptual model. When used in this way, the term usually means that the therapy in question also uses interventions used by other treatments. In practice, most experienced therapists are integrative in this sense: they use interventions from various therapies that they have found useful even though they primarily subscribe to a particular school. IMT simply takes what expert therapists do a step further by using an eclectic combination of interventions selected on the basis of effectiveness and relevance for treating a given problem.

However, integration in IMT goes beyond adopting a trans-theoretical approach. Integration is also a treatment goal. BPD involves not only unstable emotions and relationships but also difficulty integrating experiences, thoughts, feelings, and actions and constructing a coherent sense of self. Hence, a central treatment task is to foster more integrated and coherent personality functioning.

The second term warranting explanation is "modular." This refers to the fact that treatment uses of an array of modules, each consisting of a set of inter-related strategies and interventions that seek to establish a particular treatment process (e.g., the treatment alliance) or target a specific impairment (e.g., unstable emotions). Based on the analyses of outcome studies, IMT uses two kinds of intervention modules: (i) general intervention modules that implement common change principles and (ii) specific intervention modules based on strategies and interventions selected from all treatments to treat specific impairments. This modular structure permits individualized therapy.

1.4 The Structure of Integrated Modular Treatment

The evidence indicates that treatment is most effective when based on a clearly defined model that specifies how therapy is organized and delivered.[15] This principle led to the development of two conceptual frameworks for IMT that describe the nature of BPD and the structure and process of treatment, respectively.

1.4.1 Framework for Describing Borderline Personality Disorder

The framework for understanding BPD, described in detail in Chapters 2–4 (see Box 1.1), is used to organize clinical information, plan treatment, and select interventions.[16] It is also intended to provide a framework for teaching patients about their disorder. Patients are often puzzled about why they are so upset, which adds to their distress and makes psychoeducation a necessary part of treatment.

The framework has three components. The first is based on the idea that personality is a complex system with multiple interacting components: traits, regulation and modulation mechanisms that control the expression of emotions and impulses, interpersonal structures, and self/identity. BPD affects all parts of the system. This idea is used to organize the multiple features of BPD into four domains of problems and impairments (see Chapter 2):

1. Symptoms: anxiety, fearfulness, emotional distress, rapid mood changes, self-harming behaviour, quasi-psychotic symptoms, dissociative behaviour
2. Regulation: impaired emotional control, tendency to act with a sense of urgency leading to self-harming behaviour

BOX 1.1   The Structure of Integrated Modular Treatment

I. Framework for Describing Borderline Personality Disorder

1. Personality as a complex system involving the trait, regulation and modulation, interpersonal, and self subsystems that give rise to four domains of impairment:
   a. Symptoms
   b. Regulation and modulation
   c. Interpersonal
   d. Self
2. Two-component structure:
   a. Core features common to all personality disorders:
      i. Interpersonal problems:
         - Inability to establish lasting intimate attachment relationships
      ii. Self problems:
         - Poorly developed sense of self
         - Unstable and fragmented self system
   b. Emotional dependency constellation of traits:
      i. Emotional traits:
         - Anxiousness
         - Emotional lability
      ii. Interpersonal traits:
         - Insecure attachment
         - Submissive dependency
         - Need for approval
      iii. Cognitive traits:
         - Cognitive dysregulation
3. Origins and development:
   a. Biological:
      i. Genetic predispositions
      ii. Other biological factors
   b. Psychosocial: clinically important factors
      i. Attachment problems
      ii. Invalidating environments

4. Clinical consequences of aetiological and developmental factors:
   a) Impaired regulation and modulation mechanisms
   b) Maladaptive schemas
   c) Maladaptive cognitive processes
   d) Core interpersonal conflict
   e) Distress without resolution
   f) Self system problems
   g) Conflict and functional incoherence

3. Interpersonal: attachment insecurity, submissive-dependent behaviours, conflicted and unstable relationships; maladaptive interpersonal relationships; maladaptive interpersonal beliefs

4. Self-Identity: boundary problems, poorly developed sense of self, unstable self and identity structure, maladaptive self-narrative, maladaptive self-schemas (e.g., "I am unlovable"), and problems with self-directedness.

Domains organize a patient's diverse impairments in a way that facilitates treatment planning and delivery. In general, each domain is treated with a different set of specific intervention modules. For example, symptoms may be treated with medication, and specific cognitive interventions and problems in the regulation domain are best treated with cognitive-behavioural modules that enhance skills in self-regulating emotions such as emotion recognition, distress tolerance, and attention control.

The second component of the framework is based on the idea that any personality disorder is best understood for diagnostic purposes as having two components: (i) *core features* common to all forms of personality disorder and (ii) a *constellation of traits* that differentiates a given disorder such as borderline from other personality disorders (see Chapter 3). This distinction reflects a current trend in the diagnostic classification to distinguish the features of general personality disorder from the traits that differentiate the various kinds of disorder. The features common to all personality disorders are chronic interpersonal dysfunction and an impaired sense of self and identity. With BPD, these core features are expressed as difficulty in establishing lasting intimate, attachment relationships and problems establishing a stable and coherent sense of self or identity.

Three kinds of traits define BPD: (i) emotional traits such as emotional lability and anxiousness, which give rise to unstable emotions and moods; (ii) interpersonal traits such as insecure attachment, submissiveness, and need for approval/fear of disapproval, which give rise to the conflict between neediness and fear of abandonment and rejection; and (iii) cognitive dysregulation – the tendency for thinking to become disorganized when stressed, which may progress to quasi-psychotic symptoms and dissociation. Interaction among these traits gives rise to the various kinds of instability described earlier.

The third component of the framework is a description of the origins and development of BPD and their implications for treatment (Chapter 4). Finally, an understanding of the lasting effects of adversity is used to define major impairments that are likely to be encountered in treatment and some of the major treatment strategies of IMT.

1.4.2 Framework for Organizing Treatment

IMT has two main components: (i) intervention modules and (ii) a stage model of how personality pathology changes during therapy (see Box 1.2). As noted earlier, intervention modules consist of *general treatment modules* based on change mechanisms common to all effective therapies and *specific treatment modules* consisting of interventions drawn from the various specialized therapies that target specific problems and impairments. The distinction between general and specific modules is important. General modules form the basic structure of treatment: they are used with all patients throughout treatment whereas specific modules vary according to the needs of individual patients and the problems that are the focus of therapeutic effort at any given moment.

This distinction implies a hierarchy of interventions. Priority is given to interventions needed to ensure safety of the patient and others.[17] Once safety is assured, general treatment

---

BOX 1.2   The Structure of Integrated Modular Treatment

II. Framework for Organizing Treatment
1. Treatment modules:
   a. General treatment modules:
      i. Structure: establish a structured treatment process
      ii. Relationship: build a collaborative working relationship
      iii. Consistency: maintain a consistent treatment process
      iv. Validation: establish a validating treatment process
      v. Self-reflection: increase self-knowledge and self-reflection
      vi. Motivation: build and maintain a commitment to change
   b. Specific modules:
      i. Crisis modules
      ii. Regulation and modulation modules
      iii. Interpersonal modules
      iv. Self modules
2. Phases of change:
   a. Safety: primary focus on the symptom domain
   b. Containment: primary focus on the symptom domain
   c. Regulation and modulation: primary focus on the symptom and regulation and modulation domain
   d. Exploration and change: primary focus on the interpersonal domain
   e. Integration and synthesis: primary focus on the self and identify domain and on building a satisfying life

---

methods are used to engage the patient in therapy, build an effective alliance, and establish conditions for change. When these conditions are met, specific interventions are used as needed to treat the problem at hand. This is an important practice point: specific interventions are only used when there is a good treatment relationship and a motivated patient. The only exceptions are when action is needed to ensure safety and when medication is indicated to address an immediate problem.

The second component of the treatment framework, the *phases of change model*, proposes that treatment progresses though five phases: (i) safety, (ii) containment, (iii) regulation and modulation, (iv) exploration and change, and (v) integration and synthesis. Each phase addresses a different domain of borderline pathology. Hence each phase involves the use of a different set of specific intervention modules.

1.4.2.1 General Treatment Modules

Generic strategies and interventions are organized into six general treatment modules: (i) structure, (ii) treatment relationship, (iii) consistency, (iv) validation, (v) self-reflection, and (vi) motivation. The first four modules are primarily concerned with establishing the within-therapy conditions necessary for change whereas the last two modules are more concerned with establishing the within-patient conditions needed for change to occur. The following section provides a broad overview of these strategies (Chapters 7–12 describe each module in detail).

Module 1: Establish a Structured Treatment Process: All effective treatments for BPD emphasize the importance of a structured process based on an explicit treatment model and a well-defined treatment frame consisting of the therapeutic stance and treatment contract. The stance refers to the interpersonal behaviours, attitudes, responsibilities, and activities that determine how the therapist relates to the patient. Based on current evidence, IMT adopts a supportive, empathic, and validating stance.[18] A key ingredient of structure is the therapeutic contract established prior to treatment that defines collaborative treatment goals and the practical arrangements for therapy.

Module 2: Establish and Maintain a Collaborative Treatment Relationship: If there is an essential ingredient to successful treatment, it is the establishment of a collaborative working relationship between the patient and the therapist. This is given priority because a collaborative relationship provides support, builds motivation, and predicts outcome. With most patients with BPD, it takes time and effort to build a truly collaborative relationship: in many ways collaboration is more the result of effective treatment than a prerequisite for treatment.

Module 3: Maintain a Consistent Treatment Process: Effective outcomes also depend on maintaining a consistent treatment process. Consistency is defined simply as adherence to the frame of therapy. This is why the treatment contract is so important: it provides a frame of reference that helps the therapist to monitor treatment and identify deviations from the frame by either the patient or the therapist. Violations of the frame are relatively common when treating BPD and it is important that they are addressed promptly and supportively.

Module 4: Promote Validation: Validation is defined as recognition, acceptance, and affirmation of the patient's mental states and experiences. Validating interventions make an important contribution to treatment by providing the empathy and support needed to build a collaborative alliance. At the same time, they counter the self-invalidating way of thinking, which is often instilled by invalidating developmental experiences.

Module 5: Enhance Self-Knowledge and Self-Reflection: Most therapies encourage patients to develop a better understanding of how they think, feel, and act, and become more aware of the links between their mental states and problem behaviour. The extent and depth of self-knowledge and self-understanding depend on self-reflection: the capacity to think about and understand one's own mental states and those of others. Impaired self-reflection hinders the development of important aspects of the self that are constructed by reflecting in depth on one's own mental processes. Self-reflection also underlies the capacity for self-regulation and effective goal-directed action.

Module 6: Build and Maintain Motivation for Change: A second within-patient factor necessary for effective outcomes is motivation of change. Patients need to be motivated to seek help and work consistently on their problems. Unfortunately, passivity and low motivation are common consequences of psychosocial adversity. For this reason, motivation cannot be a requirement for treatment. Instead, therapists need to become skilled in building motivation and to make extensive use of motivation-enhancing techniques.

Implementation of the general modules means that treatment is organized around a strong therapeutic relationship characterized by support, empathy, consistency, and validation. Priority is given to the relationship due to the serious problems most patients have experienced with attachment relationships and their consistent difficulties with interpersonal relationships. The objective is to establish a treatment process that provides a continuous corrective therapeutic experience to counter the lasting effects of psychosocial adversity. This is an important aspect of therapy: change is brought about not only by interventions of one kind or another but also by the way therapy is organized and delivered.

Phases of Change Model: The overall course of treatment is divided into safety, containment, regulation and modulation, exploration and change, and integration and synthesis phases that are used to guide the use of specific intervention modules. A challenge for integrated treatment is how to coordinate the use of specific interventions so as to avoid confusion arising from the use of multiple interventions. The phases of change model reduces this problem because each phase addresses a different domain of impairment and hence requires different specific intervention modules. Thus the model describes the sequence in which problems are addressed and specific interventions are used with a general progression from more-structured to less-structured methods.

The first two phases, safety and containment, primarily deal with the symptom domain. The third phase, control and modulation, continues the focus on symptom resolution but deals primarily with emotional dysregulation and associated suicidal and self-harming behaviour. Phase four, exploration and change, focuses primarily on the interpersonal domain using a diverse array of interventions, and phase five, integration and synthesis, deals with the self/identity domain.

The sequence for addressing domains partly reflects the clinical priority given to symptoms including suicidality and self-harm and partly the degree to which problems associated with a given domain are amenable to change. In general, the sequence of symptoms, regulation and modulation, interpersonal, and self/identity reflects increasing stability and resistance to change.

Phase 1. Safety: When treatment begins with the patient in a decompensated crisis state, the immediate concern is to ensure the safety of the patient and others. This is largely achieved by providing structure and support that may be delivered through outpatient treatment and a crisis intervention service, or occasionally through brief in-patient treatment. Interventions are largely generic and non-specific – providing the support and structure as needed to keep the patient safe until the crisis resolves – although medication may also be used with some patients.

Phase 2. Containment: The brief safety phase usually gives way quickly to containment where the goal is to contain and settle emotional and behavioural instability and restore behavioural control. The objectives are to return the patient to the pre-crisis level of functioning as quickly as possible and lay the foundation for further treatment. As with the previous phase, change is achieved through support, empathy, and structure, supplemented if necessary with medication.

Phase 3. Regulation and Control: Crisis resolution and increased stability are usually accompanied by an improved treatment relationship. This makes it possible to begin focusing on improving emotional dysregulation and reducing symptoms including deliberate self-harm, suicidality, and the consequences of trauma. Specific interventions are used to: (i) provide psychoeducation about emotions and emotional dysregulation; (ii) increase awareness, acceptance, and tolerance of emotions; (iii) improve emotion regulation; and (iv) enhance the capacity to process emotions. Emphasis is placed on cognitive-behavioural interventions because of evidence of the effectiveness of these interventions in reducing deliberate self-harm and increasing emotion-regulating skills.[19]

However, skill development is not considered sufficient: it is also important to improve the ability to process emotions more adaptively. Although cognitive-behavioural interventions are also useful for this purpose, they usually need to be supplemented with methods that help patients to construct meaningful narratives about their emotional life. Inevitably, this work begins to involve interpersonal impairments linked to intense emotions and hence treatment gradually moves to the next phase.

Phase 4. Exploration and Change: The focus of this phase is to explore and change those aspects of personality that underlie symptoms and dysregulated emotions, especially interpersonal problems. Particular attention is given initially to self and interpersonal schemas associated with emotional instability and deliberate self-harm. This focus gradually extends to the core interpersonal conflict between neediness and fear of abandonment and rejection and the interpersonal experiences that contributed to the development of this conflict. Discussion of these problems usually generates considerable distress, which is why consistent work on these themes is deferred if possible until emotion regulation increases and the patient is able to tolerate the stress involved. Change is achieved through the continued use of cognitive interventions to explore and restructure maladaptive schemas, but these usually need to be supplemented with methods drawn from interpersonal and psychodynamic therapy. During this phase, the treatment relationship becomes a major vehicle for examining and restructuring interpersonal schemas involving distrust, rejection, abandonment, self-derogation, and shame forged by early adversity. At the same time, the relationship with therapist provides the patient with a new interpersonal experience that challenges many of the maladaptive schemas that have shaped their interpersonal lives.

Phase 5. Integration and Synthesis: The final phase of treatment deals primarily with the self/identity domain. Broadly speaking, the goal is to help patients to "get a life" – to develop a more adaptive life script, create a more satisfying and rewarding way of living, and acquire greater purpose and direction to their lives. Although only a few patients reach this stage, all patients need help with building a more congenial lifestyle to help them to maintain changes made in treatment. Throughout treatment, therapists need to be mindful of the importance of helping patients to construct a personal niche that allows them to express their personal aspirations, talents, interests, and traits and avoid situations and relationships that activate vulnerabilities and conflicts. Nevertheless, the formulation of a more adaptive sense of identity is largely achieved in the latter part of treatment when more distressing problems move to resolution. The development of a more coherent self-structure is often difficult to achieve and there is little empirical research to help identify effective strategies. However, consistent application of the general therapeutic strategies creates a treatment environment that challenges core schemas and promotes self-understanding by providing consistent and veridical feedback. Narrative methods also seem useful in building a more adaptive self story.[20]

1.5 The Other Ingredient of Integrated Modular Treatment

Thus far the focus has been on the structure of therapy – what to do and when. However, there is another aspect of therapy that is just as important: what might be referred to as the tone of therapy. What matters is not just what therapists do but how they do it. This is more nebulous and difficult to describe. It is captured in part by the emphasis on an empathic, supportive, and validating therapeutic stance. But this is only part of what matters. Other features of the therapeutic interaction that therapists need to create are the following: respect, compassion, acceptance, attentiveness, involvement, and empathic attunement. These features characterize a treatment process that offers new experiences to challenge old ways of interacting with the interpersonal world. We need to get this part of therapy right: technical competence may be necessary but it is not sufficient.

1.6 Comment

The IMT framework is designed to provide the structure needed to deliver the cohesive and consistent treatment needed for successful outcomes while also being sufficiently flexible to allow therapists to tailor treatment to their specific style, patient need, treatment setting, and the modality of treatment delivery. Consequently, the principles of IMT are relevant to short-term crisis intervention lasting at most a few months; medium-term treatment lasting perhaps a year or so, which is primarily concerned with increasing emotion regulation and decreasing self-harming behaviour; and long-term treatment lasting several years, which is intended to change interpersonal patterns and promote more integrated personality functioning.

Notes

1. For treatment manuals and descriptions of these therapies, see: DBT (Linehan, 1993), TFT (Clarkin et al., 1999), SFT (Young et al., 2003), MBT (Bateman and Fonagy, 2004, 2006), CBT (Beck et al., 1990, 2004; Davidson, 2008), CAT (Ryle, 1997), and STEPPS (Blum et al., 2012). The randomly controlled studies supporting these treatments include: DBT (Linehan et al., 1991, 1993), TFT (Clarkin et al., 2007; Doering et al., 2010; Levy et al., 2006), SFT (Bamelis et al., 2014; Giesen-Bloo et al., 2006), MBT (MBT, Bateman and Fonagy, 1999, 2000, 2001, 2008, 2013), CBT (Davidson et al., 2006), CAT (Chanen et al., 2008), and STEPPS (Black et al., 2004; Blum et al., 2002, 2008).

2. The prevalence estimates noted are for the DSM-IV/DSM-5 diagnosis (see Morgan and Zimmerman, in press). Estimates for DSM-III-R diagnoses differ slightly. See also review by Torgensen (2012).

3. Paris et al. (1987); Paris and Zweig-Frank (2001).

4. Schmideberg (1947).

5. The trait component of BPD as described in this volume is based on empirical studies of personality disorder traits. This means that although there is substantial overlap between the way BPD is described here and in DSM-IV/DSM-5, there are several differences. First, the DSM criterion of affective lability is divided here into emotional lability and anxiousness to reflect the results of empirical studies. Second, the criterion describing a pattern of unstable and intense relationships is replaced by a description of a core conflict between neediness and fear of rejection because this captures the core interpersonal problem associated with BPD better. This conflict is not referenced in the DSM criteria although it is central to understanding the interpersonal behaviour of these patients. Third, here reference is also made to the dependent-submissive features of these patients, which are often expressed in a hostile-dependent way. These differences are reflected in treatment strategies that target behaviours that are not included in the DSM criteria set. However, the approach described is equally applicable to treating BPD diagnosed on the basis of DSM criteria.

6. Crawford et al. (2011), Verheul et al. (2008), Tyrer and Johnson (1996), Hopwood et al. (2011).

7. See reviews by Bartak et al. (2007), Budge et al. (2014), Leichsenring and Leibing (2003), Leichsenring et al. (2011), and Piper and Joyce (2001).

8. This outcome study by Giesen-Bloo et al. (2006) reported differences between SFT and TFT. However, these differences were relatively small and largely offset by concerns that the quality of therapy was not comparable across the two treatments (Yeomans, 2007).

9. Three specialized therapies compared with good clinical care are: DBT (McMain et al., 2009) MBT (Bateman and Fonagy, 2009), and CAT (Chanen et al., 2008; Clarke et al., 2013).

10. Cottraux et al. (2009).

11. Jorgensen et al. (2013), despite that fact that the supportive therapy group received only about one-third the amount of therapy as the MBT group: one 90-minute group session every two weeks versus 90 minutes of group treatment and 45 minutes of individual therapy each week.

12. The results of this study are also consistent with an earlier study showing that the long-term supportive therapy was as effective as that of more intensive TFT and DBT (Clarkin et al., 2007).

13. Livesley (2012).

14. Castonguay and Beutler (2006b).

15. Critchfield and Benjamin (2006).

16. This framework is an extension and elaboration of the model described in Livesley (2003), and the box modifies the general model described by Livesley and Clarkin (2015a) to treat BPD.

17. Most therapies prioritize interventions required to ensure safety (see Linehan, 1993; Clarkin et al., 1999).

18. Livesley (2003).

19. Randomized controlled trials of treatments such as DBT (Linehan et al., 1991), STEPPS (Blum et al., 2008), and CBT (Davidson et al., 2006; Evans et al., 1999) demonstrate the effectiveness of cognitive-behavioural interventions in treating deliberate self-harm and emotional dysregulation. In addition, evidence suggests that specific problem behaviours are best treated directly with cognitive-behavioral interventions (see Lipsey, 1995, 2009).

20. See for example, cognitive analytic therapy developed by Ryle (1997).

Chapter 2

Understanding Normal and Disordered Personality

This chapter begins to develop a framework for understanding borderline personality disorder (BPD) by describing the structure of normal personality and how this structure is impaired in BPD. However, first I am going to introduce the case of Anna, which will be used throughout the book to illustrate assessment, treatment planning, and intervention strategies. Here the case is used to discuss the range of problems and psychopathology seen in BPD.

2.1 The Case of Anna

Anna was 36 years old, married with three children, when she was assessed following a brief hospital stay due to a serious drug overdose. Anna said that the overdose was triggered by a fight with her husband that caused intense distress and she became afraid that he would leave her. Feeling overwhelmed and unable to cope, she took an overdose. Such crises were common and she had several previous admissions for self-harming behaviour. Most of the time her feelings were "all over the place," and she felt depressed and persistently worried "about every little thing." Although, there were times when she wondered if these feelings were real. She also had uncontrollable rages, especially with her husband. She also had chronic thoughts of suicide.

Anna's upbringing was characterized by family dysfunction, physical and emotional abuse, and childhood sexual abuse. Her marriage was unstable. She and her husband fought constantly and he was emotionally abusive. The relationship was typical of many previous relationships. Anna commented that she always seemed attracted to the wrong kind of men but she was unable to leave her husband because she did not have the financial resources. She later explained that she was also afraid to live alone and that she was terrified of being abandoned and needed to feel loved. As a result, she became very dependent on the men she was involved with. Currently, she was afraid of being abandoned and constantly sought her husband's reassurance that he would not leave. This fear caused her to submit readily to his demands and go out of her way to placate him.

Anna had few friends and she felt uncomfortable with people because she worried that they found her uninteresting. This was a problem because she was easily bored and needed company. Despite this need for excitement, Anna also had mild obsessional traits – she liked things to be tidy and organized. Anna had no real plans for her life apart from caring for her children. She noted that she had always drifted through life unsure about herself and what she really wanted.

Anna's multiple problems included symptoms such as anxiety, suicidality, unstable emotions, interpersonal problems, maladaptive traits, and self/identity problems. To treat this array of problems, it is not sufficient simply to diagnose BPD based on DSM-5 criteria. Instead, we need a scheme that would help us to make sense of her diverse problems and organize them in a systematic way that can be used to plan treatment, select interventions, and help Anna to develop a new understanding of her life and circumstances. This chapter begins to develop such a framework by describing the main features of normal personality. Although this may seem an unusual starting point because most conceptions of BPD pay little attention to normal personality, it reflects the assumption that we cannot fully understand personality disorder without understanding normal personality, much as a cardiologist cannot understand heart problems without knowledge of the normal cardiovascular system. Also, as I hope to show, knowledge of normal personality can enrich our understanding of BPD and guide treatment strategies.

2.2 The Normal Personality System

We can begin imposing structure onto Anna's problems by thinking of personality as a complex system of interacting components.[1] This idea is useful because it forces us to think about personality as a whole rather than a list of criteria and about how Anna's problems interact with each other. We need to do this to achieve the integrated modular treatment (IMT) goal of promoting more integrated personality functioning. Four components or subsystems of personality are important in understanding the clinical features of BPD: (i) the regulatory and modulatory system used to manage emotions and impulses; (ii) the trait system; (iii) the interpersonal system; and (iv) the self system (see Figure 2.1). The self and interpersonal systems overlap more than other systems because both are

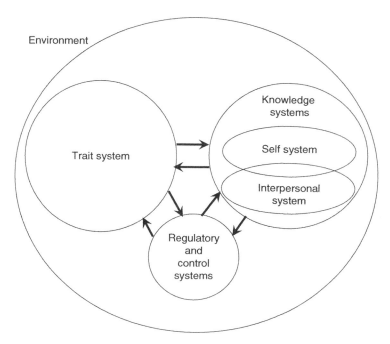

Figure 2.1 The Personality System

influenced by the same developmental experiences. Both are essentially knowledge systems that store and process slightly different domains of information.

Anna's problems encompass all subsystems. Besides symptoms such as anxiety, suicidality, and deliberate self-injury, her personality problems include difficulty in self-regulating emotions and impulses, maladaptive traits such as emotional lability and insecure attachment, interpersonal difficulties including attachment and intimacy problems, and a poorly developed sense of self or identity. Before discussing the personality subsystems in detail, I need to introduce another idea that is fundamental to the conceptual framework of IMT: that each personality subsystem consists of cognitive structures that are used to organize information, interpret experience, and guide action.

2.3 The Cognitive Structure of Personality

The various theories of BPD describe these cognitive structures using terms such as "schemas," "early maladaptive schemas," "object relationships," and "working models." Despite the different labels, all theories share the idea that these cognitive structures are the basic units of personality and that treatment is largely concerned with restructuring them.

Despite this commonality, theories differ in one important respect – whether these constructs are purely cognitive in nature, as assumed by cognitive-behavioural therapy (CBT), or whether they also have an emotional component as assumed by object relationship theory; object relationships are considered cognitive and emotional representations of the characteristic relationships established between self and others. Here, these fundamental units of personality will be referred to as personality schemas or schemas for brevity. The term "schema" is used because it has a long tradition in psychology and cognitive science. In IMT, schemas are considered cognitive-emotional personality systems – constellations of related ideas, expectations, memories, and emotions. The emotional component is integral to the concept, and emotions are assumed to play an important role in schema activation and expression. Hence the concept of schema as used in IMT differs from that used in cognitive therapy.

The brief account of Anna's problems suggests that she has a wide variety of maladaptive schemas involving attachment and dependency needs, rejection fears, submissiveness and the need to placate others, the importance of order and structure, ideas about risk-taking and excitement-seeking, and so on.

The personality schema is an important trans-theoretical construct that is assumed to be the basic building block of the trait, regulatory, interpersonal, and self systems. The idea that schemas are basic to our interpersonal and self systems is probably readily understandable – in everyday life we use a wide range of constructs to describe ourselves and others. The idea that schemas are also integral to traits and regulatory mechanisms may be less obvious but this will be discussed later.

Several aspects of schemas are important to bear in mind when treating BPD. First, schemas are both "frames" and "cages."[2] Like a lens, schemas frame and colour our understanding of the world. However, schemas can also cage us in, forcing us into rigid ways of looking at ourselves and others and hence to stereotyped behaviours. Inflexibility is common in people with BPD: they have a limited repertoire of schemas that they use in fixed ways. This is illustrated by the rigid way that Anna's intense sensitivity to abandonment influenced how she perceived and understood the relationships that dominated her life.

Second, people differ in the number of schemas they have. Generally, the more schemas we have, the more adaptive our behaviour, because we have more options in how we construe and respond to events. Having too few schemas limits our understanding of ourselves and others. This is a problem with people with BPD – many have relatively few schemas. Hence their understanding of self and others is often limited. Third, schemas differ in importance. Some are core constructs that play a central role in how we perceive and react to events and how we think about ourselves and others, whereas others are more peripheral and have less influence on our actions.

Fourth, schemas are organized into systems such as the trait, regulatory, interpersonal, and self-schemas. Within each subsystem, schemas are further organized into more specific systems. In the case of the trait system, schemas are organized around individual traits and they influence the way the trait is expressed. Within the self system, self-schemas are organized into different images of the self. Similarly, interpersonal schemas are organized into different representations of others.

The richness of connections among schemas is important: the more extensive the interconnections among schemas, the greater the integration and flexibility of the overall structure. Peripheral schemas have relatively few connections with other schemas, whereas core schemas have extensive linkages with other schemas. Consequently, core schemas are more difficult to change and any change is usually anxiety provoking. For example, Anna's abandonment schemas had extensive connections with multiple interpersonal and self-schemas. As a result, they were frequently activated by interpersonal events, and they structured many of her interactions with others and defined important aspects of her sense of self.

Given the important role schemas play in all aspects of personality functioning, I will discuss in detail the schemas associated with different personality subsystems and how schemas are shaped by developmental experiences. The central role of schemas means that a general treatment task is to help patients to recognize and restructure maladaptive schemas across the different subsystems of personality and to understand how these schemas are linked to symptoms and recurrent problems. However, this is not the whole story. As we will see later, schemas are also used to construct narratives that give meaning and structure to our experience. Thus an important part of therapy is also to help patients construct more adaptive narratives about all aspects of their experience. But now we return to exploring the subsystems of personality with the concept of personality schema in mind as an integrative construct.

2.4 Trait System

It is convenient to begin describing the personality system with traits because traits are familiar concepts that are useful in describing clinically important differences among patients; this is because traits have a major influence on adjustment, health, and well-being, and on the development of other personality structures. Traits are enduring characteristics that change little after early adulthood. They are also universal characteristics – like height and weight, they apply to everyone although to different degrees. Hence the traits delineating BPD are the same as those that characterize normal personality, although they differ in degree and how they are expressed.

2.4.1 Trait Structure in Normal and Disordered Personality

Empirical studies suggest that normal traits are organized into five main clusters – the Big Five – consisting of (i) neuroticism (anxiousness, dependency, self-consciousness, and vulnerability); (ii) extraversion (active, outgoing, and sociable); (iii) openness to experience (imaginative, curious, open to ideas, and artistic); (iv) agreeableness (straightforward, compliant, cooperative, and tender-minded); and (v) conscientiousness (orderliness, dutifulness, dependability, and self-discipline).[3]

Personality disorder traits are organized similarly although only four clusters are usually identified: (i) emotional dependency, (ii) dissocial or antisocial, (iii) social avoidance, and (iv) compulsivity.[4] Openness to experience is not found in studies of personality disorder traits probably because it does not directly affect the development of personality pathology. Table 2.1 lists the main traits defining each cluster based on studies of the phenotypic and genetic structure of personality.[5]

The emotional-dependent cluster consisting of emotional lability, anxiousness, insecure attachment, submissive dependency, need for approval, and cognitive dysregulation will be used to describe BPD traits because it provides a more detailed and clinically useful description of the disorder than the global DSM-5 diagnosis. Also, the four-factor structure is supported by extensive evidence and hence its use is consistent with the evidence-based focus of IMT. This cluster of traits will be described in detail in Chapter 3. However, it is also important to evaluate other trait clusters because these often affect treatment. For example, Anna showed compulsivity and sensation-seeking, both of which influenced how she has managed in therapy.

Table 2.1 Personality Disorder Traits

Emotional Dysregulation	Dissocial	Social Avoidance	Compulsivity
Anxiousness	Hostile-dominance	Low affiliation	Orderliness
Emotional lability:	Sadism	Avoidant attachment	Conscientiousness
Emotional reactivity	Egocentrism	Restricted expression	
Emotional intensity	Exploitiveness	Inhibited sexuality	
Pessimistic anhedonia	Conduct problems	Self-containment	
Generalized hypersensitivity	Sensation seeking	Attachment need	
Insecure attachment	Impulsivity		
Submissiveness	Narcissism		
Need for approval	Suspiciousness		
Cognitive dysregulation			
Oppositional			

2.4.2 The Internal Structure of Traits

Although traits are useful ways to describe personality, it is not always apparent to clinicians that an understanding of a patient's traits is useful in therapy. This is because traits are usually considered stable characteristics that are unlikely to change. However, traits are complex structures with an elaborate cognitive component composed of schemas that mediate between an event and behavioural responses to that event. An understanding of schemas associated with traits is useful in helping patients to use their traits more effectively and in helping to modulate the expression of maladaptive traits by restructuring the schema component.

Although traits are heritable entities – about 50 per cent of the variation among individuals is due to genetic influences – they are also shaped by environmental events. These events lead to the development of schemas consisting of beliefs that influence how the trait is expressed.[6] For example, anxiousness, an important borderline trait, is based on a genetically based mechanism for managing threat that constantly scans the environment for threats.[7] When a threat is detected, anxiety is triggered to signal that there is a problem requiring attention. Ongoing behaviour is halted so that attention can be focused on evaluating the threat and initiating an appropriate response, typically either flight or fight. Thus if you hear footsteps behind you when you are walking on a quiet street late at night, momentary alarm occurs and all thoughts stop so that you can concentrate on what is happening, appraise the situation, and decide what to do.

Repeated experiences of threatening events during development give rise to schemas consisting of beliefs about how threatening the world is and self-appraisals of the ability to manage threat. These schemas influence the expression of anxiousness by affecting how often situations are considered threatening and hence how frequently anxiousness is activated. Anna, for example, believed that the world was a threatening place that she could not manage. Consequently, her threat system was almost chronically aroused. Since similar processes occur with other traits, an understanding of the cognitive component of traits allows therapists to intervene to modulate the frequency and intensity with which traits are expressed. For example, therapists may help highly anxious patients to change their interpretation of events so that fewer events are considered threatening and to re-evaluate their ability to manage threat.

2.4.3 Traits, Environment, and Adaptation

Although traits are relatively enduring, healthy individuals express their traits in flexible ways. Traits are dispositions that bias us to respond in particular ways. The higher the level of a given trait, the more likely we are to express that trait. However, trait expression is context dependent. In most instances, the situation has to be appropriate for a given trait to be expressed – even roaring extraverts are quiet at funerals and the most disagreeable person can be amicable when the need arises. The importance of the situation to trait expression means that over time, we create a personal niche – an environment and a way of living that provides opportunities to satisfy our traits and use them adaptively. In general, the better the fit between our basic traits and the circumstances of our lives, the better our adaptation and feelings of well-being. This idea is also useful in managing maladaptive traits. Given the genetic basis of traits and their consolidation by developmental experiences over many years, it is often more effective to help patients to change how they express their traits and to encourage them to develop lifestyles that allow them to use their traits more adaptively rather than to try to help them to change their traits in more radical ways.

Thus socially avoidant individuals may be helped to build a lifestyle that allows them to manage their level of social interaction and meet their need for solitude. Or, highly dependent individuals who are compulsive caregivers can be helped to channel this need by helping others in a planned and structured way, for example, by volunteering or working in a caregiving role for a fixed time each week as opposed to always feeling obliged to meet the needs of others. These kinds of interventions were needed in the treatment of Anna. She also needed help in developing interests and activities that allowed her to meet her needs for excitement and stimulation without resorting to maladaptive behaviours such as creating crises with her husband because she was bored. Therapies for BPD have largely neglected the idea of working with traits (as opposed to changing them) and helping patients to build a satisfying personal niche.

2.5 Self System

The self system is also crucial to understanding BPD: self-pathology is a core feature of any personality disorder. To understand self-pathology and how it relates to other features of the disorder, we need a framework for conceptualizing the self. This is where an understanding of normal personality is helpful. The study of personality disorder has largely neglected the task of constructing a coherent and evidence-based approach to self and identity.[8] However, contemporary study of the self offers a rich array of constructs that we can use to understand self pathology and identify possible treatment strategies. I am going to spend a little time discussing the self system because an important part of therapy is to help patients construct a better understanding of themselves – a self-narrative – that helps them to live more contented lives and to build an environment – a personal niche – that meets their needs and provides opportunities for growth and personal satisfaction.

We can think of the self as a higher-order system that helps to integrate, coordinate, and direct personality functioning. Contemporary descriptions of the self focus on three main features: (i) the self as experiencing subject or knower – our subjective experience of ourselves; (ii) the self as known to the individual – the various qualities and characteristics we attribute to ourselves; and (iii) the self as agent and centre of self-regulation and self-direction.[9] This structure will be used to describe self pathology in BPD and to organize its assessment and treatment.

2.5.1 The Self and Knower

This aspect of the self refers to our experience of ourselves. Most people feel that there is something inside their heads that notes experiences, thinks, and feels and that this "thing" is who they really are.[10] This aspect of the self is fundamental to adaptation: it grounds us in our world, and its absence in patients with BPD is a serious impairment. At least four aspects of our experience of ourselves are important for mental well-being: (i) personal unity – a sense of wholeness, coherence, and integration; (ii) continuity – a sense of personal continuity through time and the realization that one has a past and an anticipated future; (iii) certainty and clarity about self-knowledge and mental states; and (iv) authenticity – the conviction that our basic feelings and wants are "real" or genuine.

These features are apparent if we ponder the question "Who am I?" Besides the various attributes, beliefs, and values that spring to mind, we are also acutely aware of a profound sense of personal unity, coherence, and continuity. This experience is the hallmark of an adaptive self system. It provides a sense of stability, direction, and control. However, the development of a coherent self also depends on the clarity, certainty, and authenticity of self-knowledge – it requires that we accept and trust our basic experiences, especially emotions and needs, and the labels we apply to them.

As we will see in the next chapter, this certainty and trust is impaired in BPD: patients are uncertain about even their basic emotions and wants, which seriously impairs self-development. Anna, for example, consistently wondered whether her distress and anger were "real." Certainty about emotions is necessary for us to experience the world as stable, and this in turn is needed to construct a stable understanding of ourselves and our place in the world.

The importance of certainty and authenticity for mental health does not mean that the interpretations placed on experiences are necessarily valid or that we should never question them. However, it is not possible to function effectively unless we initially accept the authenticity of our experience of basic emotions and needs. In a sense, this certainty has to be the default mode. One needs to be sure about these basic experiences to interact with the environment effectively. Continually doubting basic feelings and needs is paralysing.

2.5.2 The Self as Known

The self as known to ourselves is best understood as a body of self-referential knowledge – an organized collection of self-schemas that represent our traits, values, beliefs, goals, hopes, and aspirations along with memories of personally significant events. The self as knower may be thought to develop through simultaneous processes of differentiation and integration.

2.5.2.1 Differentiation and Integration of Self-Knowledge

Self-knowledge progressively differentiates during development as new understandings arise and new schemas are constructed. Some schemas develop because they are part of our salient traits. In this sense, our traits help to structure our understanding of ourselves. Other schemas are acquired through our interactions with others. Hence many self-schemas are also part of the interpersonal system and are used to understand both self and others. At the same time, schemas become organized into different self-images. People see themselves differently in the various roles they occupy – parent, spouse or partner, son or daughter, clinician, friend, and so on. These images in turn are organized into increasingly higher-order conceptions culminating eventually in an overarching self-view or self-narrative.[11] If questioned, most healthy individuals could provide an autobiographical account of themselves and the events that shaped their lives.

In general, adaptive self systems are more differentiated and integrated. A well-differentiated system with multiple schemas allows a nuanced understanding of ourselves and our lives. And, the sense of personal unity and coherence that are integral to mental well-being are the experiential consequences of the links among self-schemas – the more extensive these links, the greater the sense of unity and integration.[12]

Self-schemas also differ in importance. Some are core concepts central to the individual's sense of self with rich connections with other self-schemas whereas others are peripheral to the individual's sense of self with fewer connections with other schemas. Core schemas contribute to a sense of identity which defines our place in the social and cultural groups to which we belong.

2.5.2.2 Self as Stable and Dynamic

Thus far the structure of the self as known has been assumed to be relatively stable. It was suggested that peripheral schemas may change but that core schemas change little and that the connections among schemas form a stable network. This structural model is consistent with clinical concepts of self, which also view the self as a stable structure. In the case of BPD, this structure is considered to be disjointed, leading to distinct and poorly integrated conceptions of the self. However, this traditional clinical conception differs somewhat from current research, which views the self as both stable and dynamic. Current models propose that important aspects of the self are temporary constructions generated to match the situation in which we find ourselves. This creates a problem. How are we to understand the apparent inconsistency between the self as both stable and dynamic and how can we reconcile this idea with traditional clinical concepts?

Consider this vignette.

It is a warm, sunny day and I am playing on a beach with my young granddaughter Mia making sandcastles that she promptly destroys with squeals of delight. I feel happy and playful but also caring and tolerant. Suddenly, she decides to go into the water. I take her hand and she jumps the waves with glee. I am intrigued by her excitement and curious about how fresh everything seems to her. I also feel protective and vigilant. Then she decides that she would like to return to playing in the sand. As we head to the beach, a larger wave causes her to lose her balance. Her face gets splashed. After I have dried it, she turns to me and, wagging her finger at me, she tells me, "Don't ever let that happen again, granddad" and runs off to play with Oliver, her older brother. I feel thoroughly scolded but also amused. I walk to my chair in the shade and pick up the book I had been reading, an academic tome about the self. My sense of self changes instantly. I am no longer the benevolent, kindly, tolerant, and protective grandfather but rather a scholar trying to understand something that intrigues me. I am analytic and critical, dissecting the material to test the argument and evaluate the evidence supporting it. But, at the same time, I am inquisitive and play with the ideas to see how they fit other conceptual positions. Absorbed by the task, I do not notice that my wife is calling. She wonders if I want to go for a walk. I join her and wander contentedly along the beach, enjoying the companionship and simply being there. As we walk, I suddenly realize just how much my sense of who I am has changed in only a short time, yet it feels quite natural and genuine. My different self-images seem to fit together.

How are we to understand the apparently stable but obviously dynamic nature of the self? A possible solution emerges if we adopt the metaphor of the self as a matrix with the self-schemas forming nodes that are linked to form a network. The nodes themselves and the strength of the links between them are relatively stable. However, the matrix is also a functional structure. The nodes that are activated at any moment vary with the situation and the roles and personal projects generated in response to the situation. In the vignette, my sense of who *I am* varied with context because I constructed different *momentary working selves* to meet the requirements of each situation and the roles and goals I established for myself in each situation.[13] These momentary working selves guided and coordinated my actions so that they fit the situation but only within the constraints imposed by the overall matrix of the self, which is relatively stable.

The vignette and the idea of momentary working self illustrates another aspect of the self – that the self is a mechanism for managing the relationship between the person and the environment, an idea that is important in understanding and treating BPD. To be proactive, we need a mechanism to link internal states, especially wants and emotions, to environmental circumstances and to manage the interaction with the immediate environment. The momentary working selves we construct are context sensitive but they are not created by that context. They are generated to coordinate and direct our interaction with the situation, the demands it makes, and the roles and projects we establish for ourselves in that situation. The interaction between situation and working self is not static or unidirectional but rather dynamic and reciprocal. In a sense, the working self helps us to manage our relationship with our environment more effectively.

This model of the self forms the basis for describing and treating self pathology. As we will see in the next chapter, BPD involves an impoverished and poorly integrated set of self-schemas leading to an unstable self. A task of longer-term therapy is to help patients develop a more differentiated and integrated self-structure – the stable matrix in the analogy above. However, patients with BPD also lack the ability to generate momentary working selves that fit the situation. They rely instead on a relatively few self-states that function in fixed ways somewhat independently of context. Anna, for example, saw herself as anxious and unable to cope, fearful of rejection, and incompetent in most situations. She lacked the ability to construct momentary working selves that could be adapted to the situations in which she found herself. Hence an additional therapeutic task is to help patients to use the matrix elaborated in therapy more flexibly to generate a variety of momentary working selves that are sensitive to the situations of their lives. These are the themes of Chapters 21–24.

2.5.3 Self as Agent

The self is not just a body of knowledge: it also includes the self as agent and centre of self-regulatory function.[14] An important part of who we are is defined by our goals and aspirations and even the person we want to be. Our goals are important: they energize, create direction and purpose, and hence give meaning to our lives.[15] In the process, they contribute to the cohesiveness of personality by drawing together different aspects of personality – they link needs and wishes with the qualities and abilities needed to attain them. It is striving towards a goal, not its attainment, that confers integration.[16]

2.6 Interpersonal System

The interpersonal system also consists of schemas that are organized into both representations of specific individuals and a generalized understanding of other people and how they are likely to behave. Representations of another person organize information about that person's qualities along with memories of experiences with that person. With casual acquaintances, these representations consist of a few salient qualities such as whether the person is friendly or honest. In contrast, a representation of someone well-known is more detailed and may recognize different facets to their personality. For example, a person may be thought to be friendly, kind, and cheerful on most occasions but irritable and disagreeable on others. Usually an attempt is made to integrate these apparent discrepancies, for example, by recognizing that a person is normally friendly but irritable when stressed.

Interpersonal schemas tend to be self-perpetuating because they lead us to interact with others in ways that reinforce the schema. For example, we tend to be cautious in our dealings with people we consider suspicious. This may lead them in turn to respond with equal mistrust, which we then interpret as evidence that our suspicions were justified.

As noted, self and interpersonal systems are not totally independent of the trait system. The initial precursors of traits influence the child's interactions with the environment from an early age and these interactions affect the environmental inputs that shape the self and interpersonal systems. Thus, a highly outgoing child will elicit very different environmental responses than a more reserved child and these differences will inevitably influence the child's self-image and interpersonal constructs. Also, traits such as insecure attachment and submissiveness represent propensities to show particular patterns of interpersonal behaviour. In a sense, traits bias our interpretation and responses to events.

BPD involves extensive interpersonal pathology that includes maladaptive interpersonal schemas such as distrust (or a lack of what Erikson[17] referred to as basic trust), intimacy and attachment fears, and rejection and abandonment sensitivity. It also includes interpersonal problems linked to difficulty in understanding the mental states of others. As a result, representations of others, like the self, are often impoverished and poorly integrated.

2.7 Regulation and Modulation System

Effective functioning requires mechanisms to control and modulate emotions and impulses, coordinate action, inhibit impulses, and delay the satisfaction of needs until the situation is appropriate. Self-regulation is also essential for goal-directed behaviour. Goal attainment requires the ability to inhibit or frustrate short-term needs and wants when they are likely to impede the achievement of longer-term goals and the ability to monitor and regulate progress towards goal attainment.

The regulatory aspect of personality also includes metacognitive processes[18] – higher-order cognitive processes that enable us to reflect on our own experiences and those of other people. Our ability to reflect on our mental activities allows us to understand the mental states of self and others, monitor our reactions to situations, regulate our responses, and change our interpretation of self and others. Many aspects of personality, especially the self and identity and interpersonal systems, are dependent on self-reflection – important aspects of personality are constructed by reflecting on experience.

2.8 Basic Processes

Personality does not exist in isolation from other mental structures. Effective personality functioning depends on an infrastructure of cognitive mechanisms involving memory, attention, and information processing. For example, the capacity of the regulatory mechanisms, discussed previously, to control and switch attention depends on the integrity of underlying neuropsychological structures. Impairments to these processes often adversely affect personality functioning and contribute to the risk of developing BPD.

The formation of many personality structures including schemas requires the ability to combine and integrate multiple sources of cognitive and emotional information. Any impairment of this aspect of information processing inevitably affects personality development, which possibly explains why some patients with BPD have a history of mild neurological trauma.

2.9 Environmental Factors

Although the environment is usually considered to be independent of the person, the environment is in fact an integral part of the personality system. As noted, people construct personal niches that fit their personality, talents, interests, and values that help to shape their behaviour and maintain adaptive functioning. Much of the structure and organization of everyday behaviour reflects the regularities and expectations of the environment. The behavioural disorganization seen in many patients often reflects a lack of structure in their environment besides internal problems regulating emotions and impulses, and the repetitive maladaptive behaviour that characterizes BPD is often perpetuated by a social environment that encourages and facilitates such actions.

Recognition of the importance of the environment to personality functioning has clinical implications. In the early stages of therapy, patients often need help organizing their day and in structuring their environments. Later, they may also need help in managing their environments more effectively and in constructing a personal niche that supports adaptive rather than maladaptive behaviour.

2.10 Defining Personality Disorder

With this understanding of the personality system in mind, we are now in a position to consider what we mean by personality disorder. We need a definition that distinguishes personality disorder from the far more common personality dysfunction. We all have personality quirks that cause occasional personal discomfort or more often irritation to those around us. We may be more anxious, irritable, or shy than we or others would like. Usually, we cope with these difficulties and they have little impact on our overall well-being because they only involve a limited part of our personality and only cause occasional problems. Personality disorder is different: as we saw with Anna, her problems encompassed most aspects of her personality. Nevertheless, it is difficult to define exactly what it is about her behaviour that indicates that she has personality disorder. The idea of personality as a system offers a solution.

The personality system, like any system, is not just a set of different components – traits, the self, schemas, and so on; it also has structure or organization. With most healthy people, personality functions in a coherent way. The different parts work together harmoniously to enable individuals to reach their goals and accomplish the personal projects they set for themselves. This is not the case with personality-disordered individuals. The different parts of their personality do not work in harmony. As a result, their behaviour is disorganized and even chaotic. We saw this with Anna. Her behaviour was erratic and her life lacked coherence and direction.

This raises the question of what markers can we use to differentiate an organized from a disorganized personality system. The two features currently used are (i) a profound disturbance of the sense of self and (ii) chronic interpersonal dysfunction.[19] This idea has been around for some time but recently gained traction when it was incorporated into DSM-5. Subsequent chapters will expand on this definition and discuss simple ways to assess these features. For now, we can note how Anna meets this definition. Self pathology is illustrated by a poorly developed self, uncertainty about who she is, and difficulty setting meaningful long-term goals. She also had chronic interpersonal problems. Truly intimate relationships eluded her. Her interpersonal life was characterized by strife and conflict, and she lived in constant fear of rejection and being alone.

This definition of personality disorder is consistent with the idea introduced in Chapter 1 that personality disorder diagnoses have two components: core self and interpersonal pathology, and a constellation of traits which in the case of BPD consists of the emotional dysregulation cluster. This structure will be used in the next chapter to describe BPD in detail. However, there is another useful thing to note about the idea of personality as a system, namely that it helps to organize the diverse features of BPD into domains that can then be linked to specific intervention modules, an idea that directly links assessment to specific interventions.

2.11 Personality System and Domains of Personality Pathology

Borderline pathology falls into four domains of impairment:

1. Symptoms: anxiety, fearfulness, low mood, dysphoria, suicidality, deliberate self-injurious behaviour, disorganized thinking, quasi-psychotic symptoms, and dissociation
2. Regulation and Modulation: problems with self-regulatory mechanisms, difficulties regulating and modulating emotions and impulses, intense unstable emotions, and frequent mood changes
3. Interpersonal: problems with intimacy and attachment, conflicted and unstable relationships, abandonment fears, rejection sensitivity, problems with submissive dependency, and maladaptive interpersonal schemas
4. Self: maladaptive self-schemas; poorly developed, fragmented and unstable sense of self; and difficulty establishing long-term goals

Domains 2, 3, and 4 represent impairments in three personality subsystems: regulation and modulation, interpersonal, and self. The remaining personality subsystem discussed earlier – the trait system – is not represented directly as a domain because the consequences of maladaptive traits are manifested though the four domains. For example, anxiousness and emotional lability are manifested through symptoms, unstable emotions, emotional distress, and fearfulness, and insecure attachment is expressed through interpersonal problems.

The idea of domains of impairment is used to select and sequence the use of specific intervention modules. Treatments of BPD typically focus sequentially on symptoms, regulation and modulation, interpersonal, and self-domains because the sequence reflects both clinical priorities – crises, distress, and suicidality need to be managed before other problems can be addressed – and differences across domains in stability and responsiveness to treatment.[20]

In general, symptoms are relatively plastic: most symptoms vary naturally over time and consequently they often improve early in treatment. An early focus on symptoms is likely to lead to some improvement that can then be used to build motivation and the treatment alliance. Impairments in regulation and modulation mechanisms are more stable than symptoms but respond readily to treatment resulting in significant decreases in deliberate self-harm and emotional distress.[21] Problems in the interpersonal domain tend to respond more slowly and only become a primary treatment focus following substantial improvement in emotional control. Finally, core self-schemas are highly stable and change relatively slowly.

This sequence for treating domains maps onto the phases of treatment. Symptoms are the main focus of intervention during the safety, containment, and regulation and modulation phases. The latter is also increasingly concerned with emotion regulation. Finally, the exploration and change and integration and synthesis phases focus primarily on the interpersonal and self-domains, respectively.

2.12 Concluding Comments

This chapter is intended to form the foundation for understanding the psychopathology of BPD by showing how the different features of the disorder relate to normal personality constructs. The intent is to provide a context for defining the kinds of changes needed for effective outcomes. Throughout therapy, when dealing with specific problems, opportunities also arise to promote more effective and integrated personality functioning. To use these opportunities, therapists need to understand the nuances of personality functioning and recognize how the different components of personality function as an integrated whole.

Notes

1. Livesley (2003), Mayer (2005), Vernon (1964).

2. Ryle (1975).

3. The two main five-factor descriptions of normal personality traits are the Big Five (Goldberg, 1993) and the Five-Factor model (FFM). The version described here is the FFM (Costa and McCrae, 1992), which has been proposed as a model for describing personality disorder (see Costa and McCrae, 1990; Costa and Widiger, 2002; Widiger et al., 2002).

4. For reviews of the structure of personality disorder traits, see Mulder et al. (2011), Ofrat et al. (in press), Widiger and Simonsen (2006).

5. Livesley (1998, 2011), Livesley et al. (1998).

6. Livesley (2008), Livesley et al. (2003), Livesley and Jang (2008).

7. Gray (1978, 1987), Livesley (2008).

8. Traditionally within psychiatry and the study of personality disorder, self and identity have largely been discussed from a psychoanalytic perspective (see Clarkin et al., 2015; Jorgensen, 2006, 2009, in press; Kernberg, 1984). More recently, metacognitive and narrative approaches to treatment have discussed the importance of self-narratives (see, for example, Dimaggio et al., 2012; Salvatore et al., 2015).

9. The tripartite structure of the self has been reviewed by Leary and Tangnay (2012). This structure reflects an earlier distinction by William James (1890) between self as knower and self as known – a distinction that has stood the test of time. Research from about 1970 onwards also focused on the self as agent, that is, the self as the centre for self-regulation, an aspect of the self that includes self-directedness.

10. Olson (1999).

11. McAdams and Pals (2006), Singer (2004).

12. Toulmin (1978), Horowitz (1998).

13. See Walton et al. (2012) for a discussion of the concept of the working self.

14. This aspect of the self became more prominent from about 1970 onwards with increasing attention to cognitive processes in personality, for example, Baumeister (1998), Carver and Scheier (1981), Hamackek (1971), Sheldon and Elliot (1999).

15. Carver (2012), Carver and Scheier (1998), Shapiro (1981), Baumeister (1989).

16. Allport (1961).

17. Erikson (1950).

18. Fonagy et al. (2002), Dimaggio et al. (2007).

19. The definition of personality disorder in terms of core self and interpersonal pathology is based on the adaptive failure definition of personality disorder that I proposed some years ago (Livesley, 1998, 2003a, 2003b; Livesley and Jang, 2005; Livesley et al., 1994). The ideas were derived from social cognitive approaches to personality and an evolutionary perspective. The conception assumes that effective personality functioning requires the development of a coherent sense of self and the capacity for intimacy and effective attachment relationships and prosocial behaviour. This proposal formed the basis for the DSM-5 definition of personality disorder and hence the A criteria for typal diagnoses, although DSM-5 modified the way self pathology was defined in the original adaptive failure definition.

20. Tickle et al. (2001), Livesley (2003).

21. Evaluations of dialectical behaviour therapy (DBT) and CBT show that deliberate self-harm and emotional distress respond well to treatment.

Chapter

3

Understanding Borderline Personality Disorder

This chapter uses the idea of the personality system to develop an empirically based description of borderline personality disorder (BPD) organized around the idea introduced earlier that BPD has two main components: the emotional dependency constellation of traits and core self and interpersonal pathology.

3.1 Borderline Traits

The emotional dysregulation cluster of traits may be divided into three groups: emotional, interpersonal, and cognitive (see Table 3.1).

3.1.1 Emotional Traits

Underlying unstable emotions are two major traits: anxiousness and emotional lability. Other less-common traits, namely, pessimistic-anhedonia and generalized hypersensitivity, also contribute to the clinical picture in some patients.

3.1.1.1 Anxiousness

Although most theories emphasize emotional lability, patients with BPD are anxious and fearful. They tend to describe themselves as life-long worriers who see the world as threatening and malevolent and themselves as vulnerable and powerless,[1] which makes them hyper-vigilant for indications of threat, especially loss, rejection, and abandonment. Consequently, emotional crises involve fear, panic-like anxiety, and rumination about painful experiences. The current framework for understanding BPD assumes that anxiousness is the cornerstone trait that influences the expression of other traits.[2]

Table 3.1 Traits Characterizing Borderline Personality Disorder

Emotional	Interpersonal	Cognitive
Anxiousness	Attachment insecurity	Cognitive dysregulation
Emotional lability:	Submissive-dependency	
Intensity	Fear of rejection/disapproval	
Reactivity	Passivity	
Pessimistic-anhedonia		
Generalized hypersensitivity		

At this point, you may be wondering why I am emphasizing anxiousness when many patients show little overt anxiety and seem more angry than anxious. This is often the case. One reason is that the threat mechanism underlying anxiousness offers the option of responding with either fight or flight. Since anxiety increases feelings of vulnerability, many patients rapidly convert it into anger (fight), which is more tolerable. This occurred with one patient who rushed her young child who had suddenly become very ill to the local emergency room whereupon she immediately quarrelled with staff trying to treat the child. The intense anxiety about the child's safety was overwhelming and hence quickly expressed as anger. It was only later, when discussing the event in therapy, that she acknowledged her fear. This reaction is common in forensic settings where it is important not to appear weak lest this is exploited by others. However, despite the propensity to convert anxiety into rage, it is important to treat the underlying fearfulness by teaching stress management skills and restructuring appraisals of threatening situations. The idea that BPD involves impaired functioning of the threat system and hyper-vigilance for signs of threat is consistent with research showing heightened sensitivity to social threat and a tendency to perceive interpersonal situations as threatening and angry[3] and with theories that consider attachment insecurity a key component of the disorder.

3.1.1.2 Emotional Lability

Emotional lability has two components: emotional reactivity, which involves rapid emotional arousal leading to irritability, intense anger, and frequent, unpredictable emotional changes; and emotional intensity, which involves strong emotional reactions that often seem exaggerated to others and a slow return to the baseline state. Since all negative emotions are probably regulated by the same general mechanism, multiple negative emotions tend to be activated simultaneously, as occurs in crisis states.

3.1.1.3 Pessimistic-Anhedonia

Some patients with BPD have a pessimistic attitude that is often combined with difficulty experiencing pleasure. The pessimism goes beyond the gloominess of depressed mood to include a pervasive tendency to expect the worse so that even positive events are considered indications that something disastrous is likely to occur. When present, pessimistic-anhedonia is important because it increases emotional reactivity and suicidality. Although empirical studies are lacking, my impression is that many patients who die by suicide show high levels of this trait. Patients with this trait are also difficult to treat: since nothing is pleasurable or satisfying, there is little to interest or motivate them.

3.1.1.4 Generalized Hypersensitivity

Generalized hypersensitivity involves a tendency to experience any form of stimulation as intense, intrusive, and overwhelming. It is as if the volume is too high on everything: sounds are too loud, colours are too intense, and people are too overwhelming. This is an important but neglected trait that amplifies emotional and interpersonal reactivity.

3.1.1.5 Emotional Traits and Inner Experience

Before leaving the emotional traits, we need to consider what it is like to have BPD and experience intense unstable emotions. An understanding of subjective experience is helpful

BOX 3.1 Characteristics of the Subjective Experience of Emotions in Patients with Borderline Personality Disorder

Undifferentiated emotional experience
Limited emotional awareness
Fusion of emotions and self
Narrowing of attention
Difficulty decentring
Escalating thoughts and self-talk
Rumination
Emotional avoidance

because there is often a discrepancy between the way patients present themselves to others and how they feel inside. Patients frequently come across as angry and demanding, and all too often other people, including health care professionals, take this at face value. Focusing only on the external presentation, they fail to empathize with patients' underlying feelings of vulnerability, distress, and pain. We came across this idea earlier when discussing how anxiety is often expressed as anger. As therapists, we need to be aware of this discrepancy and try to understand patients' subjective experience. The characteristic features of the subjective experience of emotions in patients with BPD are listed in Box 3.1.

Undifferentiated Emotional Experience and Limited Emotional Awareness Probably the most obvious feature of the emotional life of patients with BPD is the undifferentiated and chaotic nature of their emotions, which consist of an excruciatingly painful mixture of distress, panic, sadness, anger, and rage that is difficult to describe and label. As a result, there is limited awareness of the actual emotions involved. This is explained by the distinction between self-focus and self-awareness. Patients with BPD have an intense self-focus: they are acutely aware of their inner experience including the physiological sensations associated with emotions but have limited awareness of the nuances of these experiences. Being unable to describe their distress, patients often resort to simple labels like "depressed," which can create misunderstanding about what they are actually experiencing. Consequently, an early step in treatment is to "unpack" these experiences by helping the patient to progress from an acute self-focus to greater self-awareness of specific feelings.

Fusion of Emotions and Self Patients' subjective experience is also dominated by difficulty separating themselves from their feelings.[4] This idea is a little difficult to explain. It is as if their intense emotions define who they are. When healthy individuals feel sad or distressed, they can usually separate themselves from their feelings and recognize that their feelings are transient. They do this by standing back and seeing their current state within a broader context. The exception is when a devastating event such as a bereavement occurs. The intense distress is engulfing and feels as if it occupies one's whole mind and will never go away. This is what happens to patients in a crisis. Rather than distancing themselves from their emotions, they "fuse" with them.[5] As a result, intense feelings are not treated as states that come and go but rather as enduring conditions that define who they are. Instead of feeling angry or ashamed, they see themselves as angry or shameful persons. Fusion leads patients to assume that they always have and always will feel this way even if they had felt very differently only a short time previously. Consequently, all that matters is their current distress. In the process, the capacity for self-reflection is lost.

Narrowing of Attention and Difficulty Decentring The fusion of self and experience and difficulty reflecting on experience lead to a progressive narrowing of attention with reduced awareness of surrounding events. This leaves patients trapped in a distraught state that they cannot process or understand, leading to an urgent need to end the distress. Consequently, there is a tendency to react to emotional events without thinking. Thus a second task is to help patients to decentre from their feelings and to process feelings as opposed to simply reacting to them. This helps to reduce the tendency to react instantly when emotions are aroused by creating a delay between an event and the ensuing response.

Escalating Thoughts and Self-Talk The subjective experience of dysregulated emotions is usually accompanied by ruminative thoughts that escalate distress.[6] When upset, patients often tell themselves that their feelings are intolerable or that they will kill themselves if the feelings continue. This kind of self-talk is often accompanied by strong self-criticism, so an additional therapeutic task is to help patients feel greater self-compassion and self-acceptance.

Emotional Avoidance Emotional avoidance is common because patients often conclude that emotions are harmful and should be avoided or suppressed. In the long-term, this gives rise to behavioural restriction because patients limit their activities to avoid situations that may activate painful feelings.[7] It also contributes to crises by creating a conflict between what the patient is experiencing and beliefs that he/she should not have such feelings.

When an understanding of the subjective experience of intense emotions is combined with recognition of how intense emotions impair cognitive control, it is readily understandable why emotional crises are so intense and why patients are so often unresponsive to many interventions – an issue discussed in Chapter 16.

3.1.2 Interpersonal Traits

The tumultuous interpersonal life of individuals with BPD arises from conflict between intense neediness and desire for closeness and fear of rejection, abandonment, and disapproval. Three heritable traits underlie this conflict: insecure attachment, submissiveness, and need for approval. This depiction of the interpersonal impairments of BPD differs to that of DSM-5, which also emphasizes attachment insecurity but neglects submissiveness and dependency and the conflict between neediness and fear of rejection, which are critical to understanding and treating patients.[8]

3.1.2.1 Insecure Attachment

Attachment insecurity is characterized by intense fear of losing or being separated from significant others and an intense fear of being alone. It is as if important aspects of the attachment system did not develop effectively, leading to difficulty functioning effectively in the absence of significant others. Whereas most healthy individuals are able to maintain cognitive connections with loved ones when separated from them by thinking about them and recalling memories of joint experiences, many patients with BPD remain dependent on the physical presence of significant others to cope effectively. Consequently, they actively protest separation from attachment figures and urgently seek proximity to them when stressed.

Attachment insecurity due to dysfunctional early attachment relationships can give rise to disorganized attachment behaviour, a pattern that is common in BPD. Difficulties arise because attachment figures that the child naturally turns to for help when distressed also cause the threat and distress and hence become the focus of conflict – the child naturally wants to approach them but is also afraid of doing so, a conflict that will be discussed further in the next chapter.

3.1.2.2 Submissiveness

Patients with BPD have a strong tendency to be subservient and unassertive, which is often coupled with dependency needs that lead to a constant need for support, reassurance, and guidance. As with anxiousness, patients with BPD do not seem submissive because it is often hidden by an angry demanding demeanour. However, an inherent part of human nature is a mechanism that leads us to appease and be subservient to those we consider to be more important or of higher status. Since most patients have low self-esteem, they tend to see other people as more important than themselves. One patient, for example, always let people go before her in supermarket queues because they seemed in a hurry and she assumed their needs were more pressing.

Submissiveness probably evolved to enable our remote ancestors to manage the dominance hierarchies that are characteristic of primate groups and avoid the anger and disapproval of more-dominant or higher-status individuals. This required the evolution of a mechanism that is sensitive to status differences and the development of a repertoire of behaviours to placate, appease, and submit to more dominant individuals. Abuse leads to the chronic activation of this mechanism. Since abusers are usually adults, or at least older than the child, they are automatically considered of higher status. Early abuse and adversity also lead to low self-esteem or, in evolutionary terms, low status that leads to chronic activation of the submissiveness and to a tendency to subordinate one's own needs to those of others. Consequently, patients with BPD tend to form relationships in which they are primarily concerned with fulfilling the needs of others,[9] and they often find themselves trapped in abusive relationships from which it is difficult to extricate themselves because of a fear of being alone. Anna provides a classical example of this pattern.

3.1.2.3 Need for Approval

Need for approval and, conversely, fear of disapproval are closely linked to submissive dependency. Most patients with BPD are overly dependent on the approval of others and on reassurances of acceptance and affection. Despite expressions of anger, they are people-pleasers anxious to do what others want lest they become angry and rejecting.

3.1.2.4 Oppositionality

Although oppositionality is not a central feature of BPD, when present it tends to increase interpersonal difficulties, resulting in passive-aggressive and disorganized behaviour that can cause problems inside and outside treatment. Passivity reduces motivation and leads to the use of oppositional behaviour to exert control without evoking the wrath of others. Lack of organization makes it difficult to execute plans and structure time effectively. Passivity also reinforces submissive tendencies and often leads to hostile, dependent behaviour, which adds to the conflicted nature of personal relationships.

3.1.2.5   Neediness versus Fear of Rejection: The Interpersonal Core of Borderline Pathology

The interaction among the interpersonal traits in the context of adversity creates a conflict between neediness and fear of rejection, and to the development of generalized rejection-sensitivity that involves fear of rejection by both significant others and the wider social group. Rejection-sensitive individuals are highly vigilant about the possibility of rejection, react strongly to rejection, and easily feel rejected because they misinterpret social cues and readily interpret situations in terms of rejection, humiliation, or embarrassment.[10] This creates rigidity in how interpersonal situations are interpreted and difficulty seeing people's behaviour from different perspectives. Consequently, these fears are repeatedly confirmed.

3.1.2.6   Interpersonal Traits, Interpersonal Conflicts, Anxiousness, and Threat

Anxiousness and the interpersonal traits are closely related. It will be recalled that anxiousness is based on the mechanism for managing threat. The interpersonal traits of insecure attachment, submissive-dependency, and fear of disapproval (need for approval) are also linked to threat; in this case, different kinds of social threat. Insecure attachment involves the threat of separation from, or abandonment by, attachment figures and significant others. Submissiveness is related to threat arising from the disapproval, anger, or rejection from higher-status individuals. Finally, the need for approval is related to fear of being rejected by the social group. Thus the threat mechanism helps to regulate the interpersonal component of BPD, and association between anxiousness and the social traits creates a general sense of social apprehensiveness that is often one of the more subtle features of BPD.

3.1.3   Cognitive Traits

Many individuals with BPD show mild cognitive impairment especially when negative emotions are aroused. The mildest disturbance and impairment is in normal thinking and problem-solving that causes patients to note that their thoughts are fuzzy, that they feel confused, or that they have difficulty thinking. These changes reduce cognitive control of emotions, leading to a further increase in emotional arousal. The adverse effect of intense emotions on cognitive functions explains why intense emotions are destabilizing for many individuals with BPD. The occurrence of high levels of cognitive dysregulation suggests that emotional arousal needs to be regulated carefully until emotion-regulating skills improve.

The impact of cognitive dysregulation on coping may also lead to regression, depersonalization, and derealization. High levels of the trait are associated with quasi-psychotic symptoms such as illusions and pseudo-hallucinations in which a voice is heard usually saying an abusive word. Unlike true auditory hallucinations, the patient recognizes that the voice is "in their head" rather than arising from an external source. A few patients also report mild suspicions that others are watching them. For example, one patient thought that her therapist arranged for the police to patrol past her home when she was upset. She knew this was not the case but she was not entirely sure. Hence, unlike psychotic disorders, insight is retained. However, a few patients with severe BPD experience more intense psychotic symptoms as part of a transient psychotic episode that usually lasts from a few hours to a few days. The persistence of symptoms beyond this time frame suggests that the diagnosis should be reviewed.

Other cognitive impairments that are important in treating BPD are difficulties understanding and reflecting on one's experiences and impaired mentalizing capacity. Mentalizing and other meta-cognitive abilities have both trait-like and state-like characteristics depending on the severity of a patient's difficulties. Some patients show marked problems that are highly stable across a wide range of situations. With others, the problem is more variable, and, like other cognitive functions, the level of impairment is influenced by the intensity of emotional arousal.

3.1.4 Self-Harm

The remaining feature of the emotional dysregulation constellation is self-harm. This has two components: a behavioural component consisting of deliberate self-injurious acts and a cognitive component involving chronic suicidal ideation that appears to be aetiologically and functionally distinct. Chronic suicidal ideation appears to be more heritable that deliberate self-harm,[11] a finding that is consistent with the clinical observation that self-harming behaviour tends to remit long before chronic suicidal ideation. Deliberate self-harm and chronic suicidal ideation are also functionally different. Deliberate self-harm is primarily a way to self-regulate emotions as evidenced by patient reports that self-injury relieves tension in an emotional crisis. Chronic suicidal ideation, however, is often more a way of life. The person finds comfort in the idea that no matter how bad things get there is always a way out.

Deliberate self-harm is usually considered to be a feature of impulsivity. However, it is useful clinically to distinguish between behaviours such as deliberate self-harm and the trait of impulsivity which involves acting on the spur of the moment without regard for the consequences. Not all actions that appear impulsive are manifestations of trait impulsivity. Self-harming behaviours are essentially actions performed with a sense of urgency. This is seen in crises when painful emotions create an urgent need for relief from distress, which is achieved by a deliberate act of self-injury. This is why deliberate self-harm correlates with anxiousness and emotional lability whereas trait impulsivity correlates with dissocial/antisocial traits.

3.2 Core Self and Interpersonal Problems

Personality disorder was defined in the previous chapter in terms of core self and interpersonal problems. With BPD, self pathology affects all components of the self but interpersonal pathology is confined to difficulty maintaining intimate relationships.

3.2.1 Core Self Problems

The self pathology ubiquitous to BPD[12] involves the three aspects of the self: the self as knower, known, and agent (see Box 3.1).

3.2.1.1 Impairments in Self as Knower

BPD involves an impaired sense of personal unity, coherence, and continuity, which leaves patients without the sense of permanence needed to anchor them to their world. Most patients live in the moment and have difficulty integrating experiences across time. It is as if their lives are lived in episodes with little continuity between them. As one patient noted, "My life is a series of snapshots not a movie."[13] Most patients are also uncertain about their personal qualities because they question the authenticity of even their most basic feelings and wants and wonder whether their feelings are real.

3.2.1.2   Impairments in Self as Known

Patients with BPD also have limited self-knowledge and self-understanding. Their knowledge about themselves does not increase and differentiate as it does with healthy individuals, and they have difficulty organizing this knowledge into a coherent self-narrative and adaptive working selves.

3.2.1.2.1   Problems with the Differentiation of the Self

Impaired development of the self results in poor interpersonal boundaries and impoverished self-knowledge. Poor boundaries create a sense of vulnerability in social settings due to fears of being swamped by the other person, being unable to resist their demands and needs, and a fear of losing oneself in other people. As one patient noted, "I feel terrified when my partner comes home. I seem to lose myself in him. It's as if I no longer exist." Difficulty separating oneself from the demands and intrusiveness of others is illustrated by a patient with an intrusive neighbour who incessantly demanded help with routine tasks who noted that "when she comes into my apartment, I can't say no because she is in my head – her needs become mine." Poorly defined boundaries also lead to a tendency to disclose personality details inappropriately, difficulty recognizing that one's inner experience differs from that of other people,[14] and a tendency to assume that other peoples' thoughts and experiences are identical to one's own.

Besides poorly defined interpersonal boundaries, most patients with BPD have an impoverished repertoire of self-schemas. The simple question, "what sort of person are you?" often elicits a puzzled and vague response even from highly articulate patients. As a result, self-descriptions are usually a simple list of a few features such as interests and general, global evaluations. As one patient commented, "I am not sure who I am. I would not harm anyone. I like pretty clothes and my favourite colour is mauve. That's all I can say about myself."

3.2.1.2.2   Problems with Integration of the Self

Integration problems are almost a hallmark of BPD. Even those with reasonably well-developed self-knowledge have difficulty forming an integrated and stable sense of self (14). Patients often note that they do not feel "whole" or that they feel "fragmented." As one patient noted, "it is as if there are many different me's." For such patients, their sense of who they are can change dramatically with mood and circumstance as if their self-knowledge is organized into separate and unrelated self-images that they switch between.

Even healthy people feel differently about themselves on different occasions but they can usually explain why these differences occur. With BPD, the ability to reconcile different images of the self or self-states is severely limited. Some patients even have difficulty recalling events that occurred when in a different self-state. One patient oscillated between two radically different self-states. In one state, he felt happy and optimistic, and that he was a competent person who cared deeply about his family. In the other state, he experienced an intolerable sense of inner emptiness and felt worthless and contemptuous towards himself and resentful towards his family. When in this state, he was unable to recall feeling very differently even a short time before and therefore the state felt permanent and everything seemed hopeless.

The combination of impoverished self-knowledge and equally impoverished links among self-schemas lead to problems constructing a coherent self-narrative and to difficulty forming flexible working selves that allow the individual to tailor his or her behaviour to the needs of the situation. Most patients have a limited repertoire of working selves and hence tend to relate to situations in rigid and stereotyped ways. This occurred with Anna who saw herself as vulnerable and incompetent in most interpersonal situations and hence reacted defensively to most people, which seriously handicapped her social life.

3.2.1.3 Impairments in Self as Agent

Impairments in the third aspect of the self, the self as agent, are manifested as an impaired sense of agency and autonomy, and difficulty setting and attaining goals. Patients feel as if they have little control over their lives. These difficulties are not surprising: goal setting is difficult when one is unsure about personal qualities, interests, and abilities and when wants and hopes are continually questioned and change frequently. Impaired self-directedness adds to problems with the integration of the self because meaningful, long-term goals help to integrate different aspects of personality.

3.2.2 Core Interpersonal Problems

The interpersonal component of core pathology is manifested in BPD through chronic difficulties with intimacy and attachment, and inability to sustain close, intimate relationships. The typical pattern is to establish relationships quickly. Romantic relationships in particular are rapidly idealized and romanticized, creating powerful and unrealistic expectations for the relationship. Inevitably, the other person eventually fails to meet such expectations, which evokes equally strong feelings of disappointment and angry withdrawal. Consequently, most relationships are conflicted, chaotic, and unstable, and the social lives of these patients are punctuated by crises triggered by interpersonal disappointments.

3.3 Core Pathology and Borderline Traits

Thus far, the core self and interpersonal impairments and the traits of BPD have been described independently. However, the two are closely interwoven. Traits influence the development and expression of core pathology. It is difficult to form stable images of self and others or to be certain about personal characteristics when unstable emotions lead to ever-changing experiences of oneself and one's interactions with others. However, the relationship between traits and core pathology is not unidirectional: core pathology also influences the way traits are expressed. A coherent self-narrative, for example, is a powerful organizing and stabilizing force that provides a "top-down" regulatory function that helps to regulate emotions by influencing the way events are interpreted and putting them into a broader perspective. With severe self pathology, this regulatory function is lost and emotional reactions are more intense and unstable.

3.4 Concluding Comments

This chapter uses the idea of personality as a system to describe the basic structure of BPD in terms of (i) core self and interpersonal pathology and (ii) the emotional-dysregulation constellation of traits. It is these traits that differentiate borderline from other forms of personality disorder. The interaction of core pathology and borderline traits creates an unstable structure that gives rise to multiple impairments. In the previous chapter it was suggested that these impairments fall into four domains: symptoms, regulation and control problems, interpersonal dysfunction, and self and identity problems. These domains will be discussed further in the chapters on assessment and treatment planning (Chapters 5 and 6). But first we need to complete the framework for understanding BPD by considering its origins and development – the themes of the next chapter.

Notes

1. Beck et al. (2004).

2. The idea that anxiousness is central to understanding BPD is based on factor analyses showing that anxiousness has the highest loading component of the emotional dysregulation factor (see Livesley et al., 1998; Livesley, 2008) and clinical observation that these patients are fearful and easily feel threatened. The next endnote provides additional support for this assumption.

3. Pretzer (1990) suggested that BPD involves hyper-vigilance to signs of threat. This is confirmed by several lines of empirical research into sensitivity to threatening stimuli (see for example, Arntz et al., 2000; Barnow et al., 2009; Staebler et al., 2011; Wagner and Linehan, 1999). For example, faced with weak or ambiguous stimuli, patients with BPD show a bias to interpret anger in the facial expression (Domes et al., 2008; Domes et al., 2009).

4. For acceptance-based behavioural therapies, see, for example, Roemer and Orsillo (2009).

5. Hayes et al. (1999).

6. Leahy (2015).

7. Roemer and Orsillo (2009).

8. A problem with the DSM approach to BPD is the focus on external manifestations of the disorder in pursuit of reliable assessment. Although reliability is a necessary feature of any diagnostic system, it lacks merit if achieved at the expense of validity. The focus on relatively specific criteria means that the criteria set does not capture key features of the disorder such as the dependent-submissive component or the core interpersonal conflict between neediness and fear of rejection that is central to understanding and treating the interpersonal problems that are hallmarks of the disorder. The DSM approach and the conceptualization of BPD also lead to an emphasis on the more hostile and angry features without recognition of the complexity and conflicted nature of these behaviours.

9. Meissner (1984).

10. Romero-Canyas et al. (2010), Ayduk et al. (2000, 2002, 2008), Downey and Feldman (1996), Downey et al. (2004).

11. Jang et al. (1996).

12. Adler et al. (2012), Bradley and Westen (2005), Jorgensen (2006, 2009, 2010).

13. Case cited in Livesley (2003).

14. Kernberg (1984), Akhtar (1992).

Chapter 4

Origins and Development

This chapter is not intended to provide a detailed exposition of the many risk factors for borderline personality disorder (BPD). Instead, it provides a broad overview of how aetiological and developmental factors shape both borderline pathology and treatment strategies.

4.1 General Conclusions

Although knowledge of the aetiology and development of BPD remains rudimentary, some general conclusions are clear. First, the disorder arises from the interplay of multiple genetic and environmental influences. Second, individual risk factors have only a small effect: disorder arises from the accumulative effects of multiple factors. Both conclusions differ radically from earlier assumptions that BPD was largely caused by psychosocial adversity, especially childhood sexual abuse. However, BPD does not have a single "big cause," which needs to be kept in mind when assessing and treating patients to avoid a pointless search for major "causes."

Third, the disorder develops along multiple pathways so that the combination of factors giving rise to BPD differs substantially across cases. Some cases arise from an array of genetic and environmental factors. With others, genetic factors appear to predominate: it is relatively common to encounter patients with no history of severe adversity. In such cases, family members often report that the child had a "difficult temperament" from birth and was anxious and emotionally reactive from an early age. Other patients, however, have a history of such severe adversity that a high level of genetic predisposition is probably not necessary for the disorder to emerge. However, even with these cases, genetic factors probably play a role because not all individuals who experience extreme adversity develop psychopathology.

4.2 Genetic Influences

Studies of twins show that genes and environment contribute approximately equally to the variability in BPD. The amount of variability in a personality phenotype explained by genetic influences is referred to as heritability. Heritability estimates for BPD range from about 40 per cent to 70 per cent.[1] The different estimates are probably due to differences in sample size: a large sample is required to give stable estimates. Large-scale studies of borderline traits report heritabilities in the 40–55 per cent range.[2] Since these estimates are similar to values reported for other personality traits, we can be reasonably confident about them.

4.2.1 Genetic Influences on Trait Structure

Genetic factors also explain why traits are organized into the four clusters described in Chapter 2.[3] Traits forming each cluster hang together because they are all influenced by the same general genetic factor. This means that the organization of traits into clusters is not influenced by environmental factors but rather represents the pattern of genetic influences. Hence even after treatment, these patterns are likely to persist although hopefully in a more adaptive form. These general genetic factors are not the only genetic influences on traits. Most traits are also influenced by a second factor specific to that trait. For example, the submissiveness is influenced by the general genetic factor that influences all other borderline traits and a specific genetic factor that predisposes to submissive behaviour.

These findings reveal a complex genetic architecture to BPD, which helps to explain why patients with the disorder are so heterogeneous.[4] All patients with BPD probably have a high loading on the common genetic factor affecting all borderline traits. However, the magnitude of specific genetic factors will differ across individuals. For example, some may also have a high loading on need for approval or submissiveness whereas others may have a low loading on these traits causing differences in interpersonal fearfulness or subservience even among those with a *DSM* diagnosis of BPD.

4.2.2 Implications of Genetic Research for Psychotherapy

What are the implications of findings on the genetics of personality disorder traits for psychotherapy? Do they matter? And, do they affect therapeutic strategies? In each case, the answer is yes. But before explaining how and why they matter, I need to dispel two misconceptions about the findings of behavioural genetic research that have influenced ideas about treatment. One misunderstanding is that because genes and environment contribute approximately equally to personality traits, personality features can be divided into those features that are influenced by genes (temperament) and those that are influenced by the environment (character). This led to the suggestion that psychotherapy should focus primarily on the characterological aspects of BPD and that temperament should be treated with biological interventions such as medication. The idea is appealing because it appears to simplify treatment. Unfortunately, however, genetic and environmental influences do not operate in this way: all personality features are shaped by the interplay between genes and environment so that it is not possible to identify features that are either primarily genetic or primarily environmental in origin.

A second misconception is that heritable traits cannot be changed. Genetic influences contribute to a bias towards showing certain kinds of behaviour but they do not determine these behaviours in an absolute sense. Moreover, environmental factors including treatment can substantially change how genes are expressed. This is illustrated by phenylketonuria, a metabolic disorder leading to mental disability that is caused by a recessive gene that creates problems metabolizing the amino acid phenylalanine. Provision of a diet low in the amino acid substantially reduces the effects.

Genetic influences on BPD have several treatment implications. First, they draw attention to the basic structure of the disorder, which is often masked by the way these features are modified during development. This is helpful in planning interventions. For example, it is useful to know that unstable emotions involve both anxiousness and emotional lability and that marked submissive tendencies may underlie angry demanding behaviour. Second, genetic influences may constrain the extent to which traits can be changed with treatment.

Many therapies give the impression that all personality characteristics are highly plastic and amenable to change. This is probably not the case. The combination of genetic predisposition and repetitive consolidation of traits during development may limit the changes that can be achieved with current techniques. For example, there is little prospect of patients with high levels of anxiousness and emotional lability or submissiveness such as Anna becoming phlegmatic and highly assertive, but it may be possible to modulate the expression of these traits and help Anna to use them more effectively.

4.2.3 Environmental Influences

Twin studies also provide strong evidence of the importance of the environment, which accounts for slightly more than half the variability in traits. Environmental influences are divided into *shared influences*, that is, environmental factors that affect both members of a twin pair such as family values, and *non-shared influences* that affect only one twin such as parental favouritism, different treatment by peers, and life events affecting only one twin. Environmental effects on personality are largely confined to non-shared effects. Common environmental influences have little effect on BPD although they do affect the development of antisocial personality disorder. These findings suggest that people are remarkably sensitive to being treated differently from others. Hence clinicians should be attentive to whether patients feel that they were treated differently from their siblings because these factors are likely to have had a substantial impact.

4.2.3.1 What Does the Environment Do?

Environmental influences appear to: (i) amplify or attenuate the intensity of a trait and (ii) influence the specific ways a trait is expressed.[5] The first mechanism is illustrated by how the environment affects anxiousness by increasing or decreasing the level of threat needed to activate the threat system and the intensity of the anxiety response. These environmental effects may be either biological or psychological in nature. For example, severe childhood trauma may lead to biological changes in stress responsivity whereas attachment problems may impair the acquisition of emotion regulation skills. The environment also affects the way traits are expressed. Not all individuals with high levels of a given trait express that trait in the same way. For example, some highly submissive individuals may become compulsive caregivers whereas others may attach themselves to dominant and controlling individuals with whom they have a hostile-dependent relationship.

These ideas suggest two general strategies for treating maladaptive traits. First, the intensity and frequency of trait expression may be reduced by modifying the cognitive component. For example, risk-taking and recklessness may be modulated by restructuring beliefs of invulnerability ("bad things only happen to other people") that often accompany recklessness. Emotional traits such as anxiousness and emotional reactivity may also be modified with medication, by teaching emotion regulation and anxiety management skills, by helping patients to change their appraisal of events, and by enhancing beliefs about their ability to manage problems. Second, patients can be encouraged to find more constructive ways to express their traits. For example, patients with strong sensation-seeking tendencies who engage in drug abuse or reckless activities may be helped to find more adaptive ways to satisfy their need for stimulation. These strategies will be discussed further in chapters on emotion regulation and interpersonal problems. For now, we simply need to note that aetiological research is beginning to suggest alternative treatment methods.

4.3 Other Biological Factors

Environmental influences may be biological in nature such as intrauterine events and minor head injuries. A few patients with BPD give a history of minor head injury or of other features that are suggestive of minimal brain dysfunction. In many cases, it is difficult to determine what role these factors play in the genesis of the disorder. However, any neuropsychological impairment in the capacity to self-regulate emotions and impulses or the ability to integrate information may contribute to borderline pathology since these processes are necessary for effective personality development and functioning.

4.4 Psychosocial Adversity

Diverse psychosocial factors influence the development of BPD including: (i) family factors such as family breakdown, dysfunctional relationships, parental loss, and attachment problems; (ii) trauma and deprivation such as neglect, privation, and physical, emotional, and sexual abuse; and (iii) social and cultural factors including societal change.[6] Individual psychosocial factors have relatively small effects and none seem either necessary or sufficient to cause BPD.

Although earlier explanations of the causes of BPD focused especially on trauma, most notably childhood sexual abuse, current evidence suggests that sexual abuse has less impact than originally thought, although when it occurs it obviously has considerable clinical significance. This means that BPD is more than a complex form of post-traumatic stress disorder. The features of the disorder are not confined to the sequelae of trauma and many patients do not have a history of major trauma. Nevertheless, there is good evidence that harsh treatment in early childhood,[7] abuse, neglect, and an unstable early environment increase the risk of BPD.[8]

Cultural factors also appear to contribute to the development of BPD – there is evidence that the disorder is becoming more prevalent probably due to societal and cultural change. Self pathology increases vulnerability to the effects of societal change wrought by increased mobility and a decline in institutionalized values because these changes require individuals to have a clear sense of self and a well-defined sense of identity to function effectively. In the past, when people were less mobile and institutional values were more widely accepted, people spent most of the lives in smaller local communities that provided the structure and support needed for many individuals with mental health problems to function reasonably well. Some cultures also provided a type of prescribed identity in the form of expectations about each person's role and place in the community. The combination of support and prescribed identity probably made it possible for those with self pathology to cope in ways that are not possible in contemporary society.

Although the diverse psychosocial risk factors for BPD operate in a variety of ways, two broad pathways are through attachment problems and the creation of a persistent invalidating environment.

4.4.1 Attachment Problems

Many forms of adversity are linked to dysfunctional attachments. When childhood attachments are satisfactory, contact with attachment figures decreases emotional distress and opens up communication channels with them. This relationship becomes the prototype for interpersonal relationships generally. In contrast, dysfunctional attachments involving neglect, indifference, and empathic failure lead to insecure and disorganized attachment patterns in adulthood.[9]

Dysfunctional attachments have widespread consequences because early attachment relationships are the vehicle for acquiring multiple capacities needed for healthy personality development. Especially important is the role attachment figures play in helping the child to structure and organize experience and in developing the capacity to understand the mental states of self and others. The attachment relationship is also the vehicle for learning to self-regulate emotions. Consequently, attachment insecurity is associated with impaired emotional regulation, distrust, cognitive rigidity, intolerance of ambiguity, dogmatic thinking, and a tendency to cling to, and defend, existing ideas, assumptions, and points of view.[10] These factors reduce the ability to learn and change. This is an additional reason for a strong focus on building the therapeutic alliance – trust and collaboration are the vehicles for decreasing rigidity, increasing communication, and promoting greater openness to new experiences and new learning.

Impaired childhood attachments are sometimes due simply to a poor fit between the child's temperament and the caregiver's personality rather than pathology or inappropriate caregiver behaviour. They also occur because some children have difficult temperaments from birth that make them difficult to manage and soothe. This seems to occur when there are strong predispositions to emotional traits. In other cases, problems arise due to caregiver behaviour involving neglect, withdrawal, or avoidance (sometimes subtle and almost imperceptible), or abuse (physical, emotional, or sexual) with emotional neglect and abuse seeming to have the greatest impact. It should be noted, however, that the pathways to disorder are multiple, and some patients report relatively little obvious psychosocial adversity.

4.4.2 Invalidating Environments

A common assumption across therapies is that invalidation and inaccurate mirroring have crucial roles in the development of BPD and that effective treatment requires a therapeutic stance that emphasizes validation and mirroring.[11] Simply put, the child needs caregivers to validate feelings and experiences and to reflect and mirror these experiences in an accurate and sustained way.

Invalidation takes many forms: the child's experiences may be ignored, rejected, criticized, trivialized, or dismissed. For example, the child may be told to mask distress by "putting on a happy face," that there is no reason to feel the way the child does, and that "nice girls do not get angry" or "big boys don't cry." Invalidation may also extend to needs, interests, and opinions that are dismissed as unimportant, inappropriate, or silly. In the process, the child's initial attempts to show agency and autonomy are stifled. Abuse is by definition invalidating because it violates the needs, wishes, and rights of the person.

Problems arise because invalidation undermines the child's understanding of him- or herself and confidence in his or her own feelings that extends to other aspects of mental life. This creates profound distrust and uncertainty about basic experiences and conflict between what is felt and what the child is told he or she should feel. In the struggle to conform to the demands of the significant other, the child is forced to suppress or deny his or her feelings, wishes, and natural reactions, which undermines the authenticity of the experience and creates confusion about what he or she actually feels. Thus an important source of information about the world is lost. When we cannot trust our feelings we feel a profound sense of uncertainty that adds to a general, almost existential mistrust of all things, even one's own existence.

4.5　Enduring Effects of Adversity

The important question for therapists is probably not what psychosocial events are risk factors for BPD but rather why adversity influences behaviour long after it occurred. An understanding of the mechanisms involved helps to identify targets for change and potential treatment strategies. The effects of adversity on personality are widespread and patients react to adversity in idiosyncratic ways. Nevertheless, the following consequences are common among patients with BPD: (i) impaired regulatory and modulatory mechanisms, (ii) maladaptive schemas, (iii) maladaptive ways of thinking, (iv) conflict between neediness and fear of rejection, (v) states of distress without resolution, (vi) self pathology, and (vii) pervasive conflict and functional incoherence.

4.5.1　Impaired Regulation and Modulation

As noted above, adversity often disrupts the development and functioning of mechanisms used to self-regulate emotions and impulses. Severe trauma can also increase vulnerability to stress probably due to biological influences on the threshold and intensity of the stress response.

4.5.2　Maladaptive Schemas

Adversity exerts a lasting effect on adjustment through the formation of maladaptive schemas that shape the person's understanding of self, others, and the world. Four sets of maladaptive schemas are common in BPD: (i) distrust; (ii) unpredictability and unreliability of others and the world; (iii) lack of personality efficacy and agency involving powerlessness, passivity, and vulnerability; and (iv) low self-esteem, inferiority, and incompetence.

4.5.2.1　Distrust

Adversity, especially attachment trauma, leads to negative schemas about relationships and a pervasive, almost existential, distrust of the world.[12] As Anna commented about her physically abusive mother, "Why would I trust anyone? If your mum is abusive who can you trust?" These beliefs are treated by providing a treatment experience that challenges them by consistently demonstrating therapist availability and responsiveness and more directly through the use of standard cognitive methods.

4.5.2.2　Unpredictability

Abuse often creates beliefs that people are unpredictable because abusive individuals are inconsistent, being abusive on some occasions and loving on others. A common example is the experience of patients with alcohol-misusing parents who recall feeling intense fear throughout childhood when they waited for a parent to come home from the bar not knowing whether he or she would be loving or abusive. This kind of anxious uncertainty creates the powerful impression that people, indeed life generally, are unpredictable and offers little opportunity to learn how to relate to others in consistent and predictable ways, thereby laying the foundation for a chaotic interpersonal life.

Not surprisingly, distrust and unpredictability schemas lead to expectations of therapist unpredictability and unreliability, which need to be countered by ensuring a consistent therapeutic process that is not derailed by the patient's conflicting demands and unstable emotions. It is also important to ensure that these schemas are not inadvertently reinforced. This requires the therapist to be as consistent as possible in relating to the patient and managing the treatment process and to avoid sudden changes to the treatment frame.

4.5.2.3 Powerlessness and Lack of Personal Efficacy

The unpredictability of abuse and the child's inability to control mistreatment creates a sense of powerlessness and beliefs that power and control lie outside the self. The result is a sense of passivity and the feeling that everything is pointless because nothing can be done to control one's own destiny. This belief adds to emotional distress because people deal with stress better when they feel in control.[13] This is also an obstacle to treatment – there is little point in working on problems if things are unlikely to change.

4.5.2.4 Low Self-Esteem, Inferiority, and Incompetence

The lasting impact of many forms of adversity is mediated through the development of negative self-schemas of inadequacy, inherent badness, and low self-esteem, which create a pervasive sense of worthlessness and shame. Adversity in the form of neglect, deprivation, and verbal abuse can also lead to beliefs that one is unimportant and unworthy of care and attention. Abusive individuals often maintain that the abuse was the child's own fault or that it was for their own good, which often leads the child to conclude that he or she is bad and to blame for what happened. These effects are compounded when the child is told not to tell others about what happened because no one would believe them or when the child confides in an adult who then either blames the child for what happened or accuses the child of lying. Individuals with low self-esteem automatically see themselves as less worthy and less important than other people, perceptions of the self that are intensified by the shame felt by many abused individuals.

4.5.3 Maladaptive Cognitive Processes

Repetitive adversity influences both *what* people think (schemas and associated beliefs) and *how* people think. Three maladaptive thinking styles are commonly associated with BPD: self invalidation, catastrophizing, and categorical thinking.

Repetitive invalidation leads to the formation of self-invalidating thinking that causes patients to doubt and question the authenticity of their feelings, ideas, and experiences. Thus the invalidating environment is internalized to exert an ongoing effect on how mental states are understood and processed, which forms a persistent obstacle to self-development. An understandable consequence of abuse is the tendency to expect the worst in most situations. Many adverse experiences must have felt disastrous to the child and the tendency to catastrophize may have been adaptive if it reduced exposure to abusive situations. Nevertheless, its continued use adds to the escalation of distress in crises. Patients with BPD also tend to think in black-and-white terms and to switch between extreme positions. This is related to rigid thinking involving a tendency to cling to existing ideas so that ideas and assumptions become frozen and difficult to change.[14]

4.5.4 Core Interpersonal Conflict

Threatening or stressful events activate the threat and attachment systems, leading to a strong desire to approach attachment figures. However, in patients with BPD, activation of the attachment system does not lead to expectations of relief as it does in healthy individuals. Instead, the attachment system itself becomes a source of threat instilled by previous experiences with attachment figures, leading to an approach-avoidance conflict regarding attachment figures that generalizes to other relationships. Consequently, any interpersonal encounter has the potential to create intense inner turmoil arising from the conflict between neediness and fear of rejection or humiliation. This leads to unstable relationships because feelings of closeness to another person evoke strong fears of rejection and hence prompt withdrawal.

4.5.5 Distress without Resolution

When life events take their toll and cause intense stress or distress, we turn to others, especially loved ones, for comfort, help, and support. Contact with another person makes us feel better regardless of any instrumental or emotional help they may give. As the old adage goes, "misery loves company." This natural proclivity to seek out others at times of stress is thwarted in BPD, closing down the major avenue used to reduce distress and increasing feelings of isolation and aloneness, which are difficult for people with insecure attachment to manage. This creates a distressed, confused, and disorganized state without any means to resolve it. This is what happens in borderline crises – irresolvable distress escalates, creating an urgent need for relief that often results in self-injurious behaviour. Add to this mix emotional instability and it becomes readily understandable why emotional crises are so overwhelming and why patients feel so desperate and powerless. To treat distress without resolution, therapists need to be empathically attuned to the patient's inner world and to use this understanding to align themselves with the distress and help the patient begin to structure his or her experience.

4.5.6 Self System

Previously it was noted that repetitive adversity affects both the *contents* of the self through the development of maladaptive self-schemas and the *structure* of the system. Briefly, persistent invalidation undermines the self as knower by creating uncertainty about the authenticity of emotional experiences with downstream effects on other aspects of self-development. At the same time, dysfunctional attachments fail to provide the consistent feedback needed to understand and organize inner experience. Invalidation also makes it difficult to understand or "read" the mental states of others and undermines the child's confidence in the intuitive processes that guide social interaction. This in turn hinders the emergence of a sense of personal autonomy and agency.

Equally problematic are experiences with significant others whose behaviours are inconsistent and chaotic as occurs when caregivers switch unpredictably between being abusive and loving. For example, when Anna was upset as a child, she did not know whether mother would comfort or scold her. As a result, she used to try to find her father because he was more consistent but he was rarely around. This meant that she did not learn to self-soothe because this is learned in the context of attachment relationships. It also led to fragmented images of herself and mother: it was almost impossible for her to reconcile experiences of a caring, loving mother with the angry, violent mother. It was also difficult to integrate the image of herself as highly independent and angry with that of being extremely needy and dependent.

The coping strategies commonly used to cope with adversity and abuse also contribute to the ensuing problems. Patients often attempt to suppress memories of traumatic experiences and some also dissociate. Both responses compartmentalize their experiences, leading to a divided and poorly integrated self.

4.5.7 Conflict and Functional Incoherence

The various consequences of adversity combine to create a personality structure riddled with conflict. This is obviously the case with the core conflict between neediness and rejection. However, it also occurs with submissiveness because tendencies to be subservient and please others conflict with anger aroused by abuse and deprivation. The conflict experienced is both internal and external: it is internal in the sense that the individual struggles to manage conflicting needs, wants, and feelings, and external in the sense that any social contact is a potential source of strife. Conflict also occurs between overt actions and inner experience. This occurs with both anxiousness and submissiveness: both lead to overtly angry behaviour that masks the feelings of vulnerability and dependency. These conflicts create inner turmoil and persistent interpersonal conflict. As one patient noted, "I am always at war with the world. I'm angry and confrontational. I have an in-your-face attitude but inside I feel vulnerable and weak. I would never let anyone see that and I don't even let myself feel that way. It's only at two in the morning when alone in my bed that I break down and sob for hours but I would never let anyone know."

The inner and external conflicts generated by adversity produce such a confusing array of feelings and actions that there is little sense of coherence to experiences of the self in interaction with others. Thus the lack of coherence to self is not just a cognitive problem arising from difficulty linking disparate parts of self but also an experiential phenomenon arising from diverse and incoherent experiences of the self in significant relationships. Patients experience what might be called "functional incoherence." And, they do so repeatedly in their main relationships. It is not surprising, therefore, that the establishment of a sense of personal unity and coherence is so elusive to patients with BPD or that their experience of the self is confusing.

The conflict and turmoil that characterizes the patient's inner world is increased by the rigid ways he or she interprets and responds to situations and the coping strategies used to manage distress. Being unable either to see or to respond to situations differently, they remain trapped in their inner world. At the same time, efforts to cope by denying or suppressing their feelings add to the feelings of inner conflict and hence to their sense of alienation and confusion. It is this confusion that therapy seeks to address by helping the patient to construct a meaningful narrative about his or her life and experience.

4.6 Concluding Comments

The rather commonsense analysis of the diverse consequences of the various factors found to influence the development of BPD described in this chapter identified major targets for change, and the implications of these targets in turn help to identify some of the more important treatment strategies. For example, schemas related to distrust, unpredictability, invalidation, and powerlessness point respectively to the importance of a treatment process that provides support and empathy, provides consistency, provides validation, and builds motivation, competency, and mastery. The analysis also points to the central role of increasing emotion regulation in the change process and the importance of fostering more integrated personality functioning. Interestingly, the basic structure of therapy suggested by this examination of aetiological factors largely coincides with the basic structure of therapy established by the review of effective change mechanisms described in Chapter 1.

Notes

1. Distel et al. (2008), Torgersen et al. (2000).

2. Jang et al. (1996).

3. Livesley et al. (1998).

4. Livesley (2008).

5. See Livesley (2003) for a discussion of how genetic influences affect personality and their implications for treatment.

6. See Paris (2001, in press) for reviews of the nature and scope of psychosocial influences on personality disorder.

7. Carlson et al. (2009), Crawford et al. (2009).

8. Helegeland and Torgersen (2004).

9. Cicchetti et al. (1990).

10. Mikulincer (1997).

11. Therapies based on different conceptual models agree that inaccurate mirroring and invalidation contribute to the development of personality disorder; see for example, Bateman and Fonagy (2004, 2006), Kohut (1971), and Linehan (1993).

12. Allen (2013), Jovev and Jackson (2004), Meyer et al. (2005), Young et al. (2003), Heckhausen and Schulz (1995), Skinner (1996), Taylor (1983), Thompson and Spacaman (1991).

13. See Kruglanski and Webster (1996) and Pierro and Kruglanski (2008) regarding rigidity. Empirical evidence also supports the suggestion that patients with BPD show high levels of categorical or dichotomous thinking in emotional situations (De Bonis et al. (1998), Moritz et al. (2011), Napolitano and McKay (2007), Sieswerda et al. (2013), Veen and Arntz (2000)).

14. Liotti (2004, 2009, 2011) makes the point that trauma produces a sense of threat without resolution because of its effects on the attachment system and the creation of an approach-avoidance conflict regarding attachment figures.

Chapter

5

Diagnosis and Assessment

The goal of assessment is to establish a diagnosis and collect the information needed to construct a formulation to use in establishing the treatment contract and planning therapy. Integrated modular treatment (IMT) usually requires a slightly longer assessment than some therapies because the process is also used to engage the patient in treatment. This is important because many patients drop out either during assessment or before therapy starts. Dropout is reduced when clinicians also use the assessment interviews to build rapport and make a connection with the patient.[1] This usually enhances the assessment because patients feel more involved and more open and communicative. The focus on engagement requires therapists to avoid being so focused on collecting information that they forget to monitor rapport. It also requires therapists to intervene promptly when rapport is poor or the patient is overly distressed, even if the assessment is to be put on hold until the problem is resolved.

5.1 Clinical Interview

Clinical assessment covers five major areas: (i) current symptoms, problems, and concerns; (ii) family history including details of parents, siblings, and family relationships; (iii) personal history including developmental history and current functioning; (iv) mental state; and (v) personality. Although most clinicians have a preferred way to cover these areas, a practical sequence is to follow the above order. Since the first four areas are part of a standard assessment, they will only be discussed briefly.

Current symptoms, problems, and concerns. Most assessments begin with an open-ended question about the reasons for seeking treatment. This provides information relatively quickly and engages the patient by focusing immediately on his or her current concerns. Open-ended questions also reveal the patient's capacity to organize thoughts, which is helpful in assessing the severity of his or her disorder. An immediate focus on current concerns also promotes the treatment alliance. Hence it is useful to work with the patient to compile a list of symptoms, problems, and concerns and explore the extent to which these difficulties have been present throughout the patient's life. The latter information helps to differentiate personality disorder from other mental disorders because personality disorders usually begin in adolescence or even earlier.

Family history. Information about the nuclear family and what it was like to grow up in the family is always helpful as is information about parents even if this only consists of thumbnail sketches of their main features and the relationship between them and the patient.

BOX 5.1 Family and Personal History: Major Themes and Illustrative Questions

Family History:
   Could you tell me about your family?
   Could you tell me about your parents? What were they like?
   Do you have brothers and sisters? Tell me about them.
   What was it like growing up in your family?
   Have your parents ever mentioned any particular problems that occurred when you were
      little?
Childhood and Schooling:
   What sort of memories do you have of childhood?
   Did anything traumatic or painful ever happen to you?
   Could you tell me what school was like?
   What was elementary school like? High school?
   Did you have many friends at school? How did people treat you?
   What did you do after school?
Romantic Relationships:
   Could you tell me about the romantic relationships that you have had?
   When did you start dating?
   What were these relationships like? How did they work out?
Work History:
   Could you tell me about the jobs you have had? What have they been like? Have you had
      problems holding down a job?
   How do you find people at work? Are they easy to get on with? Do you find the people
      that you worked with difficult to get along with? Have you had any problems?
Current Circumstances:
   Could you tell me about your current life?
   Could we talk about your current relationships?
   What sort of social life do you have?
   What are your days like? What do you do on a typical day?
   Do you find your life stressful? In what way? Has anything particularly upsetting and
      stressful happened to you recently?

Personal history. Ideally, the assessment should include developmental history and present functioning. However, when time is limited, an evaluation of current adjustment and life situation is more useful because IMT focuses primarily on current functioning. Evaluations of current circumstances should include current social circumstances including degree of social support, family and relationship problems, the nature and effects of the patient's social network, and so on. Box 5.1 outlines key themes related to personal history and examples of the open-ended questions used to explore each theme. This component of assessment is also intended to provide an understanding of critical life events and how the individual managed major life transitions.

Mental state. The clinical interview should also include a systematic evaluation of mental state in order to make a careful assessment of any co-occurring mental disorders.

Personality assessment. A full evaluation of personality will cover: (i) diagnosis of personality disorder and assessment of severity; (ii) assessment of major traits; and (iii) assessment of impairment across the four domains: symptoms; regulation and modulation problems; interpersonal difficulties; and self/identity.[2]

Sidebar 5.1 presents Anna's personal history to complement the information provided in Chapter 2. Sidebar 5.2 provides similar information about a second patient, Madison, who will also be discussed in subsequent chapters.

SIDEBAR 5.1 The Case of Anna

Anna was introduced in Chapter 2. The initial assessment was short due to the need to start treatment because she was in a severe decompensated state.

Current Symptoms, Problems, and Concerns: Anna said her main concern was unstable moods, intense anger, and feeling depressed and that she had felt this way for as long as she could remember. She said that her life was a mess and that it felt as if she was running around like "a chicken without a head" as she lurched from crisis to crisis, each involving deliberate self-injury and suicidal thoughts. Her marriage was unhappy and she and her husband fought constantly. She ruminated endlessly about being abandoned by a previous husband who was the only person she had loved. When upset she was filled with intense uncontrollable rage.

Family History: Anna's parents were in their mid-60s. Mother was described as anxious, unpredictable, angry, and abusive. All her life, Anna had longed for her mother to love her. Father was more loving but he often left the family, sometimes for several years although he always moved back. Anna had a much older brother and two older sisters. The brother sexually abused her when she was in her early teens as did a neighbour.

Personal History: Anna was raised in a small farming community. Anna described her childhood years as unhappy and family life as chaotic and unpredictable. She never knew whether mother would be abusive or loving or whether father would be there or not. It felt as if all she had ever known was chaos and she actually found it difficult to cope when things were different. She had been a sickly child with several hospital admissions in infancy. Throughout childhood she felt closer to father but worried constantly that he would leave and never return.

Early school days were unremarkable. Her performance was adequate. During the immediate pre-teen years, Anna had more difficulties. She had few friends and frequently squabbled with other girls. At first, she got satisfactory grades but later did badly. At the age of 13 years, father left for a longer period, which was followed by Anna acting out intensely. Deliberate self-harming behaviour started at about 15 years. She was hospitalized for the first time at 17 years due to suicidal behaviour. Subsequently, she saw several therapists but never remained in treatment for long.

Anna left school at 18 years, uncertain what to do and found it hard to keep a job. Following a series of fleeting relationships, she fell head over heels in love with Marty and went to live with him and cared for his two children. Subsequently, she had a daughter with him. Although the relationship was steady, Anna's abandonment fears and Marty's emotional abusiveness caused ongoing problems until he ended the relationship, leaving Anna feeling devastated. A series of impulsive relationships followed, which resulted in her having two more children. Eventually, she met her current husband who was divorced with a daughter and son who lived with him on alternative weeks. The relationship was stormy with constant arguments and mutual emotional abuse. Anna felt unable to leave for financial reasons but she was also afraid of being alone.

Mental State: Although Anna was open and cooperative with the assessment, a full evaluation was not possible due to an intense symptomatic state and suicidality. Symptom review revealed unstable emotions, frequent feeling of sadness, and low mood that fluctuated rapidly with no consistent pattern. There was no evidence of vegetative symptoms other than sleep disturbance due to intense rumination. The frequent crises were associated with chronic suicidal thoughts and deliberate self-harm but she had no clearly formed intent or plan. The self-harm always occurred during crises and Anna usually felt better after cutting herself. She said that she cut herself because she was so desperate and not because she wanted to die. Anxiety symptoms involved constant worry and rumination often about little things ("I'm a worry wart"), and apprehensiveness so that she "never feel safe." This was intensified by fears of abandonment. Other notable symptoms were hearing a voice in her head when she was extremely distressed that said brief phrases such as "you're nothing," "you're no good," and "fat." Anna recognized that the voices were "in my head" although they felt real. At other times, she felt her head "was filled with distortions." By this she meant that she ruminated about abandonment and about being a bad person, and that she did "not deserve to be loved."

SIDEBAR 5.2 The Case of Madison

Current Symptoms, Problems, and Concerns: Madison was 22 years old, a student, single, and living alone when assessed. Her initial complaints were persistent anxiety; worry about her future, especially future relationships; and intense emotional states that she could not control. She said that she had always been a worrier. She also noted that her feelings changed a lot – she would feel fine and then get suddenly upset and distressed. When this happened, she sometimes cut herself. These incidents had occurred more frequently over the last three years, following an attempted rape. About six months earlier she was forced to discontinue her studies.

Family History: Madison's parents were in their early 50s. Mother was also a worrier and emotionally volatile. She had a small business and worked part-time. Madison described her as loving and supportive but inconsistent. This caused tension between them because mother got angry when Madison was upset. Father had a high-powered position in a large company. Although he was also anxious, he was much less emotional than mother and tried to deal with everything in a rational way; as a result Madison felt that he did not really understand her problems. Also, the combination of business demands and an enthusiasm for golf meant that he was rarely available. There also seemed to be problems with anxiety on both sides of the family. Madison had a brother two years older with whom she had a strained relationship. He considered her a "drama queen" and resented the time their parents spent dealing with her problems and tantrums.

Personal History: Madison described childhood as happy. Although, she thought that she was a difficult child who even as an infant was difficult to settle. Subsequent interviews with the parents confirmed this and they noted that she was also very anxious worrying endlessly about tiny things and needed constant reassurance. She had temper tantrums and would also lash out when anxious. From an early age, her mood was unpredictable. The parents said that she still acted in this way and they had lost track of the number of family celebrations that had been marred by her behaviour.

Madison excelled at school and was an excellent athlete. She had many friends, but as she got older, she seemed to change friends frequently because they were unable to cope with her moods. Madison matured early. She started dating when she was about 14 years.

A boyfriend attempted to rape her when she was 17. Although traumatized by the incident, she only told her parents about the incident several months later She was upset by their reaction because mother did not believe her and dismissed it as an attention-seeking manoeuver and father asked what she had done to encourage it. Madison was devastated. Her distress increased subsequently. She also developed a strong need to feel loved and wanted, which led to a series of disastrous relationships. After school, Madison went on to university. Her symptoms increased and her emotions became increasingly volatile about a year earlier following the break-up of relationship with a boyfriend she had lived with for nearly two years.

Mental State: Madison presented in an intense way that suggested engagement but seemed more superficial. Nevertheless she was frank and open. Problems were recounted in an articulate and relatively matter-of-fact way initially, but she became very distressed when describing her relationship with her parents and her fears of being abandoned by the men she dated. A relatively long-standing relationship had ended a few weeks before and she felt devastated and found it difficult to be alone. She needed to feel wanted and cared for.

Madison's primary complaint was anxiety – a lifelong problem. Mood changes were common and she described her feelings as being all over the place but her mood was not consistently low. She also experienced episodes of intense distress. On these occasions, she cried incessantly and became extremely frustrated, which sometimes progressed to uncontrollable rage. These states were also characterized by loneliness. The combination of intense distress and loneliness sometimes became so intolerable that she harmed herself, got drunk, or acted out in some other way. Madison also noted mild depressive symptoms that seemed part of the emotional lability. She did not report any other symptoms of mood disorder apart from occasional suicidal thoughts but added that she knew that she would never do it.

5.1.1 Length of Assessment

Combining assessment and alliance building usually requires multiple sessions. This is not usually a problem for most patients because they usually prefer in-depth assessments.[3] The first session typically covers personal history with a primary focus on current concerns and an alliance-building component. The second session is used to evaluate personality and discuss aspects of the personal history flagged previously as needing further exploration. If further sessions are needed, they can focus on gaining more information on current social circumstances, key schemas, and conflicted relationships. Towards the end of the assessment process, the patient's treatment goals are discussed. This is also a good time to evaluate motivation for change and to deal with any concerns the patient may have about treatment. Subsequently, the diagnosis and formulation can be discussed as the first step in negotiating the treatment contract (see Chapter 6). The remainder of this chapter deals with personality assessment and concludes with further discussion of how to build the alliance during the assessment.

5.2 Diagnosis of Personality Disorder and Assessment of Severity

The first decision related to personality is whether the patient has personality disorder based on the impairments in self and interpersonal functioning (Chapter 2) listed in Box 5.2.

BOX 5.2 Definition of General Personality Disorder as Applied to Borderline Personality Disorder

Personality disorder is characterized by (i) an impaired sense of self and/or (ii) chronic interpersonal dysfunction.

1. **Self Pathology**

Poorly developed sense of self as manifested by problems with at least one of the three main components of the self: (i) the self as knower, (ii) the self as known, and (iii) the self as agent.

(i)   Self as knower: problems with the way the self is experienced that may involve:

(a)   personal unity: does not have a sense of wholeness or cohesion; for example, "I sometimes wonder if I really exist." "I feel as if there are lots of different me's." (Note: aspects of personality unity overlap with manifestations and descriptions of problems with the integration of self-knowledge. This is because they are different ways to refer to the same phenomenon. A sense of personal unity is the subjective experience of the extent to which different elements of self-knowledge are interconnected.)

(b)   continuity: lacks a sense of continuity through time; exists in the moment and does not have a meaningful sense of having a past that is linked to the present; for example, "It doesn't feel as if I have a past. I know I have but it does not feel real to me." "My life is just a series of events and I do not know where I am in them." "It doesn't feel as if I have a future." (Note: this latter example would require an evaluation of whether this is a short-term feeling related to depressed mood or a long-term way of experiencing the self.)

(c)   certainty and clarity: uncertain about personal qualities; has difficulty identifying personal characteristics and attributes; vague and unsure about personal qualities and mental states. For example, "I do not know who I am." "I find it hard to know what I am like or what I really feel."

(d)   authenticity: doubts the authenticity of basic emotions and wants; wonders if feelings are real; lacks the conviction that feelings and wants are "real" or genuine. For example, "Sometimes my feelings don't feel real." "I'm very upset. But how do I know that I am really upset?"

(ii) Self as known: impairments with the self as known involve:

(a)   impaired differentiation of the self: poorly developed self construct with limited development of self-schemas and impaired interpersonal boundaries; difficulty describing personal qualities and attributes; descriptions limited to a simple list of a few relatively concrete features; difficulty differentiating self and other; confuses own thoughts for those of other people; assumes own thoughts and feelings are identical to those of other; worries about losing self in others; easily feels overwhelmed by other people.

(b)   impaired integration of the self: self-concept is poorly integrated leading to a fragmented and unstable sense of self and a limited sense of personal unity and continuity; experiences shifting and poorly integrated self-states; may not always recall experiences in different self-states; feels that sense of who they are

> is fragile and that ideas about the self vary markedly across situations; sense of discontinuity between the self presented to the world and the "real" self.
> (iii) Self as agent: lacks self-directedness and a sense of personal autonomy and agency; difficulty setting long-term goals; low motivation leading to difficulty attaining any goals that are established; has little sense of direction and purpose; does not make plans; passive; tends to drift through life.

> **2. Interpersonal Pathology**
>
> Chronically impaired interpersonal functioning manifested by impaired capacity for closeness, intimacy, and attachment.
> 1. Intimacy: difficulty establishing and/or sustaining intimate relationships; relationships are unstable and conflicted; shifts rapidly between idealizing and romanticizing relationships and intense disillusionment.
> 2. Attachment: Difficulty establishing adult patterns of attachment; severe problems may include symbiotic relationships.

Although this may seem a difficult and even daunting task, it is relatively straightforward. The best approach is for the clinician to become familiar with the features shown in Box 5.2 and to use these features to make an assessment based initially on information obtained during the interview and then to supplement the initial impression with the assessment methods suggested in the next section.

Most interviews provide extensive information about self and interpersonal pathology if the assessor is attuned to assessing these features. For example, patients may mention being uncertain about who they are, that they lose themselves in other people, or not knowing what they want from life. Such statements respectively hint at poor differentiation of the self, boundary problems, and low self-directedness. This initial evaluation is then easily pursued with a few specific questions to establish a diagnosis. Severity is assessed in the same way.[4] When assessing severity, it should be noted that severity refers to the level of personality impairment, not degree of symptomatic distress, because the two are often confused.

5.2.1 Clinical Assessment of Self Pathology

The assessment of self pathology is based on the three facets of the self discussed in Chapters 2 and 3: the self as knower, known, and agent. It is best to begin by assessing the self as known followed by the self as agent. In the process, information is usually obtained that permits an evaluation of the self as knower.

5.2.1.1 Assessing the Self as Known

A simplest way to assess the *self as known* is to ask patients to describe themselves.[5] A good time to do this is after evaluating the patient's mental state because it is a smooth transition to switch from asking about symptoms to asking about personality. The topic can be introduced with a comment such as: "Perhaps we could now talk about how you see yourself. Could you tell me what sort of person are you? How do you describe yourself?" This is one of the most useful questions to ask patients with suspected personality disorder because it elicits diagnostic information relatively quickly. The first thing to note is how the patient handles the question – can the patient provide a self-description or is she/he puzzled by the request and have difficulty organizing her/his thoughts?

When evaluating the patient's responses, the assessor seeks to answer four questions:

1. Does the description include a variety of self-schemas and information about the self or is it impoverished? (differentiation component of the self as known);
2. Is the sense of self fragmented and unstable and does sense of self change markedly over occasions? (integration component of the self as known);
3. Does the description and personal history show evidence of self-directedness and does the patient have difficulty setting and attaining goals? (self as agent);
4. Is there evidence of a sense of personal unity and continuity or does the description suggest that patient wonders who he/she is, and does it suggest that the patient accepts the authenticity of basic emotional experiences or wonder whether his/her basic emotional experiences are genuine? (self as knower).

5.2.1.1.1 Differentiation Problems

Patients with a poorly developed self have difficulty describing themselves. They may comment that they do not know what to say or that they are not sure who they are, or offer a simple evaluation of themselves such as "I'm a nice person" or as one patient with narcissistic features said "I am an exceptional person – there is nothing more I need to say about myself." Others list a few concrete attributes. For example, Anna initially said she could not think of what to say and then added, "I think I am a nice person. I like to help people. I can't think of anything else." Probing questions did not produce additional information. In contrast, Madison provided a longer description:

> "I think I'm great. My life is amazing. I have a lot of energy. I want to succeed and I'm going to. I am an anxious person and I'm a mess just now but I intend to get over it. Sometimes it feels as if it will last for ever but I am determined it won't. I like everything to be right and when it's not I fret … "

This account shows Madison had a more developed sense of self and a larger repertoire of self-schemas than Anna. As we will see, her self pathology took a somewhat different form.

Before evaluating patients, it is helpful to form an impression of how non-personality disordered individuals describe themselves by asking a few of them to describe themselves. Such descriptions are usually more detailed and refer to a variety of features including traits, values, beliefs, and social roles. They are also more organized and highlight features that the person considers important as opposed to being just lists. For example: a middle-aged man described himself:

> I am a fairly successful businessman. I work hard, perhaps too hard, but I'm a self-made man and believe you should work for what you want. I am also generous. This is important to me. I like to help my kids even though they are grown up. My wife says that I am too generous and help too much. But that's the way I am. I am also loyal to people and stick

with them no matter what. I am not as fit I as I should be. I exercise regularly but I indulge myself too much.

Even this brief example differs qualitatively from descriptions by patients with borderline personality disorder (BPD). It reveals a richer understanding of the self and greater insight into positive and negative attributes and their consequences.

After giving patients a few moments to describe themselves, a few probing questions may be used to see if they can provide more information. This usually reveals the extent of differentiation problems. It is also useful to ask specifically about two specific features of poor differentiation: feelings of "inner emptiness" ("Do you feel as if there is nothing inside, as if you are empty and hollow inside?") and boundary problems ("Do you ever feel as if nothing separates you from other people?" "Do you ever confuse other people's ideas with your own?" "Do ever worry that you will lose the sense of who you really are?").

Differences in differentiation of the self are useful in evaluating severity. Patients with *less-severe* BPD, such as Madison, are usually able to provide a self-description although it is usually less detailed than that of healthy individuals. Interpersonal boundaries are present but not fully developed. They also tend to feel empty or "hollow" inside. Those with more *severe disorder* such as Anna have a severely impoverished self-concept and hence they find it difficult to describe themselves in psychological terms and their descriptions are usually limited to a few concrete characteristics. Interpersonal boundaries are very permeable, leading to enmeshed relationships and the "sense of losing oneself" when the person is with others.

5.2.1.1.2 Integration Problems

Self-descriptions also provide information on the unstable and poorly integrated nature of the self in BPD. Patients comment that it is hard to describe themselves because their ideas about who they are keep changing. For example, "My ideas about myself differ from one moment to the next"; "I sometimes feel as if I am different people." These problems may be explored with questions such as: "Does your sense of who you are change a lot from day to day?" "Do you have contradictory feelings about yourself and who you are?" "Do you ever get the feeling that you are several different people, as if there are several different yous?"

Levels of severity are distinguished by the degree of disconnection between self-states. Those with less-severe disorder have an unstable sense of self and feel fragmented. Hence their sense of who they are changes across situations and time. However, they can recall what it was like to be in these different states and how they felt about themselves and others at these times. In contrast, those with severe disorder experience more extreme self-states that feel totally disconnected so that they have little sense of personal unity and continuity through time. Most importantly, it is difficult for them to remember what it felt like when they were in a different state. The following example may make this idea a little clearer. One man with severe disorder said he felt as if he were two different people – a relatively calm person who had few feelings and a very agitated person. In the agitated state he felt intense despair and totally empty inside as if there was a void within him. These states usually lasted for days. Interestingly when in the despairing state, he had little recall that he felt differently only a short time before. Hence the state felt as if it was a permanent condition.

5.2.1.2   Self as Agent

Difficulty setting long-term goals and lack of self-directedness are also readily evaluated during a standard interview. The personal history usually reveals whether patients have clear goals and a sense of direction and purpose or whether they drift passively through life. This initial evaluation can be probed with questions such as: "Do you feel as if you are in control of your life or do you feel as if there is nothing that you can do to change your life?" "Do you have difficulty setting goals?" "Do you change your mind a lot about your major goals or what you want?" "Do you know what you want out of life?"

Patients with less-severe disorder may set long-term goals but these are rarely attained and their goals often change with emotional fluctuations. Those with severe disorder are usually unable to establish goals and tend to adopt a passive attitude to life.

5.2.1.3   Self as Knower

Self-descriptions may also provide information that is pertinent to assessing the self as knower. For example, patients may note that they do not feel whole, indicating problems with a sense of unity or continuity. More information can also be obtained by asking directly about whether the patient feels "whole." They may also note that they are unsure about what they really feel and whether their feelings are real. However, much of the information needed to assess this aspect of the self is usually obtained during treatment. Patients with personality disorder usually show minimal impairment in this facet of the self although they do not have the same sense of personal unity as healthy individuals whereas those with severe pathology usually have substantial doubts about the authenticity of basic emotional experiences.

5.2.1.4   Case Examples

The assessment of self pathology will probably become clearer if we consider the assessment of Anna and Madison. Anna was determined to have severe personality disorder whereas Madison was considered to have less-severe disorder. Anna's self-description was impoverished and included few self-schemas. In contrast, Madison's self-description revealed a more differentiated body of self-knowledge and more self-schemas although these schemas suggested a grandiose self. Both had boundary problems but these also differed in severity. With Madison, boundary problems were confined to inappropriate disclosure of personal information, especially to potential partners, because she needed to feel wanted. Anna also was inappropriately self-revealing but she also said that it was difficult at times to separate herself from her husband and ex-husband. She noted that when they made demands of her, she could not refuse because it felt as if their wants became her wants, and when they said something critical or abusive, it seemed as if their words were "inside my head."

Anna and Madison both had a poorly integrated self. When directly questioned, Anna said that it sometimes felt as if she were different people. She also described several self-states and the important feature for assessment purposes was that these states were relatively extreme and disconnected. When upset, she just needed to be loved and cared for and she was terrified of being left and abandoned. In this state, she felt that she could not cope and took to her bed for days at a time. She also felt suicidal because it was as if she had always felt this way and always would. At other times, she got into an outraged state in which she was intensely resentful of the demands made of her and did not care about anyone or anything.

She also felt bored with her life but did not feel motivated to do anything about it, which caused her to become more angry and demanding. On other occasions, she felt a powerful need to care for others, especially her children, and devoted her time to them to the exclusion of everything else.

Madison also felt fragmented as if there were two different sides to her: a competent and strong side that was successful and confident about herself and her abilities and a fearful and needy side that was terrified of being abandoned and of being alone. In this state, it was hard to cope and she spent a lot of time curled up in bed as if she was afraid to face the world. She was not sure how she got into these states or how they changed.

Impairments to the sense of self as agent also differed substantially in these patients. Anna had little sense of direction and seemed to drift passively from one relationship to the next with no long-term goals apart from caring for her children. In contrast, Madison had clearly defined long-term goals of completing her studies and pursuing a professional career. At the time, she was having difficulty pursuing these goals but there was no uncertainty about them.

Even more marked were differences in the self as knower. Although this was difficult to evaluate in both patients during the initial assessment, Anna presented information that hinted about severe problems. It was noted in Chapter 2 that, on several occasions, she described feeling upset or angry only to wonder moments later whether the feelings were real. This uncertainty about the authenticity of basic feelings became more apparent as therapy proceeded. Madison did not have these difficulties: she was confident about her feelings and wants and never questioned their authenticity even though she frequently expressed puzzlement about why she was so distressed.

5.2.2 Clinical Assessment of Interpersonal Pathology

The second component of general personality disorder, chronic interpersonal dysfunction, is manifested in BPD as inability to sustain intimate relationships. This capacity is readily evaluated using information obtained when taking a history of family and sexual and social relationships. Differences in severity are less marked than those occurring with self pathology. Those with less-severe disorder usually have a history of relationships but they never seem to work out. The usual pattern with romantic relationships is rapid involvement with others who are idealized followed by equally rapid disillusionment. With more severe disorder, there is less evidence of lasting relationships although there may be a history of frequent casual relationships. Some patients also form enmeshed and symbiotic relationships and have difficulty differentiating self and other.

5.2.2.1 Case Examples

Both Anna and Madison had difficulty with intimate relationships. They had a history of unstable relationships that were romanticized and idealized with equally rapid disillusionment. The level of pathology was consistent with a diagnosis of personality disorder rather than more severe disorder although Anna's problems were more severe in the sense that she was much needier.

Based on the combination of self and interpersonal pathology, Anna was deemed to have severe personality disorder largely on the basis of the severity of self pathology whereas Madison was considered to show personality disorder. This suggested that the two patients needed to be treated somewhat differently as will be discussed in the next chapter. First, however, we need to consider the assessment of personality traits.

5.3 Assessing Trait Constellations and Primary Traits

Even if a DSM-5 categorical diagnosis is established as part of the assessment, it is useful to make a more comprehensive evaluation based on the four trait constellations because interventions are usually selected to treat specific traits such as emotional lability and attachment insecurity rather than the global disorder.[6] Medication, for example, is used to treat specific symptom clusters such as cognitive dysregulation, emotional lability, and impulsivity, not global BPD.[7] Also comprehensive assessment provides a more balanced understanding of the patient's personality that recognizes assets as well as problems.

It will be recalled that traits are organized into four clusters – emotional dysregulation, dissocial, social avoidance, and compulsivity – and that BPD is characterized by traits from the emotional dysregulation cluster (see Chapter 2). Box 5.3 provides a narrative description of each cluster and Box 5.4 provides detailed definitions of borderline traits. Traits defining dissocial/antisocial, social avoidance, and compulsivity are shown in Table 2.1.

BOX 5.3 General Descriptions of the Four Trait Constellations

Emotional Dysregulation: a pattern of intense and unstable emotions involving (i) anxiety, worry, fearfulness, and pervasive sense of threat and (ii) intense labile emotions that are easily aroused and change frequently. These emotional features are closely related to interpersonal problems involving (i) attachment insecurity involving fear of losing or being rejected by significant others; (ii) submissive and subservient behaviour and a strong need for support and guidance; and (iii) a strong need for approval and fear of social disapproval or humiliation. Interpersonal relationships are often unstable and chaotic due to conflict between intense dependency and attachment needs and sensitivity to rejection.

Dissocial: a pattern characterized primarily by callousness, interpersonal hostility or aggression, and the failure to develop prosocial behaviour. Callousness is typically expressed as lack of empathy; disregard for the feelings, well-being, and suffering of others; lack of remorse about the consequences of one's actions on others; exploitativeness and manipulativeness; an egocentric attitude; and sadism involving pleasure in humiliating, demeaning, dominating, and hurting others. Interpersonal hostility involves aggressive behaviour and a need to dominate and control others. These interpersonal traits are associated with antisocial behaviour, sensation-seeking (including risk-taking, impulsivity, and recklessness), and narcissistic tendencies, most notably grandiosity and entitlement.

Social Avoidance: a pattern characterized by avoidance of social relationships. There is little desire for social contact. Social relationships and contacts are minimized or avoided, and there is an active tendency to seek out situations that do not include other people. Opportunities to socialize are declined and little effort is made to initiate social contact. Intimate attachments are avoided and there is a general fear of intimacy and sexual closeness. Emotional expression is severely restricted and there is a reluctance to disclose personal information and a strong desire to be self-sufficient.

Compulsivity: a pattern characterized by orderliness, conscientiousness, and exaggerated perfectionism. The central features are a desire for order and precision that lead to activities being conducted in a hyper-methodical and overly detailed way. There is strong concern with details, time, punctuality, schedules, and rules.

BOX 5.4 Definitions of Borderline or Emotional Dysregulation Traits

Emotional

Anxiousness	Readily feels anxious and worried; easily feels threatened; has lifelong sense of tension and feeling "on the edge"; ruminates and broods about unpleasant experiences; is unable to divert attention from painful thoughts; tends to be indecisive and have a pervasive sense of guilt
Emotional lability	i. Emotional reactivity: frequent and unpredictable emotional changes; moody; irritable; irritable and easily annoyed; impatient; intense, easily aroused anger ii. Emotional intensity: expresses feelings intensely; experiences strong feelings; over-reacts emotionally; exaggerates emotional significance of events
Pessimistic-anhedonia	Anhedonic, derives little pleasure from experiences or relationships, has no sense of fun, feels pervasive pessimism, feels hopeless for the future, accentuates the negative, strongly adheres to negative beliefs
Hypersensitivity	Experiences any form of stimulation as intense, intrusive, and overwhelming; noises, sounds, and people are experienced as intrusive and overwhelming

Interpersonal

Submissiveness	Subordinates self and own needs to those of others; adapts behaviour to interests and desires of others; subservient and placating in relationships; submits to abuse and intimidation to maintain relationships; is unassertive; needs advice and reassurance about all courses of action; readily accepts others' suggestions; is gullible
Insecure attachment	Fears losing attachments; coping depends on presence of attachment figure; urgently seeks proximity with attachment figure when stressed; strongly protests separations; is intolerant of aloneness; avoids being alone and plans adequate activities to avoid being alone
Need for approval	Needs to be accepted and approved; has a strong fear of disapproval; needs to fit in with the social group; has a fear of exclusion; has strong fear and expectations of humiliation, ridicule, and embarrassment in social situations; constantly seeks reassurance and acceptance; is very sensitive to humiliation

Cognitive

Cognitive dysregulation	Depersonalization or derealization; schizotypal cognition; brief stress psychosis

5.3.1 Clinical Assessment of Traits

Although clinical assessment of traits is sufficient for treatment purposes, traits can also be evaluated by questionnaire. Two questionnaires specifically designed to evaluate personality disorder are available: the Schedule for Nonadaptive and Adaptive Personality (SNAP) and the Dimensional Assessment of Personality Pathology – Basic Questionnaire (DAPP-BQ).[8]

The most practical way to assess traits is to become familiar with the brief descriptions of the four clusters provided in Box 5.3 and to evaluate the extent to which the patient fits each description when taking a personal history.[9] If a given trait constellation is considered present, the next step is to evaluate each trait from that cluster using the descriptions of those traits provided in Box 5.4. If additional information is needed to evaluate a given trait, additional questions may be asked, based on the definitions provided in Box 5.4. In most cases, the information provided by this process is sufficient for planning and initiating treatment. However, it is useful to keep the four-factor structure in mind throughout treatment so that the overall assessment of personality can be refined as new information is obtained.

5.3.2 Case Examples

Anna and Madison showed features that matched the emotional dysregulation constellation of traits. Both showed high levels of anxiousness, emotional lability, insecure attachment, and submissiveness, but neither showed clinically significant levels of pessimistic-anhedonia or hypersensitivity. However, Anna was more submissive than Madison and she had stronger dependency needs presumably due to greater attachment trauma.

The major difference between these patients with respect to borderline traits was in cognitive dysregulation – the tendency for thinking to be disrupted by strong emotions. Anna showed high levels of this trait, which led to difficulty in organizing her thoughts during crises. This also occurred during the assessment. On several occasions, when distressed she lost track of what was being discussed and commented that she could not think. She also reported that pseudo-hallucinations sometimes occurred when she was very distressed. This suggested that the level of emotional arousal in therapy would need to be more carefully managed.

Both patients also showed clinically important levels of traits from other constellations. Most notably, Anna had a strong need for stimulation and excitement. She was easily bored and she thought that she sometimes started fights with her partner to create some excitement. Both patients also had moderate but helpful levels of compulsivity that were likely to prove helpful during treatment.

5.4 Domains of Psychopathology

The final step in assessment is to evaluate domains of impairment. A distinguishing feature of IMT is the emphasis on decomposing borderline pathology into functional domains that closely linked to specific intervention modules. Box 5.5 lists typical problems and impairments associated with each domain. The problems and impairments identified through domain assessment help to structure a discussion with patients about the issues they want to address in treatment. This issue is discussed in more detail in the next chapter.

BOX 5.5 Characteristic Problems and Impairments Associated with Domains
of Personality Pathology

Domain	Characteristic Problems and Impairments
Symptoms	Dysphoria, unstable emotions, anxiety, unstable moods, anger and rage, self-injurious behaviour, dissociative behaviour, regressive behaviour, cognitive impairments, quasi-psychotic symptoms
Regulation and Modulation	Under-regulation of emotions, maladaptive emotional schemas (e.g. schemas about the uncontrollability and unpredictability of emotions), impaired metacognitive processes
Interpersonal	Impaired intimacy and attachment, insecure attachment, maladaptive interpersonal patterns, unstable and conflicted relationships, rejection sensitivity, maladaptive interpersonal schemas and representations
Self	Maladaptive self-schemas (feeling unlovable, flawed, and worthless), problems regulating self-esteem, unstable sense of self or identity, poorly developed self system

5.5 Building the Alliance during Assessment

In order to reduce dropout early in therapy, the assessment interviews are also used to make a connection with the patient so that by the end of the assessment the patient feels heard and understood. Box 5.6 lists clinician activities that are related to a positive alliance during assessment.[10] Five factors are especially helpful. First, the alliance is better if the assessment is conducted in a respectful and compassionate way. Since many patients have had adverse experiences with the health care system, an encounter with a respectful clinician helps to change expectations and build confidence in treatment. Second, confidence and credibility are enhanced when the assessor is seen to be knowledgeable and competent as conveyed by a professional manner and the use of questions and summary statements that reveal an understanding of BPD. A simple example is to follow a discussion of deliberate self-injury by asking whether these acts made the patient feel better. Such questions indicate that the clinician understands that such acts reduce distress and that the clinician is not judgmental about these behaviours.

Third, the alliance is promoted by attentive listening to the patient's concerns and empathic attunement to the patient's feelings and ideas about his or her problems. This is facilitated by personalizing the interview to avoid the impression that that clinician is following a script. Fourth, rapport improves when the patient feels that the assessment is collaborative. Although the goal is to collect information, this needs to be done in a way

BOX 5.6 Clinician Activities Related to a Positive Alliance during Assessment

Factors Related to the Frame of the Assessment
  Longer and more depth-orientated evaluation
  Collaborative stance
  Attention to emotional and cognitive content while also containing emotional arousal
  Clear, concrete, experience-near language
  Adoption of the patient's own words when possible
Focus of the Assessment
  Focus on current concerns
  Encourage the patient to initiate discussion of salient concerns
  Exploration of personal concerns
  Provision of adequate time for the patient to discuss personal concerns
  Clarification of the nature and sources of distress
  Identification of key relationship themes
  Exploration of uncomfortable feelings while containing emotional arousal
  Discussion of the patient's feelings about the assessment
Feedback
  Discussion of preliminary ideas and conclusions as assessment proceeds
  Give the patient ample opportunity to discuss these conclusions
  Provide an opportunity for the patient to elaborate or modify conclusions
  Incorporation of a psychoeducational component

(Modified from Hilsenroth and Cromer, 2007)

that gives the patient ample opportunity to feel heard and understood. Finally, the alliance is fostered when the assessment increases patients' understanding of their problems. Although there are practical limits on the extent to which this is feasible, the interview often provides opportunities to note simple patterns, for example, noting that deliberate self-harm seems to follow feeling rejected. It is also helpful to provide summary statements about tentative observations and invite the patient to give his or her reactions to these statements so as to create an atmosphere of exchange and collaboration.

5.6 Concluding Comments

An important feature of an effective assessment is that patients see that the therapist is trying to understand them and how they see things rather than being primarily concerned with collecting information and following his or her own agenda. To treat BPD effectively, we have to be able to put ourselves in our patient's shoes and communicate the understanding this provides. The rapport established during assessment influences the quality of the alliance in therapy, especially during the early phases. Outcome is better if the therapist also conducts the assessment and there is evidence that therapist-conducted assessments lead to less premature termination at least during the early sessions.[11]

Notes

1. This issue was investigated by Ackerman et al. (2000). See also Hilsenroth and Cromer (2007) for a review of interventions that are useful in building the alliance during assessment.

2. Livesley and Clarkin (2015b).

3. Hilsenroth and Cromer (2007).

4. Severity is usually assessed for research purposes either by the total number of DSM personality disorders present or the total number of criteria present. Neither are very practical measures because they require an evaluation of all DSM criteria. They also equate severity with breadth of pathology (the number of criteria present) rather than degree of impairment; a patient may show a large number of criterial features, all of which are relatively mild. Fortunately, there is a simpler option for clinical purposes. It is sufficient to evaluate two levels of severity – personality disorder and severe personality disorder – based on the features described in the chapter.

5. Livesley (2003).

6. Sanderson and Clarkin (2013).

7. Soloff (2000).

8. The SNAP (Clark, 1993) assesses 16 personality disorders that were identified by exploring the structure underlying the personality terms included in the DSM. The DAPP-BQ assesses 18 scales identified through statistical analyses of the structure underlying nearly 1,000 terms used to describe personality disorder in the clinical literature (Livesley and Jackson, 2009).

9. The trait structure adopted to discuss individual differences in personality disorder traits throughout this volume is based on a series of studies on clinical, general population, and twin samples. The rationale and procedure for designating salient traits are described in Livesley (1998). The main analyses are reported in Livesley et al. (1989, 1992, 1993, 1994, 1998).

10. This section is based on studies by Ackerman et al. (2000) and Batchelor (1995) and a review by Hilsenroth and Cromer (2007).

11. Tantum and Klerman (1979), Wise and Rinn (1983).

Formulation, Treatment Planning, and the Treatment Contract

The end point of diagnostic assessment is a formulation of the patient's problems. This chapter discusses structure of the case formulation in integrated modular treatment (IMT) and its use in planning treatment and establishing the treatment contract.

6.1 Formulation

Formulations are narrative accounts of how diverse biological, psychological, social, and cultural influences coalesce to create a patient's current condition, which provide therapists with a road map for treatment and patients with an explanation of the nature and origins of their problems. This requires formulations to be expressed in clear, jargon-free, non-technical, "near-experience" language based on the patient's own language whenever possible.[1]

6.1.1 Contents

Effective formulations have descriptive and prescriptive components.[2] The descriptive component describes the origins, precipitants, and factors that perpetuate problems. The prescriptive element specifies initial treatment goals, treatment intensity, expected course of treatment, and potential obstacles. However, a formulation does not simply list important facts; it shapes this information into a narrative that welds together key factors and draws attention to salient issues.

Formulations typically include (i) an account of presenting problems including symptoms, current concerns, and contemporary situational factors (social, financial, legal, and occupational) along with a brief history of these problems; (ii) a discussion of vulnerability factors, including genetic predisposition, other co-occurring mental disorders, psychosocial influences, and any medical conditions; (iii) a developmental history organized around critical events and relationships; (iv) a description of personality; (v) a broad understanding of how personality factors and life events interacted to create and perpetuate current problems; and (vi) diagnostic information about borderline personality disorder (BPD) and other mental disorders. The formulation should also identify targets for change. This is readily achieved by organizing problems into the four domains (symptoms, regulation and modulation, interpersonal, and self/identity) described earlier. This leads naturally to the prescriptive aspects of the formulation because domains are closely tied to specific treatment modules and the sequence in which problems are addressed.

When constructing a case formulation, comprehensiveness and specificity need to be balanced against practical matters such as the length of the assessment and the need to start treatment. Comprehensiveness is often not possible when the patient is in an acute decompensated state as was the case with Anna. In these situations, what is needed is a formulation with sufficient detail to map the broad structure of therapy – other details can be added later. However, even when patients are less acutely distressed, the initial formulation should be limited to key themes and avoid excessive detail to avoid confusing the patient with a formulation that lacks clarity and focus.[3]

6.1.2　Function

The formulation serves multiple purposes. The narrative format makes it easier to recall the patient's history during therapy and provides patients with an explanation of their problems that is easier to understand. When patients do not understand why they are so distressed, a coherent, easily assimilated explanation helps to settle their distress. Later, we will see how the formulation of her crisis behaviour helped Madison to understand situations and feelings that seemed incomprehensible and how this settled her distress sufficiently to begin focusing more consistently on change.

Formulation is also an important integrative tool. With IMT, integration is both an operational task (combining an eclectic array of interventions) and a treatment goal. By giving meaning to experiences and problems, the formulation provides a blueprint for constructing a more adaptive self-narrative. Contemporary personality research documents the role of personal narratives in integrative personality functioning.[4] People construe their lives as ongoing stories that establish their identities, shape their behaviour, and help them to integrate with their culture and community. Self-narratives are seriously impoverished in people with BPD. The descriptive component of the formulation lays out the essential details of the patient's life and personality by combining a variety of facts into a coherent narrative that resembles the autobiographic self. Thus, the formulation is the first step in a therapy-long endeavour to promote integration. This is why it is important to have a collaborative discussion of the initial formulation with patients that invites their input and stimulates self-reflection. This enables them to take ownership of the formulation so that as it is subsequently revised in the light of new information elicited in therapy, the formulation is "metabolized" so that it becomes incorporated into the patient's self-narrative.

6.1.3　Form

A practical issue is whether the formulation should be written and whether the patient should receive a copy. Many authors concur that a written account is helpful[5] because it encourages clarity and conciseness and provides a more critical evaluation of the information. It is also easy to share with patients so that they can add their perspective. A further refinement is the use of diagrams to explain key themes.[6] Diagrams force the clinician to be clear. They are also often easier for patients to understand because the patients can see at a glance how different thoughts emotions and events are connected. Patients can also take the diagram with them and add to it and refine it between sessions, which will help them to assimilate the ideas.

6.2　Illustrative Formulations

6.2.1　The Case of Anna

Diagnostically, it was clear that Anna had severe BPD that arose from a wide range of genetic and psychosocial risk factors. The family history suggested that mother had similar problems and that anxiety problems were common in the family. Anna's history suggested severe attachment trauma due to abuse and separation from mother in infancy that led to attachment insecurity, problems with emotion regulation, and a self-image of inherent "badness" and self-loathing that arose because Anna blamed herself for mother not loving her. Anxieties about father leaving added to Anna's insecurity. Abuse and neglect also led to intense neediness coupled with profound distrust in everyone and everything because those who had cared for her and who she had looked to for care and attention had hurt her and failed to meet her needs. These experiences laid the foundation for both the core conflict that dominated her interpersonal relationships and the states of distress without resolution that added to the intensity of her crises. They also led to a powerful need to care for others in the hope that they would provide the love and caring that she so desperately sought. Sexual abuse probably contributed to problems created by attachment trauma that gave rise to severely disturbed interpersonal relationships and maladaptive schemas related to insecurity, powerlessness, mistrust, and self-derogation. Family dynamics added to, and continued to maintain, these problems by reinforcing schemas of self-blame and low self-worth, and consistently invalidating Anna's feelings, wants, and sense of autonomy.

Events in the adult years confirmed Anna's distrust and reinforced her dependency needs. She consistently established relationships with abusive but needy men whom she initially thought were strong and able to look after her. A long series of such relationships ensued driven by an intense need to be loved and Anna was prepared to do whatever her partner wanted to ensure affection and avoid rejection. This consolidated the need to care for others that developed initially as a way to try to gain mother's love and attention and the submissive, subservient behaviours that were acquired in this context and established a pattern of hostile-dependent relationships.

The chaotic and traumatic nature of her upbringing and the personality characteristics described in the previous chapter led to an unstable and vulnerable personality structure filled with conflict that included lack of a coherent self-structure and an adaptive self-narrative that allowed Anna to make sense of her life and experiences. As a result she seemed to lurch from crisis to crisis and from one dysfunctional relationship to another that re-enacted her developmental experiences. Several complicating factors were noted that had treatment implications. First, there was a tendency for cognitive functions to be impaired when stressed. Second, Anna also tended to dissociate when she recalled painful events. These features suggested that it would be important to regulate emotional arousal especially at the beginning of therapy. Offsetting these liabilities was the presence of moderate levels of compulsivity, which generally improves prognosis for patients with BPD.

It was anticipated that initial phase of therapy was likely to be prolonged and that it would take some time to build the alliance and engage Anna in therapy because of the severity of the pathology, profound distrust, and previous experiences in therapy.

6.2.2 The Case of Madison

Madison was assessed as having BPD. A strong family history of anxiety disorders and anxiousness on both sides of the family suggested a strong genetic predisposition. This is supported by family members' reports that Madison had difficult temperament as an infant and that she was an anxious child who ruminated and worried about everything. There is no evidence of severe psychosocial adversity during childhood. The problem seemed to be that Madison was difficult to soothe from early infancy so that there was a poor fit with mother who had her own difficulties at the time with anxiety. Mother was also under considerable stress for much of Madison's early childhood and felt that she had little support from Madison's father who was busy building his career in a rapidly growing international company, which meant that he was frequently away from home. Nevertheless, Madison felt that she had a happy childhood and she did well at school.

More problems began to emerge in the mid-teenage years and problems with anxiety and temper tantrums became more severe and emotional volatility increased. When she started dating at age 14 years, her early relationships did not last long causing her to feel abandoned and intensely distressed. Emotional difficulties increased substantially following sexual abuse at age 17 years – moods became more volatile and the anger increased. Madison' parents did not know how to help her, which led to family friction that added to her fears of rejection and abandonment.

Being interested in sports, she was attracted to other athletes, many of whom seemed to have their own ego problems that caused frequent relationship crises, adding to her sensitivity to rejection. At about the time she started university, one of these relationships became more serious and Madison and her boyfriend moved in together. It was a problematic relationship from the start. They fought constantly often because Madison, who seemed more committed to the relationship, frequently felt hurt and rejected by the way he treated her. As a result, her behaviour became more unstable and she varied between demanding that he be more caring, which caused to him withdraw further in anger, and intense needy and placating behaviour in which she was pleading that he forgive her and stay with her. During this time, the emotional volatility increased and she began to cut herself, initially superficially but later more severely. Eventually, the boyfriend ended the relationship, leaving Madison distraught. Although she started dating again soon afterwards – it was as if she did not feel complete without a partner – her university studies deteriorated, forcing her to take a leave of absence.

The interesting questions stimulated by this history is how Madison coped so well previously with anxiousness, emotional lability, and attachment insecurity and why she became so dysfunctional. The answer seems to lie in another aspect of her personality. Despite the anxiety and unstable moods, Madison was supremely self-confident and had a somewhat grandiose sense of self. She saw herself as an outstanding scholar and athlete, a self-image that was reinforced by success in both fields. This coping strategy stood her in good stead until her late teens and early 20s when it began to crumble for multiple reasons; none, apart from the attempted rape, was especially noteworthy. And, once this happened, the very things that had supported the over-confident coping strategy – academic performance and athletic success – also declined and the deterioration escalated.

Based on this formulation and current mental state, it was anticipated that Madison would engage in therapy relatively quickly although the crises were expected to continue for some time because there was little structure to her life and she was engaging in a variety of self-harming behaviours that added substantially to her distress. However, it was noted during the assessment that when she talked about her distress it began to settle, which seemed to suggest that once engaged and the reactivity was more contained, she would respond well and that specific interventions designed to improve her ability to manage crises and contain self-harming behaviour could be used relatively early in therapy.

6.3 Treatment Planning

IMT may be delivered in various settings including hospital in-patient units, day hospitals, outpatient services, community care teams, forensic services, and office practice. Whatever the setting, decisions need to be made about intensity, duration, and intervention strategies.

6.3.1 Treatment Intensity and Severity

With IMT, treatment intensity refers to the extent to which general change modules are supplemented with specific intervention modules and the anticipated rate at which this occurs. This issue is similar to the traditional psychodynamic distinction between expressive therapy and supportive therapy. The relative balance of general versus specific interventions is important because general interventions are inherently supportive and place minimal strain on the alliance and patient whereas specific interventions often cause additional strain for both because they place a more direct emphasis on change and require the patient's active participation. The level of strain increases with the effort required of the patient and the extent to which the intervention generates strong emotions.

Decisions about treatment intensity are based on severity although it is also useful to take into account factors such as cognitive dysregulation (especially any tendency to dissociate or develop quasi-psychotic symptoms when stressed) and metacognitive functioning (the capacity for self-reflection and to understand the mental states of self and others). What matters is the patient's capacity to (i) establish an effective working relationship that can withstand the strain of therapeutic work and (ii) tolerate emotional arousal without it adversely affecting the cognitive processes involved in the self-regulation. Both are related to severity. With increasing severity, emphasis is placed on containment and stabilization rather than on more definitive change. Hence treatment largely relies on generic interventions and simple specific interventions that reduce emotional distress and are easy to use such as self-soothing and distraction with less use of specific modules that are likely to generate emotional arousal and catharsis. Also the rate at which other specific interventions are incorporated into treatment is slower. The pace of therapy is discussed further when the management of the early phase of therapy is discussed in Chapter 14.

Since Anna was considered to have severe BPD and also had high levels of cognitive dysregulation, it was determined that considerable emphasis would be placed on alliance building in the early sessions with minimal exploration of issues and little use of specific interventions until the alliance was deemed satisfactory and a degree of within-session stability had been achieved. This meant a heavy emphasis on containment interventions to reduce cognitive impairment and control dissociation and the use of medication to manage emotionality and cognitive symptoms. In contrast, it was decided that since Madison had less-severe BPD and did not show symptoms of cognitive dysregulation, the use of general intervention strategies would be supplemented from the onset with exploration of the triggers and consequences of crisis behaviour and simple specific interventions to reduce distress and self-harming behaviour, providing the alliance was satisfactory. This decision was based on observations during the assessment that efforts to understand distress in the interview usually helped to settle it.

6.3.2 Duration and Frequency of Treatment

Treatment planning requires some indication about the likely duration for therapy. This volume describes long-term therapy because the intent is to provide a comprehensive treatment framework. However, IMT is applicable to treatment of differing durations. The phases of change framework (see Chapters 1 and 2) provides a structure for organizing therapies of different duration. Treatment is described in terms of five distinct but overlapping phases: (i) safety, (ii) containment, (iii) regulation and control, (iv) exploration and change, and (v) integration and synthesis, which are associated with the symptomatic (safety and containment phases), regulation and modulation, interpersonal, and self/identity domains of impairment, respectively.

Short-term therapy (approximately ten to twenty sessions) would primarily cover the safety and containment phases with a focus on treating symptoms related to emotional dysregulation and suicidality. This would essentially be a form of crisis management, designed to contain symptoms and provide some strategies for coping with future crises. Medium-term treatment (about three to twelve months) would also incorporate the regulation and modulation phase and focus on increasing the self-regulation of emotions and enhancing emotion-processing capacity (see Chapters 15–17). Longer-term therapy would have a more intense focus on interpersonal and self pathology and cover the exploration/ change and integration/synthesis phases of treatment. I will reconsider the problem of duration again in the final chapter based on a fuller understanding of the nature and scope of an integrated and trans-theoretical approach.

We have little empirical information on the optimal frequency of sessions and decisions are often based on administrative factors and clinical lore. IMT does not adopt a fixed position on this matter. My usual pattern is to see patients weekly at least in the first half of long-term therapy. However, if the patient is severely decompensated, twice-weekly appointments are made until a reasonable level of stability is achieved – anything from about two to nine months – and then appointments are weekly. When treatment begins to focus more on interpersonal issues and self pathology, sessions are usually reduced to every two weeks and then to once a month or even every six weeks. This seems to work well because patients need time to work through the issues discussed in sessions in the latter phases of treatment. However, because I work in an area where some patients have to travel a considerable distance for treatment, there have been times when it was only possible to arrange monthly appointments from the outset. This arrangement also seems to work, providing the patient is relatively stable (not having frequent crises) and the goals are to increase emotion regulation and perhaps deal with interpersonal factors that trigger distress. The patient also has to be motivated to do therapeutic work between sessions. The point is that since there is little research on how best to deliver treatment, the clinician has to rely on clinical judgement and be prepared to be flexible.

6.4 Discussing the Formulation

The assessment process typically ends with the therapist sharing his/her understanding of the patient's problems and inviting the patient to comment on and add to the formulation. Even when the formulation is written, it is best to discuss the formulation with the patient before presenting the written version to prevent the patient from being overwhelmed by too much information. The amount of information provided differs according to the severity and the patient's current state. Patients who are stable can usually be given a more detailed formulation. This is what happened with Madison although she was not stable, she was able to process the information despite being distressed. In fact, the discussion helped her understand her distress, which made her hopeful that therapy would help. In contrast, Anna was in a decompensated state and often had difficulty processing information during the assessment. Consequently, a very brief formulation was offered that concentrated on her current life situation but also noted key themes such as problems in her family of origin and abuse. Little time was spent on goal setting because she was clear that all she was concerned with was to control her distress and stop harming herself. This was simply reiterated to get a commitment to change. Hence the therapist followed a brief formulation by saying "we have talked about how difficult your life is just now and about the things that have happened to you at different times in your life but I suggest that we concentrate for now on helping you to get your mood and feelings under control so that you begin to feel better and also on helping you to manage the intense emotional states that have previously caused you to be admitted to hospital." And, the therapist then asked what Anna thought of the idea. She was happy with the idea and the therapist noted that when she felt better, they could discuss "what other things that you would like to deal with."

6.4.1 Diagnosis

When discussing the formulation, patients usually ask about their diagnosis, which needs to be dealt with openly. If a co-occurring disorder such as mood disorder or substance abuse is present, it should be fully discussed and the relationship between this disorder and BPD explained. Discussion of the BPD diagnosis is more complex but frankness is important. As noted in the preface, I do not like the term "BPD" and rarely use it in my practice. Nevertheless, patients usually ask if they have BPD because they have been given the diagnosis previously or looked it up on the Internet. In which case, I usually respond that I understand why they received the diagnosis because they show many of the diagnostic features. However, I add that it is not a term that I like or use and then go on to explain that I think that their main problem is with regulating emotions – that they have emotion-regulating disorder, which causes intense feelings and frequent mood changes, and these emotional difficulties cause problems with their relationships and how they feel about themselves. Most patients are comfortable with this explanation and it seems to make sense to them. However, some patients are also pleased with the diagnosis of BPD because it is a relief to know they have something that has a label as opposed to something that is vague and confusing and also because it means that they are not alone with this disorder – others suffer from the same problems.

Discussion of the diagnosis should include a discussion about what the patient has heard about BPD and personality disorder because misconceptions about the diagnosis are common; for example, that the disorder is untreatable or that people with this disorder are difficult or even "bad". The disorder is painful enough without the diagnosis itself adding to the distress.

Occasionally patients have strong concerns about their diagnosis and reject the idea of having BPD or personality disorder. Nothing is gained from getting into an unproductive debate about diagnosis and labels. Some concerns about labels are understandable and justified. They can often be dealt with by acknowledging the problems that labels create and by focusing on reaching an agreement about the problems that need to be dealt such as suicidality, dysregulated emotions, and interpersonal problems. Such patients are often more comfortable with a problem focus, which is why I prefer to couch problems in terms of difficulties with emotion regulation.

6.4.2 Medication

Discussion of the diagnosis also usually raises questions about whether medication would be helpful. IMT considers medication an adjunctive treatment that is helpful for some patients and that it should be used in a targeted way to treat specific symptom clusters (medication is discussed further in Chapter 14). At this stage, it was suggested to Anna that medication might help to settle her distress and reduce the difficulty she sometimes had in organizing her thoughts and hence make it easier for her to work on her problems. She accepted the recommendation and she was prescribed a low-dose neuroleptic (quetiapine 25 mg) and a selective serotonin reuptake inhibitor (SSRI). It was explained that the quetiapine was being prescribed to treat the cognitive symptoms and reduce reactivity and that the SSRI was being used to reduce the mood symptoms.

6.5 Establishing the Treatment Contract

The treatment framework or contract defines the purpose, practical arrangements, format, and limits of the proposed therapy.[7] The contract has three parts: (i) agreement on collaborative treatment goals, (ii) an explicit understanding of the roles of patient and therapist in helping the patient to attain these goals, and (iii) an agreement on the practical arrangements for therapy.

6.5.1 Establishing Treatment Goals

IMT adopts a goal-oriented approach because of evidence that it enhances outcome and reduces early dropout.[8] Goals are useful in focusing the treatment process and helping the patient to focus on change. The process of setting goals also promotes hope by changing an amorphous sense of distress into specific treatment targets.

The goal of IMT is to increase adaptive functioning through (i) the acquisition of cognitive and behavioural skills and strategies needed to reduce impairment and build competency across the symptom, regulation and modulation, interpersonal, and self domains; (ii) the construction of meaning systems to structure and restructure experience; and (iii) the promotion of more integrated personality functioning. This overarching goal provides a context for working with the patient to establish collaborative treatment goals based on what the patient wants to achieve in therapy. Since problems are dealt with in the approximate sequence of symptoms, dysregulated emotions, interpersonal problems, and self/identity problems, domains provide a way to organize goals into an orderly sequence.

The end of the assessment is a good time to explore what the patient wants from treatment. The goals established should be specific, have a clearly defined outcome, and be realistic and attainable. However, patients often identify goals that are vague such as "feeling better" or "sorting out my life." In which case, further work needs to be done on helping the patient to define these goals more precisely. This process is useful because it addresses a basic problem that most patients have in organizing their experience and establishing coherent objectives for their lives.

Madison initially said that she "wanted to feel normal so she could finish her degree." When asked what she needed to do to feel normal, she explained that she wanted to "stop having ups and downs" and frequent "crashes." She also added that she would like to "feel vibrant again" and stop worrying so much whether her boyfriend would leave her. When discussing these goals, Madison was clear that her priority was to deal with the crises because they led her to do potentially harmful things. This led to the decision to focus initially on reducing crises, learning to manage crises more effectively, and reducing self-harm. It was also agreed that a subsequent goal would be to learn to control and regulate emotions and that it would be easier to deal with abandonment fears once she felt better.

6.5.2 Establishing Patient and Therapist Roles

An important part of the treatment frame is an explicit understanding of the roles and functions of both patient and therapist. This is necessary to establish an alliance because a collaborative relationship requires both parties to have a clear understanding of their responsibilities.[9] This agreement is especially important for patients with BPD because they have significant difficulties structuring their relationships in a realistic way and have boundary problems that make it difficult to differentiate between their own thoughts and those of other people. As a result, they need considerable assistance in understanding and maintaining the structure and boundaries of treatment. Fewer problems are likely to arise if there is a clear understanding from the outset about expectations and responsibilities (see Chapters 7 and 10).

A major distinction in roles that needs to be made explicit is that the therapist's responsibility is to create the therapeutic conditions needed for the patient to change whereas the patient's responsibility is to implement changes. This requires the therapist to establish a treatment process that allows the patient to feel secure enough to examine his/her problems and to implement change and then to act as a consultant who guides the patient through the change process. The patient's role includes taking action to change and steps to deal with any behaviours or feelings that interfere with therapy and efforts to initiate change. The different responsibilities and roles of patient and therapist are discussed further in the next chapter and again in Chapter 12.

Besides discussing differences in role and responsibility, it is also useful to stress the collaborative nature of therapeutic work. It is important to explain and work though the idea that the therapist's task is to work with the patient to help him/her achieve the goals that have been established and that the patient's task is to work with the therapist to understand the problems and behaviours that the patient wants to change and then to try out and make these changes.

Some patients are reluctant to accept that treatment is a collaborative process or that change is their responsibility. Dependent or oppositional patients sometimes seek to put responsibility for change on the therapist by commenting that they need the therapist to tell them what to do because they do not know how to change, and if they did they would have done it. Some even couch their concerns in terms of the therapist being an expert who has treated many people with the same problems and hence knowing what to do. Such comments can be restructured by the therapist acknowledging that

> I know about the kind of problems you are having and how to treat them but you are the expert on you. Only you can decide what you want to do, what you want to achieve, and

how you want to live your life. So we have to find some way to combine our different knowledge and expertise to help you get better. You need to help me to understand you and what it is like to have the problem you are having, and we need to find a way for you to use my expertise to help you understand yourself better and to make the changes that we have talked about.

As part of this discussion, therapists need to be clear and open about what they can and cannot do and about their own limits.

6.5.3 Practical Arrangements

The contract includes the practical arrangements for treatment including time and place of sessions and their frequency and duration. Since these arrangements help to define treatment boundaries, therapists and patients should adhere to them and sessions should occur as planned. Discussion of such housekeeping matters should include arrangements for absences and therapist availability in crises. Since therapy needs to be as consistent as possible, patients should be told that they will be advised well in advance of any changes to scheduled appointments with the proviso that unexpected and urgent events occur. When the therapist is away fairly frequently, it is useful to provide patients with a written schedule. Strenuous effort should be made to avoid situations when the patient is advised that the therapist has to cancel the next session.

The treatment agreement should also include an understanding of therapist availability in the event of emergencies and crises. These arrangements will vary according to the treatment setting and the therapist's professional circumstances. However, the important thing is that there is a clear understanding of the arrangements and that the patient has a crisis plan. If the therapist is available should an emergency arise, he/she may wish to indicate that the patient is free to telephone and the therapist will return the call when convenient. Under these circumstances, the only additional understanding would be what the patient should do out of hours. Things are more complicated when the therapist is working in a context in which it is difficult for the patient to make contact between sessions other than by leaving a voicemail. Over the years, I have used a variety of ways to deal with emergencies and it does not make a lot of difference what procedure is adopted, providing the plan for emergencies is clearly worked out and discussed with the patient and that this discussion involves the patient's input. Nowadays, I initially ask patients what would work for them and then we work out a practical arrangement. Such plans need to be tailored to the patient and the options available. The plan may include guidelines about when to go to emergency departments, contacting a family doctor who is prepared to offer emergency care, contacting a crisis line, seeing a supportive minister or friend, attending a crisis service or group, and so on.

6.5.4 Different Approaches to the Treatment Contract

Although all therapies for BPD emphasize the importance of the treatment contract, they differ in the kind of contract established. Dialectical behaviour therapy (DBT) has more detailed expectations from those outlined above. For example, the pre-treatment period of DBT is used to get an agreement to work on stopping suicidal, self-harming, and therapy-interfering behaviour. These are not pre-therapy requirements for IMT. Instead, the therapist works with the patient early in therapy to establish a commitment to change because the process of negotiating the commitment is itself an important therapeutic activity. Another difference is whether patients who are not working or in full-time education are expected to obtain employment either before or just after treatment starts. This is an expectation of transference-focused therapy (TFT). This is a problem for severely disordered patients who are in a decompensated state with frequent crises. However, the group that developed TFT does not see patients in a crisis, which suggests that either they are treating less-severe conditions or that patients had received previous treatment that stabilized their condition. Either way, these patients seem to have less-severe BPD than the patients discussed in this volume. Similarly, some of the cognitive-behavioural therapies (CBTs) illustrate their approach with case vignettes of patients who are working in demanding professional positions despite having a diagnosis of personality disorder. Again, this suggests a relatively mild level of personality pathology. Hence the contracting process of TFT and some CBTs are not appropriate when treating patients with more severe pathology.

6.6 Patient Education

The assessment and contracting sessions are opportunities to provide information about the nature of BPD, the efficacy of therapy, and how treatment works. Although we do not want to overwhelm patients with information, patients feel more positive about assessments that are informative about the disorder. Such information reassures patients that they have a treatable condition and reduces some of their confusion about the nature of their problems. General information on the effectiveness of treatment and a positive attitude about outcomes also increase optimism and motivation for therapy. It is also useful to note evidence that BPD often improves gradually over time even without treatment and to discuss how treatment can enhance this natural process.

Patients also need to know how treatment works and what they can do to make the most of the process. This topic is largely neglected – therapists often seem to assume that patients automatically know what to do. Having identified goals, it is helpful to explain that treatment will enable the patient to understand the problems associated with these goals and that this is the first step towards changing them because it is difficult to change something without understanding it. With some patients, this can be taken a stage further by explaining that the best thing they can do to help themselves is to become curious about their own minds and how their minds work. And, this involves asking themselves how and why they think and feel the way they do and how these thoughts and feelings influence their actions. It also means thinking about what was discussed in therapy between sessions and perhaps keeping a journal to record their thoughts and reactions. It should also be made clear that treatment only works if the patient tries to do things differently and works to change thoughts and actions that cause problems.

Finally, it is also useful to give the patients some idea about the changes that can be expected and perhaps an idea about the kinds of change that are likely to occur first. The sequence of symptoms→emotion regulation→interpersonal problems→self/identity problems is a simple way to describe what is likely to change first and how things are likely to change over time. However, it is not necessary to provide a lot of detail and care is needed not to create either unreasonable expectations or the idea that change occurs in a fixed sequence. It is also helpful to draw attention to the fact that treatment is not only concerned with changing problematic feelings and behaviours but also with helping the patients to change the way they think about themselves and their experiences.

6.7 Concluding Comments

The importance of the process of discussing the formulation and establishing the treatment contract should not be underestimated. They make a substantial contribution to outcome and to the number and type of problems encountered in treatment. Sitting with patients to review the assessment and formulation is a crucial part of treatment that sets the tone for a collaborative exchange and fosters the alliance by offering new understanding and insights and by the clinician explaining the nature of the patient's problems and how therapy may be helpful.

Notes

1. Hilsenroth and Cromer (2007).

2. Eells (1997).

3. Eells (1997).

4. McAdams and Pals (2006).

5. Bateman and Fonagy (2015), Davidson (2008), Perry et al. (1987), Ryle (1997).

6. The use of diagrams to help the patient understand a formulation is described in Livesley (2003), Salvatore et al. (2015), and Ryle (1997).

7. Orlinsky and Howard (1986), Links et al. (2015).

8. Critchfield and Benjamin (2006).

9. Gunderson and Links (2008) refer to this aspect of the treatment contract as the contractual alliance, which consists of treatment goals and definitions of therapist and patient roles.

General Treatment Modules

Introduction

Each chapter in this part describes one of general treatment modules that form the basic structure of integrated modular treatment:

Module 1: Structure: establish a structured treatment process

Module 2: Treatment relationship: establish and maintain a collaborative treatment relationship

Module 3: Consistency: maintain a consistent treatment process

Module 4: Validation: promote validation

Module 5: Self-reflection: enhance self-knowledge and self-reflection

Module 6: Motivation: build and maintain a commitment to change.

Each module consists of multiple interventions. Together the six modules seek to maximize the impact of change mechanisms common to all effective therapies. These interventions are used throughout treatment regardless of duration, the theoretical orientation of the therapist, and individual differences in the patient's personality and problems. Later chapters describe how these strategies can be supplemented with specific interventions tailored to the needs of individual patients.

These general modules are designed not only to establish the conditions needed for effective treatment but also to bring about change by creating a treatment process that challenges many of the maladaptive schemas, cognitive processes, and relationship patterns of borderline personality disorder, most notably mistrust, powerlessness, unpredictability, and self-invalidating thinking.

Chapter

7

General Treatment Module 1: Structure

Establishing a Structured Treatment Process

Structure is one of the most important and neglected aspects of therapy. Although evaluations of treatment outcome note the importance of a structured, focused, and theoretically coherent approach,[1] discussion of the topic is usually confined to the treatment contract. However, "structure" in integrated modular treatment (IMT) is a broader concept. It refers to the multiple factors that organize and shape treatment: the conceptual frameworks for understanding borderline personality disorder (BPD) and treatment; the context in which treatment occurs; the daily routine of scheduled activities when treatment is hospital or residentially based; the therapeutic stance and interpersonal approach of therapists and staff; an understanding of the work of therapy; and the treatment plan and contract discussed in the previous chapter.

Description of the general treatment modules begins with structure because this module establishes the conditions for therapy whereas the other general modules address the treatment process. Structure is important because patients with BPD have difficulty structuring their lives, and indeed their inner experience, hence it is important that the therapist structures treatment.[2] The various components of structure make treatment possible by establishing treatment boundaries, creating expectations, and clarifying what is and what is not acceptable. The structure created sets the course of therapy, helps to settle and contain reactivity, creates predictability, and promotes the feelings of safety and security needed for therapeutic work.

Implementation of structured treatment begins with an explicit treatment model. This is needed to manage the complexity of BPD and the ever-changing issues raised in treatment. A clearly defined model is especially important with IMT because it provides the guidelines for coordinating the delivery of an eclectic combination of interventions. Hence the emphasis placed earlier on frameworks for understanding of both BPD and therapy. However, it is not sufficient to have an explicit treatment model; therapy also has to be delivered in a way that is consistent with its intent and design.[3]

7.1 Context of Treatment

The context in which treatment occurs varies in complexity, ranging from private offices, through community mental health and forensic services and hospital outpatient departments, to institutional settings such as hospitals or forensic facilities. No matter where the treatment is delivered, context inevitably influences the process. Patients are usually acutely aware of the treatment context and use it to glean information about treatment and their therapist. In most settings, patients interact with many staff besides their therapists, and these interactions can colour patient–therapist interaction. Consequently, considerable therapeutic time may be spent dealing with problems created by these extraneous interactions. For example, patients receiving in-patient treatment interact with other members of the treatment team who often respond to the patient differently from the therapist. This can cause inconsistency to creep into treatment and even undermine progress. Hence, it is important for all personnel (clinical and non-clinical) in contact with patients to understand the treatment model and comply with its requirements.

When treatment occurs in an institutional setting, the institution's policies, procedures, and culture need to be consistent with the basic principles of IMT. This is often not the case, especially in forensic settings. When this happens programme integrity is undermined, and therapists are placed in a conflicted situation that contributes to stress and burnout.

It is also important to be aware of another aspect of context that impacts treatment – the patient's social circumstances. Therapists need to be alert to how these circumstances can affect therapy. Sometimes significant others support the patient in seeking therapy but this is not always the case. Parents sometimes discourage patients from talking about the family and concerns about the impact of change on relationships with significant others can obstruct treatment.

7.2 Therapist Support and Supervision

Therapist support, supervision, and access to consultation are integral to good care and evidence-based practice. They contribute to the consistency needed for effective outcomes. Most therapies advocate therapist supervision. Dialectical behaviour therapy even suggests that therapists should only work as part of a team.[4] Although this is often impractical, therapists need support and regular opportunities to discuss cases to be consistent. Ideally, this should occur with a consultant. If this is not available, peer supervision is a viable alternative.

The emotional and interpersonal intensity of borderline pathology and the central role of the treatment relationship in the change process place considerable strain on therapists and evoke strong emotional reactions that need to be discussed in regular debriefing sessions. Therapists also need opportunities to ventilate and explore their emotional reactions to therapy and the patient. In institutional settings, this is one of the most important things that the institution can do to promote effective care.

7.3 Treatment Schedules and Routine

The routines of therapy help to bring structure and predictability to the patient's life. This is helpful because patients with BPD tend to have disorganized and unstructured days. In individual or group therapy, the importance of regular appointments and a fixed schedule which does not change without adequate notice is widely accepted. However, in many institutional settings, there is less understanding of the value of this aspect of structure. Ward routines and treatment schedules provide regularity and consistency, which is enormously helpful to patients who have difficulty organizing themselves. They also promote safety and security by creating predictability. Unfortunately, many institutions are lax in maintaining scheduled functions. Staff are often reassigned to other duties at the last minute with little recognition of how this upsets patients, disrupts treatment, and reinforces patients' mistrust of both the therapist and the institution. This is a simple way in which administrative decisions undermine and invalidate therapy and therapists and degrade programme integrity.

7.4 Therapeutic Stance

The therapeutic stance is a key component of structure. The stance refers to the therapist's interpersonal approach, responsibilities, and activities.[5] The stance frames patient–therapist interaction, sets the tone of therapy, and defines the therapist's role in the treatment process. The following section discusses the stance in terms of the therapist's interpersonal approach, level of activity, functions, and flexibility.

7.4.1 Interpersonal Approach

Evidence indicates that the most appropriate stance for treating BPD is to provide support, empathy, and validation. Therapy is rarely effective unless the therapist relates to the patient in a warm and empathic manner, regardless of the therapist's technical competence. Patients who do well in therapy usually describe their therapists as warm, attentive, interested, understanding, respectful, experienced, and active.[6] Essential components of the stance were captured in Carl Rogers' description of helpful therapeutic relationships: (i) positive regard, (ii) genuineness, and (iii) accurate empathy.[7] This also describes the stance that is appropriate for treating BPD.

7.4.1.1 Positive Regard

Little is achieved in therapy unless the therapist relates to the patient in a respectful and non-judgemental way that conveys unconditional acceptance. Respect is a general need that has special significance for patients with BPD, given their life experiences. Respect builds self-esteem and fosters a desire to change. A non-judgemental approach builds the relationship – we all feel supported by those who accept us uncritically. It also counters self-criticism, low self-esteem, and negative self-talk. Therapist acceptance and positive regard also provide a model that patients can use to learn to show compassion towards themselves, something that is missing for many patients.

7.4.1.2 Genuineness

Genuineness requires that therapists interact with the patients in an honest, open, transparent, and authentic way without subterfuge and deception and that they take an authentic interest in understanding their patients' problems and mental states. This means avoiding pretense, stereotyped statements, and jargon and that therapists are clear and open about what they can and cannot do and about their own limits. It also means that therapists do not hold secrets. Patients sometimes want to tell their therapists things and request that they do not share them with the treatment team or a family member may reveal something and request that the therapist does not share it with the patient. Such secrets are best avoided.

7.4.1.3 Accurate Empathy

The most important feature of Rogers' triad is accurate empathy. In everyday life, interactions with an empathic person are reassuring and comforting. Similarly for patients, empathy creates a sense of safety, strengthens the relationship, builds trust, and enhances motivation.

Empathy should not be confused with sympathy. Sympathy involves having the same feelings as someone else and being affected in the same way. Patients rarely perceive expressions of sympathy as helpful. Sympathy often evokes hostility because it is seen as patronizing or phoney. Empathy is more complex: it involves appreciating and understanding the feelings of another person. This requires the ability to put oneself in the position of others and see things from their perspective, and then to communicate this understanding in clear and direct language. The capacity to establish and communicate empathic attunement[8] with the patient is a core therapist skill that probably affects outcome more than anything else apart from severity.

Rogers noted that empathy has two components: (i) an *attentiveness component* that is conveyed by eye contact and non-verbal acknowledgement of the patient's statements, which draws the patient into a relationship by providing a tangible demonstration that the clinician "values" the patient and what he or she has to say; and (ii) a *reflective component* that involves active listening and reflecting back what the patient has said in a way that clarifies the patient's statements without imposing the therapist's own interpretation or point of view.

It is important that these reflections capture not only the facts in patients' narratives but also underlying feelings in a way that facilitates patients' exploration of their inner world. Therapists often become so caught up in the details of what the patient is saying that they neglect the emotional component. This is especially common in crisis situations. Therapists also get drawn into adding their understanding of what the patient has said and even into offering interpretations rather than simply reflecting the emotional component. This does not mean that there is no place for interpretative statements or restructuring of the patient's cognitions but rather that interpretations and restructuring should follow careful reflective statements that communicate that the therapist is attentive to what the patient is saying and feeling. It is this type of communication that creates the rapport needed for other interventions to be effective.

7.4.2 Level of Activity

Evidence indicates that therapists treating BPD should be relatively active.[9] The low levels of therapist activity associated with some psychodynamic therapies have a limited role: a more active stance is needed to engage patients in treatment and contain emotional reactivity. A high level of therapist activity that emphasizes the therapist's presence is especially helpful when patients feel overwhelmed or begin to dissociate.[10] The therapist's presence creates a holding and containing relationship that helps to anchor the patient in the present and reduce the distorted perceptions of the relationship that tend to occur when there is little structure to patient–therapist interaction.[11]

7.4.3 Functions

The kind of therapeutic stance proposed serves several functions. First, effective treatment requires the therapist to facilitate both the *exploration of problems and psychopathology* and the *development of more integrated personality functioning.*[12] Therapists are usually clear about exploratory and restructuring components of therapy but do not always recognize the importance of integration and the synthesis of new ways of thinking about self and others. However, this aspect of therapy is especially important in treating BPD. Patients' experiences of themselves and their lives are often disjointed and disconnected, so they require help with constructing more adaptive narratives that integrate their experiences.

Second, the therapist is best considered a consultant who makes his or her expertise available to pursue collaborative treatment goals. Support, acceptance, exploration, and gentle confrontation are part of this function but responsibility for change lies firmly with the patient. This aspect of the stance is important because it minimizes the polarization that can occur when the therapist is seen to be pressing for change, which is resisted by the patient. The approach is also consistent with an emphasis on building a sense of agency and personal autonomy.

Finally, therapists also have a psychoeducational function, which begins during assessment and remains an ongoing part of treatment with information being imparted in manageable amounts. The education offered ranges from brief explanations of the factors that contribute to a particular problem or way of thinking to more lengthy explanations of the nature and origins of a given problem such as deliberate self-harm or unstable emotions and how therapy works. Information may be provided in discrete chunks as is the case with specific psychoeducational sessions or incorporated into the flow of therapy. Both are useful but it is often best to simply provide appropriate information as issues arise in therapy. Thus early in therapy a patient may note that he/she cannot think clearly when upset. A brief explanation of how intense emotions interfere with thinking processes may help him/her to focus on learning to manage distress as opposed to blaming him-/herself for being confused. Or, later in therapy, patients who castigate themselves for not being able to get over abuse that occurred in early childhood may be helped to show more self-compassion by an explanation of how early abuse has a lasting effect because it influences the development of important self- and interpersonal schemas. Such explanations also help to focus attention on changing these beliefs.

7.4.4 Flexibility

IMT has an explicit conceptual framework, and adherence to this framework is assumed to contribute to successful outcomes. However, there is also evidence that therapist flexibility, open-mindedness, and creativity are related to outcome. Although these ideas may seem incompatible, this is not the case. The conceptual frameworks underlying IMT are not intended to be applied rigidly regardless of circumstances. Rather, the therapist is given considerable discretion over what interventions to use and how to handle specific situations within the broad confines of an empathic, supportive, and validating stance. In this sense, flexibility is built into the framework. This is necessary because the complexity of BPD often leads to situations in therapy that cannot be anticipated.

Therapist flexibility and creativity are especially important during crises and when the patient is frustrated by lack of progress. During crises, therapists need to be flexible about providing additional help and support. When establishing the treatment contract, sufficient latitude needs to be built into the agreement about the therapist's availability during crises to allow the therapist to respond appropriately without violating the contract.

Flexibility is also needed when the patient feels stuck and has difficulty applying what was learned in therapy to everyday situations. Here the requirements for flexibility are different – they require the ability to respond creatively in providing support and managing whatever obstacles are impeding change. This may, for example, require conjoint sessions with family members and partners to address their concerns and help them to adjust to and support changes in the patient when the patient is concerned that any change may adversely affect their relationship. Family members often echo these concerns because they are forced to accommodate shifts in the patient. Thus a partner who is used to dealing with a highly submissive and dependent person may have difficulty adjusting to one who is a little more assertive.

7.5 The Work of Therapy

Therapists need a broad idea about the work of therapy and how treatment goals are to be achieved. With IMT, the *work of therapy is to engage the patient in the collaborative description of the patient's problems and psychopathology and how they affect the patient's life and relationships, which leads to increased self-understanding and helps the patient to identify and use opportunities for change.*[13]

This depiction of therapy extends ideas about the therapeutic stance based on empathic and reflective listening. The idea combines an attitudinal position with an intervention strategy, which is intended to promote and structure the descriptive process. Self-knowledge is increased as patients become increasingly aware of their repetitive maladaptive patterns of behaviour and experience, the events that trigger these patterns, and how these patterns contribute to ongoing problems. A new understanding emerges as obstacles to self-awareness are overcome, and the patient is drawn almost inevitably into considering alternative ways of thinking and acting.

The process is guided by the therapist seeking clarification when things are unclear and details when the patient's narrative is too general and by highlighting those parts of the patient's narrative that are important for self-understanding and change. In the process, the therapist not only stimulates more detailed descriptions of problems but also structures the patient's understanding of these problems in the way specific issues are selected for further description and by providing summaries and narratives that re-frame the patient's understanding. The result is a shared understanding that expands self-awareness, re-frames patients' ideas about themselves, and reformulates problems so that they are less distressing. Hence collaborative description does not provide a historical account of events but rather a detailed reformulation of the patient's experiences and reactions, which combines the therapeutic tasks of exploration and synthesis discussed earlier.

Viewed in this way, collaborative description fits well with a supportive, empathic therapeutic stance. Patients are encouraged to work with the therapist to develop straight-forward accounts in the context of a collaborative relationship that differs substantially from many previous relationships, and offers a way of relating that challenges the maladaptive schemas that dominate their interpersonal relationships. A consistent focus on both *what* the patient thinks and *how* they think promotes self-appraisal and helps to counter self-criticism.

7.6 Concluding Comments

The ideas discussed in this chapter set the tone for therapy, shape the patient–therapist relationship, and form the foundation for the consistent treatment process necessary for good outcomes. However, they are not a set of fixed rules. Flexibility is part of the structure of therapy so that therapists are free to use their clinical judgement when responding to whatever exigencies arise in treatment with the proviso that these responses are consistent with the spirit of IMT. Finally, it should be noted that the formulation and treatment contract discussed in the previous chapter are an indispensable part of the structure of therapy. The formulation provides the road map for planning therapy and a frame of reference that helps to keep treatment on track by reminding the therapist and the patient of the main tasks of therapy. The contract establishes the boundaries of therapy and the agreement needed to ensure a consistent process.

Notes

1. Castonguay and Beutler (2006a, 2006b).

2. Roth and Fonagy (2005), Links et al. (2015).

3. Hollin (1995).

4. Robins et al. (2001).

5. Gold (1996).

6. Strupp et al. (1969).

7. Rogers (1951, 1957).

8. "Empathic attunement" is discussed by Greenberg and Paivio (1997). I have drawn extensively on their ideas when discussing the therapeutic relationship and the treatment of emotional dysregulation.

9. Critchfield and Benjamin (2006).

10. Ryle (1997).

11. Waldinger and Gunderson (1989), Ryle (1997).

12. Mitchell (1993), Livesley (2003).

13. Livesley (2003). This depiction of the work of therapy has some similarity to the idea of the therapist's role as a participant observer emphasized by contemporary interpersonal theory as described by Benjamin (2003), Horowitz (2004), Horowitz et al. (2006), Kiesler (1996), Pincus and Ansell (2012), which also reflects the early contributions of Sullivan (1953).

General Treatment Module 2: Treatment Relationship

Building and Maintaining a Collaborative Treatment Relationship

All therapies agree that the main task in treating borderline personality disorder (BPD) is to build a good working relationship and bond with the patient because these predict outcome.[1] This relationship is variously referred to as the therapeutic relationship, the working alliance, and the working relationship and hence these terms will be used interchangeably. The essential characteristic of the alliance is patient–therapist *collaboration* in working for the patient's benefit. The alliance results from the patient forming a positive bond with the therapist who is perceived as helpful, supportive, trustworthy, and reliable.[2] A good alliance is often achieved as much by the manner in which the therapist approaches the patient as by what is done and said. A warm, supportive, open manner promotes engagement.

Given the importance of the alliance, therapists need to monitor it carefully and intervene quickly when problems arise. We usually know intuitively how treatment is going. When treatment is progressing, the patient is engaged, actively participating in the process, and is open to exploring issues and trying new things. We also intuitively recognize when things are off track. The patient seems disinterested, silent, relatively uncommunicative, angry, or tetchy. Therapists also feel a little less engaged, and even bored or irritated. Nevertheless, it is the patient's perceptions of the alliance, not the therapist's, that predicts the outcome.[3] Hence therapists should not rely solely on their own impressions but also ask patients about how they see therapy and the relationship, and whether they think that they are helpful.

Without a good alliance, outcome is poor and dropouts are common[4] probably because the alliance influences motivation for treatment. A good therapeutic relationship also has a settling effect: it provides the support needed to contain distress. As distress settles, it becomes possible to work more directly on problems as opposed to struggling with unstable emotions.

8.1 Professional and Social Relationships

When thinking about an effective patient–therapist relationship, it is useful to recall how therapeutic relationships differ from social relationships established with friends and acquaintances. Many staff confuse the two. Social relationships are typically reciprocal: both parties expect to give something to, and to get something from, the relationship. When this does not happen, the relationship is experienced as unsatisfying and one-sided and most people think about ending it. Professional relationships are different. Therapists are properly concerned with helping the patient, not with meeting their own needs other than in the professional sense of engaging in a rewarding task. Hence, therapists are "deprived" of the emotional and social support provided by satisfying social relationships.

This situation is often unsatisfying for patients with BPD who try to draw clinicians into more typical social interactions. They express curiosity about their therapists' personal lives and experiences. Patients may talk about "being friends" and can be persistent in their quest to know more about their therapist. Although it is important that therapists and other staff resist this pressure, it is easy for some to get caught up in the dynamic and begin to question the need to be so "professional." As will be discussed later, boundaries are important and boundary violations are fraught with problems. Pressure to act differently may be more easily resisted by recalling that professional boundaries are a safeguard for both parties: they ensure that the relationship remains focused on the task at hand. When dealing with these problems, it is important that therapists indicate that they understand their patients' wants and needs in an empathic and respectful way while remaining firm. It is also useful to remind patients that the therapist's role is to help them to deal with their problems.

8.2 Why Is It Difficult to Establish a Collaborative Alliance?

Therapists from all conceptual orientations agree that it is often difficult and takes time to form a collaborative alliance with patients with BPD and that once formed the alliance needs nurturing throughout treatment. Even after six months of treatment, a good alliance is not achieved with most patients.[5] And, when a reasonable alliance is achieved, it usually fluctuates because any deepening of the relationship tends to evoke feelings of vulnerability and fears of rejection, which cause patients to distance themselves (the enactment of the core relationship conflict in therapy). As therapists, we should expect rapport to fluctuate and not be disappointed or alarmed when a good session is followed by one in which the patient is less involved.

When treating many other mental disorders, patient motivation and a good alliance are often considered prerequisites for treatment. This is not the case with BPD: a good alliance is often the end point, not the starting point, of treatment. Effort to build the alliance is not time wasted. It is an integral part of therapy because it involves changing maladaptive self- and interpersonal schemas.

Many factors hinder alliance formation including deficits in social skills; poor object relationships; poor family relationships; strong defensive attitudes; hopelessness (also pessimism and anhedonia); low psychological mindedness (metacognitive deficits); high levels of resistance, negativism, and hostility; and perfectionism.[6]

Pervasive distrust makes many patients cautious about interacting with others and suspicious of their intent. Trust has to be earned and fostered: it is not something that occurs automatically. Other factors add to these problems. Patients often lack the skills required for collaboration – they have difficulty working cooperatively and lack the ability to negotiate effective relationships. The tendency to be hostile when anxious or threatened adds to the problem.[7] Also, many individuals are more used to controlling rather than cooperative relationships. Negotiation and reciprocity in relationships are often alien ideas. Rigidity and the tendency to cling to ideas and opinions mean that it usually takes time to foster trust and build the alliance. These challenges are not surprising – they arise from the negative expectations about relationships created by psychosocial adversity and from beliefs that others will not provide help and support voluntarily but have to be coerced into doing so.

Emotional instability also hinders alliance formation especially early in treatment because it is difficult to focus on the alliance when emotions are chaotic and life is a constant crisis. Some patients also enter treatment with negative expectations, hostility, and reluctance to engage in the therapeutic process. Such patients usually have poor outcomes. Alliance formation can also be hindered by feelings of envy towards the therapist, conflicted attitudes towards authority, passive-oppositional tendencies, and conflict between neediness and fear of rejection.

8.3 How to Build and Strengthen the Relationship

The alliance is fostered by focusing on the patient–therapist relationship and by a collaborative therapeutic style that addresses the patient's goals and current concerns.[8] It is useful to think of the alliance as having two components: (i) an attitudinal component linked to therapist credibility that involves the patient seeing the therapist as providing help and the patient accepting it; and (ii) a relationship component wherein the patient sees the patient and therapist as working collaboratively for the patient's benefit.[9] These components are closely related although the former often develops first. It is helpful to keep the two components of the alliance in mind during each session because this makes it easier to recognize opportunities to strengthen the relationship.

The maintenance of an effective alliance requires timely intervention to deal with any breakdown in the relationship – what are often called alliance ruptures. Thus, we can think of the relationship module as having three sub-modules designed to (i) build credibility, (ii) build collaboration, and (iii) repair alliance ruptures. Many of the interventions used are based on ideas about the therapeutic stance introduced in the previous chapter.

8.3.1 Building Credibility

Patients need to believe that treatment can work and that the therapist is helpful and competent for them to form a working relationship. Credibility is built through the accumulative effects of multiple interactions, none in themselves highly significant.

8.3.1.1 Build Optimism and Confidence

An important task is to build the patient's confidence that treatment will produce the benefits sought. Optimism is built from the outset by how the therapist approaches the patient and conducts the assessment. A confident professional manner that conveys respect, understanding, and support instills hope that here is someone who may understand.[10]

8.3.1.2 Listen, Accept, Reflect

The alliance is also built on the rapport created by careful listening and thoughtful reflection of the patient's dialogue. It also helps to provide short summaries of what was discussed that amplify the patient's understanding. These summaries not only indicate that the therapist is listening but also reduce any fears that the patient may harbour that the therapist will not take their problems seriously.

8.3.1.3 Provide Information and Education

Psychoeducation is an effective way to build therapist credibility by showing that the therapist understands the patient's problems, what caused them, and how they can be treated. It also helps to build the alliance indirectly by helping to settle distress and reduce self-blame.

8.3.1.4 Support Patient Treatment Goals

Research indicates that a goal-orientated approach fosters the alliance and enhances outcome.[11] It may also help to reduce early dropout. Therapists need to support the goals patients set for themselves and be seen as helping with goal attainment. Discussion of the patient's goals and primary concerns when establishing the treatment agreement conveys the message from the outset that the therapist wants to ensure that treatment is relevant to the patient. Having established goals, regular reviews of progress serve to keep treatment on track and confirm that the therapist genuinely wants to help patients to achieve their objectives. When a patient mentions a specific event that illustrates a problem related to an agreed goal, simple comments such as "I remember that this is one of the things that you said that you wanted to deal with in therapy – perhaps we can talk a little more about it" remind patients of their goals and demonstrate the therapist's commitment.

8.3.1.5 Communicate Realistic Hope

Hope is an important ingredient of treatment. Hope that treatment will be helpful is needed to bring patients into treatment and needs to be fostered throughout therapy. Hope is instilled by explaining how therapy works, by questions that reflect a sensitive understanding of the issues, and by the therapist's willingness to work with the patient on what may seem to the patient to be intractable problems. During the early stages of treatment, exploration of the patient's reservations about treatment and the therapist's ability to help may contribute to reducing premature termination. The hope generated through such explorations counteracts demoralization and hopelessness and builds a commitment to treatment.

8.3.1.6 Recognize Progress

Nothing succeeds like success. Therapist and treatment credibility ultimately depends on the patient feeling better and making changes. Hence it is important to have some successes early in treatment, no matter how modest. This may involve an early response to medication or a modest change in how the patient handled a distressing event. Even minor changes should be highlighted and used to show that change is possible and that the patient has the ability to change. It is easier to achieve an early success if major goals are broken down into smaller, more easily achieved goals – as will be discussed in Chapter 12.

When acknowledging progress, therapists should avoid statements that could be interpreted as the therapist acting as the source of reinforcement. For example, statements such as "I am pleased with how you handled the situation" or "I am glad you were able to do things differently" are best avoided. They put the focus on the therapist rather than on the patient and hinder the patient learning to reward and motivate him-/herself. Instead, progress can be acknowledged by noting that "This seems to be a different way of dealing with things – it seems that you were able to use what we talked about last session to change how you reacted." Such statements focus on the patient and on how the patient was able to use treatment to make changes.

8.3.1.7 Acknowledge Competence

Patients often begin therapy in a demoralized state. Faced with the multiple problems of each patient, therapists often lose sight of the fact that most patients also have areas of competency. Thus a patient may be able to hold down a part-time job or care for a child despite overwhelming problems. A therapist's acknowledgement of such competencies without minimizing problems or distress helps to modulate feelings of demoralization, incompetence, and low self-esteem. Such interventions also influence the patient's perception of the therapist and the relationship because they indicate respect and that the therapist is able to see the big picture as opposed to being focused only on what patients often see as shortcomings.

8.3.2 Building Cooperation

The second component of the treatment relationship is collaboration. Although it is convenient to describe two components of the alliance as distinct entities, they are interconnected and many interventions promote both credibility and collaboration.

8.3.2.1 Create a Bond

Most conceptions of the alliance emphasize the patient–therapist bond and the importance of the patient feeling secure enough to explore problems and feelings.[12] The bond is experienced and expressed as liking, trust, mutual respect, shared commitment to the process, and a shared understanding of the treatment process and goals.[13] Hence a positive bond is created by the empathic and supportive therapeutic stance discussed in the previous chapter.

8.3.2.2 Build Trust

The alliance depends on a sense of trust about therapy and the therapist. This is a central problem because many patients are distrustful of treatment due to early adversity and the reinforcement of this distrust by previous contact with the mental health system. In any relationship, trust is built by each partner learning that they can depend on the other. Therapists can facilitate this learning by being clear and open during the contracting phase about what they can and cannot do and by being meticulously honest in responses to patients' questions and concerns. During treatment, it is also built by being consistent and following through on commitments, and by a non-judgmental stance.

8.3.2.3 Use Relationship Language

The alliance is fostered by language that captures the idea of therapy as a collaborative relationship. Statements that include words like "we," "us," and "together" are simple ways to build a connection. Patients and therapists use such words more often during successful treatments.[14] Acknowledging that "*We* were able to make some progress with that problem ... " or "In the past *we* were able to work this out *together*" promotes the idea of collaboration. Used judiciously, such statements move patients away from perceiving the relationship in terms of status or control and more towards seeing therapy as a shared venture.

8.3.2.4 Create a Shared History

In everyday life, one of the things that cements the bond in close relationships and creates a sense of intimacy and mutuality is having a shared history. When couples recall the things they have done together, it draws them together and strengthens the bond. This idea can also be used to cement the therapeutic bond by referring to shared experiences in treatment.

Therapists can recall things that have been talked about in the past, and how "we discussed this a few weeks ago." This reminds the patient of shared experiences and perhaps past struggles to deal with specific problems. As therapy progresses, more opportunities arise to refer to past experiences. In some ways, the therapist serves as an auxiliary memory or historian of the therapy, by reminding patients of what happened in therapy and how they have changed.

8.3.2.5 Search for Meaning and Understanding

Most patients are confused by the intensity of their distress and have difficulty making sense of their problems. Any action by the therapist that helps patients to understand their problems produces relief and strengthens the relationship. It helps if the therapist communicates the idea that an important part of therapy is work together in search of understanding. When discussing patient concerns or experiences, simple comments such as "we need to understand this" or "let's see if we can work this out" draw the patient into a collaborative exchange.

8.3.2.6 Explore in a Tentative and Collaborative Way

Cooperation involves searching for meaning in a way that invites the patient's participation in the process. This is achieved by the therapist making observations about the patient's behaviour and experiences in a way that leaves the patient free to accept, reject, modify, or elaborate the observation. This style of communicating models openness and invites the patient to join in. This contrasts with the experiences of many patients of people telling them who they are, how they feel, and what they should do.

8.3.2.7 Acknowledge the Use of Therapy Skills

Successful outcomes require the patient to learn the skills the therapist uses to examine problems and then to apply these skills to everyday situations. When the therapist recognizes and acknowledges instances when this has happened, the bond is strengthened because the acknowledgement creates a connection – it draws attention to the fact that the patient has learned from the therapist and now shares certain skills with the therapist.

8.3.2.8 Review Goals, Methods, and the Work of Therapy Regularly

When discussing ways to build credibility, it was noted that collaboration is promoted by regular reviews of progress towards attaining treatment goals. As therapy progresses, this can be extended to a discussion about whether current treatment methods are helpful and enquiring about other methods that the patient thinks may be useful. Such discussions demonstrate the therapist's openness to other possibilities – an important skill that patients need to learn. These discussions also foster collaboration by focusing the patient's attention on looking at, and talking about, the way he or she is working with the therapist. Although such discussions need to occur regularly, they should not be broached in a stereotyped way or made a routine part of each session lest it appears that the therapist is following a formula rather than being genuinely interested in the patient's opinions.

8.3.3 Managing Alliance Ruptures

Despite the therapist's best efforts, the alliance invariably fluctuates throughout treatment: ruptures are unavoidable and occur in most sessions. A rupture is any deterioration in the alliance that reduces collaboration between the patient and the therapist in working on treatment goals and tasks and any strain in the patient–therapist bond.[15] Ruptures result from both patient and therapist actions. Patient factors include problems with close relationships, maladaptive schemas, limited interpersonal skills, and volatile emotions and self-states. Therapist factors include lapses in empathy and support, failure to acknowledge important concerns raised by the patient, premature exploration of sensitive issues, poorly timed interventions, and so on. A critical therapist task is to identify and manage ruptures as they occur. However, therapists are not always aware of alliance ruptures. Consequently, patients should be asked regularly about how they think therapy is progressing.

Ruptures most frequently result from the activation of maladaptive interpersonal schemas in either the patient or the therapist.[16] Hence ruptures should not be viewed as negative events but as opportunities to change maladaptive beliefs. They also provide information on the patient's inner world. Interestingly, research shows that patients find that therapy is more helpful when therapists are aware of alliance ruptures and work with patients to explore them.[17] This is probably because the process highlights and explores key schemas in the there-and-now of therapy. Such actions by the therapist also indicate that he or she is highly attuned to the treatment process.

Ruptures take two main forms – withdrawal and confrontation ruptures – both of which are common with BPD.[18] *Withdrawal ruptures* involve disengagement from the therapist and therapy. They include silences, short responses, emotional withdrawal, and non-involvement in therapy. They may also involve withdrawal from the self as when emotions are denied or suppressed and when attempts are made to deceive the self about what is happening as occurs when patients refuse to acknowledge problems even to themselves and insist that all is well when it is clearly not. *Confrontational ruptures* typically involve challenges to the therapist in the form of angry comments, expressions of dissatisfaction with treatment, and attempts to control the therapist to ensure he or she responds in a certain way. All ruptures should be dealt with promptly. The following five-step process is useful for this purpose:[19]

Step 1: Notice "rupture markers" – changes in the relationship and rapport. Typical markers include affect changes, decreased involvement, a drop in rapport, disagreement with the therapist, closing the eyes, apparent disinterest, comments about feeling sleepy, changes in eye contact, a frown, a bored expression, decreased commitment to treatment, anger towards the therapist, and so on.

Step 2: Draw the patient's attention to the decreased rapport in an empathic and non-critical way. For example, "something seems to have changed, it seems as if you are a little less involved than you were. Have you noticed?" Explore the concrete details of what happened and why the rupture occurred. Avoid abstract speculations about the rupture because they are often ways to avoid dealing with specific feelings about the event. For this reason, it is best to focus on the patient's here-and-now experience and not get drawn discussing what happened in the past. It is especially important to encourage patients to discuss any negative feelings that they may have about the rupture and the therapist – something that many therapists find difficult. However, it is an important part of repairing the alliance.

Step 3: Explore further the rupture and the maladaptive schemas involved. With BPD, most ruptures occur because an event in therapy activated beliefs about rejection, abandonment, disapproval, and distrust. These need to be acknowledged and discussed. The depth of this discussion varies according to the stage of therapy: care is needed to ensure that the patient is not overwhelmed. In the early phases, the occurrence of these beliefs may simply be acknowledged along with a discussion of what triggered them. Later in therapy, they can be explored in more detail and attempts be made to change them. An important part of this process that is linked to positive outcomes is the therapist's ability to help the patient to recognize that the dysfunctional interpersonal behaviours that led to the rupture are the same as those causing problems in patient's relationships in everyday life.[20] This linkage is an important part of the change process and a further reason to view ruptures as opportunities for change rather than purely negative events.

Step 4: Validate the patient's description of his or her experience. This is also an important step. Therapists should also be frank and non-defensive in acknowledging their part in causing the rupture. If you make a mistake, acknowledge it, discuss it with the patient, apologize, accept responsibility, and change whatever created the problem. These actions provide a corrective experience that strengthens the patient's acceptance of, and trust in, his or her own feelings and impressions. They also help to disconfirm maladaptive schemas such as beliefs that the therapist cannot be trusted or will be angry at being criticized. Patients with BPD are often ready to find fault with their therapists. However, there is often a grain of truth to these criticisms even if exaggerated. Therapists should be scrupulously honest in acknowledging mistakes and promote joint reflection on the reasons why things went awry and how to re-establish a collaborative bond. In this way, the therapist models how to manage and resolve interpersonal problems and conflicts. This is helpful for patients who see relationships in black-and-white terms and do not understand the give and take of good relationships in which both parties are open to discussing their mutual problems and concerns.

Step 5: If these steps are not effective, discuss how the patient is avoiding recognizing and exploring the rupture.

The value of this strategy is that a potentially negative event is used as an opportunity to apply several change processes. By drawing attention to the rupture, the therapist demonstrates empathy and validates the patient's feelings and concerns. At the same time, the patient's attention is drawn to aspects of the self and behaviour that may not be fully recognized. This recognition opens up the possibility that these behaviours can be controlled and changed, thereby promoting self-efficacy and agency. At the same time, the patient's awareness of the therapist is increased. The process provides a new interpersonal experience that can be generalized to other relationships.[21]

The repair process also builds collaboration because the rupture can only be resolved through patient–therapist collaboration. By drawing attention to the rupture, the therapist invites the patient to look at what has happened and work with the therapist to understand it. This also teaches how to solve interpersonal problems by modelling cooperation and acceptance of responsibility. The therapist's preparedness to discuss problems communicates the idea that relationships are not fragile and that relationship problems can be discussed, understood, and resolved.

8.4 Managing Other Alliance Problems

Alliance problems include initial difficulties establishing an alliance, the formation of a pseudo-alliance where the patient fails to improve despite forming an apparently compliant alliance, and persistent failure to form a bond.

8.4.1 Difficulty Establishing an Alliance

Although it usually takes time to build an effective working relationship with patients with BPD, persistent difficulty establishing an alliance is cause for a careful review of the problem with the patient. This discussion should note the difficulty establishing a working relationship while taking care to avoid attributing blame and responsibility by presenting the problem as a joint therapist–patient issue and broaching it in a matter-of-fact way that invites the patient to talk about the difficulty. Sometimes simply noting the problem is sufficient to trigger a productive discussion.

When reviewing the reasons for alliance failure, it should be borne in mind that not all problems originate with the patient. Unclear treatment goals, discrepancies between the patient's and the therapist's understanding of these goals, and disagreements about how goals should be attained contribute to alliance problems. Alliance problems may also occur because the roles of patient and therapist were not discussed adequately when establishing the treatment contract. For example, strong dependency needs and passive features may hinder alliance formation because they are associated with powerful expectations that the therapist is largely responsible for what happens in therapy that were not adequately addressed when discussing the process of therapy and the patient's role in the process. Or the patient may not have processed the implications of this discussion so that further discussion and clarification may be needed to help the patient to understand and accept the necessity of a collaborative process.

Managing alliance failures is often difficult and solutions differ widely across patients. What is clear, however, is what does not work. Therapists are often tempted to become more confrontational at these times. Such methods rarely work and usually make matters worse – patients cannot be coerced into developing a relationship. Nor does it help to blur boundaries – therapists sometimes feel pressured into less professional exchanges in an attempt to build trust. The best course of action is to maintain a supportive, empathic, and enquiring stance.

Difficulty establishing an alliance should not be confused with a negative-oppositional alliance in which the patient struggles with the therapist over everything, including treatment goals, the contract, and treatment methods. Such negative reactions to treatment do not invariably indicate a poor alliance as long they are expressed directly and dealt with early in treatment. In fact, overtly angry patients are sometimes easier to engage than purely negativistic patients. Although this type of alliance may be uncomfortable for the therapist, it does not prevent good outcomes if patients can be encouraged to stay in treatment.[22]

8.4.2 Managing the Pseudo-Alliance

Situations sometimes arise where treatment seems to be progressing – there are no obvious problems with the treatment relationship and the patient is agreeable and apparently compliant – but nothing really changes. In these situations, patients form a compliant alliance. They adhere to the treatment contract by attending consistently and punctually but they do not really collaborate with the treatment plan. It often takes time for the therapist to recognize what is happening because sessions are easy to manage without obvious disruptions or difficulties. Then, it suddenly becomes apparent that nothing is changing. There is a counterintuitive aspect to the problem because therapists need to be more cautious about patients who are compliant in a passive, supplicating manner than those who are actively hostile and oppositional. Therapists should be especially wary of patients who eagerly agree with everything the therapist says.

It also takes time to recognize these problems because progress is usually slow when treating BPD. However, when progress is slow but the alliance is satisfactory, the patient is seen to be working. In each session, the patient makes an effort to understand his/her problems and to act differently. He/she also recalls what was talked about in previous sessions. With the pseudo-alliance, this work is absent. Although these patients usually talk about their strong desire to change and how they plan to implement the ideas discussed in therapy, this somehow never happens. A telling feature is that they usually are unable to recall the content of the previous session.

This pattern is seen in highly submissive-dependent patients with oppositional tendencies who give the impression of working collaboratively because they overtly agree with the therapist and are even deferential but nevertheless continue doing their own thing. They are compliant because of their dependency and their regard for the therapist and they often deceive the therapist into believing that they are doing well when they are not. Occasionally, there is a narcissistic element to this pattern: the patient is overtly compliant but continues as before as if he/she secretly knows that he/she is right. Some highly deprived and neglected individuals also form this kind of alliance – as if they want the emotional support that therapy provides but do not want to change either because they feel there is no point or because they are afraid that therapy will end if they improve.

Compliant non-compliance is difficult to manage. At some point, sooner rather than later, the therapist has to confront this behaviour. The term "confront" as used in psychotherapy is often misunderstood. It tends to be assumed that it involves a forceful, and even coercive, challenge. In integrated modular treatment (IMT), the term is used simply in the sense of "pointing out" what is happening in a firm way that may indeed be challenging but which is also supportive and understanding. The therapist draws the patient's attention to the fact that nothing seems to change in a way that invites the patient to reflect on what is happening. The therapist might ask if the patient has also noted the same thing and wonder what the patient thinks about it. This also needs to be done in a way that does not invalidate the patient by making him/her feel bad or useless or that it is the patient's fault.

8.4.3 Persistent Failure to Form an Alliance

Sometimes an effective alliance proves elusive. Not a lot is known about patient characteristics associated with major alliance problems. However, there is some evidence that patients with poor motivation who form a superficial involvement from the outset often remain difficult to engage.[23] Since the ability to form a good alliance is related to the ability to relate to others,[24] it is useful to evaluate the capacity to form effective relationships when assessing patients so that potential difficulties can be identified early in the treatment process.

Difficulty forming an alliance formation is often seen in patients who have been severely abused and neglected and who become extremely passive and feel that nothing can be done to deal with their problems while at the same attributing all blame to their abusers. This can lead to a help-rejecting stance with the patient persistently seeking help but then either rejecting all attempts to help or dismissing them as inadequate.[25] This is often a difficult pattern to manage and alliance building under these circumstances requires considerable time and patience. Considerable support is needed to allow patients to voice their understandable anger at the injustice of having to deal with problems created by their abusers while also helping them to accept that the only way forward is to begin to take charge of their lives by addressing the problems created by the abuse.

8.5 Concluding Comments

The relationship module lies at the heart of IMT – without a good relationship, little is achieved. Hence, therapists need to keep a template of the module at the forefront of their minds throughout treatment, especially in the early stages, because each session offers multiple opportunities to enhance the alliance but many slip by unnoticed because they are relatively minor events. The following example illustrates one such incident in the treatment of Madison who described how she had managed not to cut herself the previous evening after being disappointed by a friend. This was early days in treatment and the therapist used the incident as an opportunity to strengthen what was still a fragile working relationship.

THERAPIST: When this happened, you were able to control the urge.

MADISON: Yes, I was. It was surprising … I did not really think I could do that.

T: I remember, when you first came to see me a few months ago, you said that you thought that you would never be able to control the urge to hurt yourself.

M: I know (smiling). It's so strong.

T: Was it as strong last night?

M: Yup and I thought I had to do it … then I seemed to stop.

T: Oh! What happened? What do you think helped you to stop last night?

M: Not sure. It just happened.

T: Really?

M: Well, I think I remembered how you asked me if I could distract myself and I thought about how I said sometimes music helped. So I just played something I really like. I just sat and listened and it got less.

T: So you remembered some of the things we talked about and they helped.

M: Yer … but I don't know if it will next time. Oh! I forgot, I also thought that maybe I was wrong. You know … er well she did not turn up because maybe something happened. You know, I sort of thought that maybe I got it wrong. I don't really think she hates me. Later on she phoned – her car wouldn't go.

M: That's important isn't? At first, you thought that she didn't turn up because she was mad with you and didn't like you. We talked last week how you always think people don't like you. But this time you could argue with yourself about whether you were right … whether you were interpreting things properly and whether you were jumping to conclusions

M: Yer … …

T: It seems as if two things helped last night. You were able to distract and soothe yourself and then you were able to argue with yourself. What do you think?

M: That's right.

T: That's a big change isn't it? The important thing is that you were able to control these feelings ... they don't always have to win.

The vignette shows the therapist using the incident to employ a variety of simple interventions to build the patient's confidence in therapy and to communicate the idea that therapy is a collaborative process. The example illustrates the key point that when treating BPD, progress largely arises from the accumulative effect of multiple minor interventions, each having a modest effect. Like water dripping on a stone, they gradually change the shape of therapy and patient pathology.

Notes

1. Hirsh et al. (2012).

2. Gaston (1990), Hatcher and Barends (1996), Horvath and Greenberg (1994), Luborsky (1984, 1994).

3. Hartley (1985), Horvath and Greenberg (1994).

4. Research indicates that weakened alliances are correlated with unilateral termination (Frank (1992), Safran et al. (2000), Samstag et al. (1998), Tyron and Kane (1990, 1993, 1995)).

5. Frank (1992).

6. Fernandez-Alvarez et al. (2006).

7. Muran et al. (1994).

8. Bordin (1979, 1994), Critchfield and Benjamin (2006), Hatcher (2010), Horvath and Greenberg (1994), Luborsky et al. (1988).

9. Luborsky (1984).

10. Batchelor (1995).

11. Critchfield and Benjamin (2006).

12. Allen et al. (1984), Luborsky (1976, 1984), Orlinsky et al. (1994), Orlinsky and Howard (1986).

13. Borden (1994).

14. Luborsky et al. (1985).

15. Eubanks-Carter et al. (2010).

16. Sommerfeld et al. (2008).

17. Sommerfeld et al. (2008), Tufekcioglu and Muran (2015).

18. Harper (1989) cited by Tufekcioglu and Muran (2015).

19. The scheme for managing alliance ruptures is based on the work of Safran et al. (1990), Safran et al. (1994), Safran and colleagues (1994, 2002), Eubanks-Carter et al. (2010) with additional ideas about the importance of working on maladaptive schemas. See also Bennett et al. (2006).

20. Bennett et al. (2006) found that therapists with good outcomes were able to help the patient to recognize that the dysfunctional interpersonal behaviours that led to alliance ruptures also caused problems in the patient's relationships outside of therapy.

21. Safran and Muran (2000).

22. Frank (1992)

23. Gunderson et al. (1989).

24. Hoglend et al. (1993), Piper et al. (1991).

25. Yalom (1985).

Chapter

General Treatment Module 3: Consistency

Maintaining a Consistent Treatment Process

This chapter is short but important. The importance of consistency is stressed by most therapies and that failure to maintain consistency is a common cause of treatment failure. Research shows that consistency is necessary for effective outcomes[1] and interestingly patients who benefit from treatment frequently mention therapist consistency as a major factor in their improvement.[2] However, the maintenance of consistency is challenging when treating patients with boundary problems, unstable emotions, ever-changing self-states, and difficulties with cooperation and collaboration. As a result, substantial frame violations are relatively common, occurring in about nearly 50 per cent of patients with borderline personality disorder (BPD) in the first six months of treatment.[3]

9.1 What Is Consistency?

Therapy needs to be as predictable as possible, which means that it needs to be delivered in adherence to the therapeutic frame and treatment contract discussed in Chapter 7. Consistency has a practical component to do with the routine arrangements for therapy and an interpersonal component that concerns the way the therapy is conducted. The practical component requires adherence to the therapeutic contract in terms of frequency and duration of appointments and that changes in the agreed arrangement are discussed with the patient well in advance. This is a necessary part of therapy for patients who are often in a disorganized state with strong feelings of distrust and attachment insecurity. Failure to maintain these practical requirements confirms patient expectations and undermines treatment. Although this principle is widely understood, it is violated surprisingly frequently. Individual therapists often announce absences such as vacations without warning and in institutional settings treatment sessions are all-too-often cancelled at the last minute or therapists changed without prior warning. Punctuality is also important. It is an indication of the therapist's commitment to the process, and it is unreasonable to expect patients to be committed to their treatment if the therapist does not show an equal commitment. The interpersonal component requires that the therapist uses the same basic approach throughout therapy and interacts with the patient in a consistent way.

9.1.1 Consistency Is Not Rigidity

Being consistent is not the same as being rigid in maintaining the treatment frame. Discussion of structure (Chapter 7) noted the importance of therapist flexibility in dealing with the complexity of borderline pathology and especially when managing crises and when the patient feels stuck. Successful management of these situations may require changes to the treatment frame such as additional appointments or telephone contact. What matters is that the frame is not changed lightly and then only after careful consideration of whether the change is actually necessary, and the likely short- and long-term impact of the change on the patient, the treatment relationship, coping capacity, and so on.

In contemplating changes, it is important to ensure that boundaries are maintained and that the basic stance of support, validation, empathy, and a consultant role is not disrupted. We also need to be careful that we are not fostering dependency. This is an important issue when treating patients with intense dependency arising from emotional deprivation because these needs can easily increase substantially in intensity in ways that are not helpful to treatment (see Chapter 20). Nevertheless, there have been occasions when I have given the sandwiches that were to have been my lunch to a patient who was feeling weak and possibly mildly hypoglycaemic because she had no money for food or I have gone to collect a patient who was dissociating in the car park outside my office. These things do not happen often and they were certainly discussed later in treatment.

What we need to avoid are extreme interpretations of what consistency means and acting in ways that lack compassion and appear ungracious. Illustrative examples that I have encountered are confronting a patient about being late for an appointment when the patient has hobbled in on a crutch following an accident that occurred since the previous session and refusing to talk to a patient who is clearly anxious when walking with him/her from the waiting room to the office because this is "outside the boundaries of therapy."

9.2 Therapeutic Benefits of Consistency

Besides providing the assurance and safety needed for patients to engage in therapeutic work and the stability needed to implement other interventions, consistency also facilitates the attainment of specific treatment goals. Early in treatment, consistency contributes to the improvement many patients experience on starting therapy by helping to contain unstable emotions and impulses. The predictability and stability of therapy contrast with the chaos and turmoil of the rest of the patient's life, so the therapy provides a safe haven and respite. Consistency also contributes to a therapeutic process that counters maladaptive schemas related to distrust and unpredictability. Perhaps the most important of all, it provides patients with a stable experience of themselves in relationship with the therapist, which can contribute to a more coherent self.

9.3 Strategies for Maintaining Consistency

Establishing and maintaining consistency require therapists both to act in ways that maintain the frame and to intervene promptly when the frame is violated.

9.3.1 Maintaining the Frame

Consistency is maintained by multiple interventions that continually and quietly adjust the treatment process. Most sessions, especially early in treatment, require some kind of simple intervention to maintain boundaries. Patients often deal with their anxiety about therapy by acting as they would in any social relationship. Hence they ask whether the therapist is well or had a good weekend as they would in any social encounter. These interactions need to be handled graciously while also helping the patient to recognize that therapy differs from everyday social interaction. A simple "thank you" followed by a similar query about how the patient is feeling is usually sufficient to keep things on track.

9.3.1.1 Explicit Structure

Consistency begins with a clear understanding of the disorder and the treatment process. Subsequently, therapists need a frame of reference for gauging compliance. This is provided by the therapeutic stance, treatment plan, and treatment contract. Consistency is simply adherence to this framework. Inconsistency suggests either that this framework is not in place or that the therapist is having counter-transference problems that are hindering the maintenance of the frame.

9.3.1.2 Maintain Interpersonal Boundaries

Consistency requires the therapist to manage interpersonal boundaries. The boundary problems that are part of self pathology of BPD lead to demanding and intrusive behaviour and inappropriate revelation of personal information. These behaviours contribute to interpersonal difficulties because people are uncomfortable when their boundaries are violated. A benefit of a consistent treatment process is that it helps patients to establish boundaries and monitor the extent to which they respect those of other people. Much of this learning occurs by observing how the therapist establishes and maintains boundaries. Patients often note that they disliked therapist consistency in the early days of treatment and often went to great lengths to test it. However, over time they come to appreciate it for the stability it provided. They then begin to copy the therapist and use the same methods to establish and maintain boundaries in everyday life.

9.3.1.3 Resist Pressures to Act Differently

Boundary problems, anxieties about therapy, and demanding in-your-face attitude of some patients can put therapists under considerable pressure to act differently, an issue discussed when considering the difference between therapeutic and social relationships (Chapter 8). This pressure needs to be resisted in a firm but understanding way by recognizing the pressures patients feel to know more about the therapist but reminding them that the purpose of treatment is to focus on the patient's problems. It may also help to offer a quiet reminder that this was something agreed when discussing treatment and that anything else distracts from this task. These incidents show the value of establishing boundaries before treatment begins. It is difficult enough to maintain boundaries under the pressure of the multiple events occurring in therapy without having to negotiate them.

9.3.2 Setting Limits

Limit setting is integral to treating BPD and the failure to set limits in a timely and effective way is a common reason for failed treatment. A therapeutic skill required to treat BPD is the ability to set limits in a supportive and understanding way while also adhering to the principle that anything that threatens to disrupt treatment should be dealt with promptly. The goal of limit setting is to help the patient recognize violations of the treatment agreement and to get treatment back on track without adversely affecting the treatment relationship.

9.3.2.1 How to Set Limits

Effective limit setting typically incorporates the following features:

1. Draw attention to the problem: The first step is to help the patient recognize the frame violation, for example, being consistently late for appointments, seeking more time at the end of sessions, and arriving under the influence of alcohol or drugs.

2. Get the tone right: The patient's attention needs to be drawn to a frame violation in a calm, matter-of-fact way that invites the patient to recognize what he/she is doing. Besides getting the tone of voice right, it is also important to ensure other non-verbal communications are consistent with the tone and do not leak any feelings of anger or uncertainty that the therapist may have.

3. Act promptly: Therapists often wait too long to address frame violations. Although it is easier to deal with problems when they first arise before intense feelings are aroused in both parties, several factors lead to a delay. First, hesitancy in limit setting is sometimes wishful thinking on the therapist's part who hopes that the problem will simply go away. This is rarely the case. Second, therapists often worry that limit setting will cause further deterioration in the alliance and that the patient may terminate therapy in anger. However, the opposite is usually the case. Effective limit setting usually strengthens the alliance by reassuring the patient that the therapist can handle his or her problems. Third, therapists do not understand or believe that limit setting can actually help to contain aggressive and self-destructive behaviour or emotional reactivity. Finally, the intense, almost raw quality of the anger of many patients can be intimidating, causing therapists to avoid actions that may arouse the patient's anger. This combination of factors often leads therapists to act only after therapy has been disrupted by which time it is often too late.

4. Explore the reasons for non-compliance: Patients are more likely to respond positively to limit setting if the therapist explores the reasons for the frame violation rather than simply seeking to ensure future compliance.

5. Explain the purpose of the limit: Acceptance of the limit is also more likely if the reasons for the limit are explained and the patient is given the opportunity to discuss this explanation offered. Patients need to understand that the limit is not just a matter of the therapist's personal rules or convenience but rather a part of effective treatment and that the violation can adversely affect therapy. The explanations provided may be brief and obvious, for example, that being late consistently means there is less time to deal with problems. Sometimes more complex explanations may be given because the violation provides an opportunity to address a significant issue. For example, Anna repeatedly asked her therapist personal questions. This behaviour reflected problems with interpersonal boundaries. However, it also seemed to serve other purposes. It was used to avoid talking about things that were painful and as a way to express painful feelings as anger because she berated the therapist about the unfairness of her having to talk about personal matters but the therapist did not. Early in therapy when the primary task was to settle things down and contain distress, the therapist simply explained the limit by saying that talking about his personal life would leave less time to deal with Anna's distress and that it was important to have sufficient time to help her to manage it. Later, the therapist noted how Anna asked personal questions when she wanted to avoid dealing with something painful and that the limit helped to keep therapy focused on major issues and not to get sidetracked.

6. Provide support and validation but be firm: Limit setting is more effective and less likely to evoke an angry oppositional reaction or impair the alliance if done in an empathic and respectful way that recognizes the reasons for non-compliance. Nevertheless this has to be done firmly without any hint of hesitancy or ambiguity about the therapist's intent.

7. Do not argue or debate: Discussion of limits should quietly but firmly restate earlier discussions of how therapy works. Nothing is gained from arguing or debating the issue because limits are not a matter of negotiation (unless of course the issue was not clarified when establishing the treatment contract). The patient's frustration and desire to change a limit need to be acknowledged without compromising the limit. Similarly, nothing is gained by getting angry or frustrated no matter how persistent the patient is. Occasionally, therapists react with frustration to repeated violations and state that it may be difficult to continue therapy if the violations continue. Such interventions are rarely successful – they are too confrontational and tend to activate either outright anger or a passive oppositional response.

Under most circumstances, the multiple components of limit setting are incorporated into a single intervention. For example, if a patient arrives late for several sessions, the therapist may simply comment: "I notice that you have been a little late for the last few sessions. Is something happening that prevents you getting here on time? I am concerned about this because it gives us less time to deal with the things that are concerning you." Subsequent discussion usually provides opportunities to support and validate. This slightly lengthy process is better than simply pointing out the frame violation and its consequences.

9.4 Managing the Counter-Transference

Consistency and effective limit setting are dependent on therapists' ability to manage their reactions to patients. BPD tends to elicit intense counter-transference responses that include anger and frustration, pain and distress evoked by the harrowing events that have happened to many patients, and deep concern and sympathy. Negative reactions are common and they are probably the most talked about since most therapists are acutely aware of them. To treat BPD, therapists need to able to tolerate criticism, anger, rage, devaluation, and other verbal attacks without retaliating or withdrawing.[4] Beginning therapists and other professionals involved in the care of these patients often find this difficult. Both retaliation and withdrawal disrupt the alliance and they can have consequences that are difficult to reverse.

The lives of many patients with BPD are populated with sad events. The patient's recounting of abuse, neglect, and losses is often painful to hear. Most people have experienced sadness and loss and even if we think we have dealt with them, the patient's recalling these events and the intense distress that he/she experiences with the retelling can resonate with the therapist's own experiences and active old pains. Sometimes, this can lead the therapist to violate the frame in response to these personal reactions.

9.4.1 Learn to Recognize "Red Flags"

To maintain consistency, therapists need to monitor the treatment process to ensure it is on track. This includes an ongoing assessment of one's own reactions both to therapy and to the patient. Although we usually know intuitively when things are not as they should be, we also need to review our own reactions on a regular basis. We each have our own "red flags" that can warn us that our reactions to the patient may lead to management problems. It is often much easier to manage our counter-transference reactions and reduce their impact on treatment if we become aware of these flags and reflect on why they occur.

Although many counter-transference reactions are idiosyncratic, there are also some common issues that therapists struggle with. Perhaps the commonest is feeling angry, frustrated, or irritated with the patient. In more muted form, this may involve not wanting the see the patient or dreading the next session. Less common, and sometimes less obvious, are feelings that denote excessive concern about the patient that goes beyond the normal professional response. In institutional settings, this may be expressed as intense irritation with colleagues about the way they treat the patient or concern that the patient is not being managed properly. Of course, these may be genuine concerns. In many settings, there are staff who do not like patients with BPD and react negatively to them. Nevertheless, the fact that one has these thoughts is cause to pause and reflect. More problematic are feelings that other staff do not understand the patient as well as you do. This feeling is sometimes associated with looking forward to talking with the patient. Again, these reactions may be understandable and even useful but they can also lead to the therapist's being blind to the underlying factors that may contribute to these feelings.

Other warning signs are things that the patient may say or do that triggers a strong reaction in the therapist. Important here is feeling flattered by the patient and patients who make us feel good about ourselves. When treatment is progressing, most patients comment from time to time that they are feeling better and express gratitude towards the therapist for the help provided. Such statements are important and need a gracious response followed by enquiry about what has changed and what the patient thinks helped in order to use the event to consolidate change. Such statements also reveal the patient's recognition of the benefits of working collaboratively with the therapist. This is an important contrast to the caution and possibly distrust of the early days of treatment. Such statements usually have the ring of sincerity to them. This contrasts to statements that are more gushing and "over-the-top" in which the patient seeks to flatter the therapist by saying things about how wonderful he/she is and how he/she is the best therapist the patient has ever seen, and so on. The problem here is not that the patient is saying these idealizing things – such statements can be explored in the usual ways. Problems arise when therapists believe these comments and respond in ways that inadvertently encourage them as opposed to seeking to uncover what lies behind them.

9.4.2 Handling the Counter-Transference

Therapists need to recognize that strong feelings are simply part of treating BPD and need to be managed like any other therapeutic event. Within sessions, there are three main things that therapists can do to manage their counter-transferences and minimize their impact on treatment:

1. Accept, examine, and reflect: Therapists need to manage their own feelings in the same way they manage patients' feelings. This means that their feelings have to be accepted rather than suppressed or avoided no matter how intense or disconcerting. This is sometimes difficult especially for beginning therapists who think that it is unprofessional to react so strongly. However, like our patients, we cannot control the thoughts and feelings that come to mind; all we can do is manage them when they occur. Also there is something about borderline pathology that generates intense feelings in others, including therapists. It is probably linked to poor boundaries that make patients appear intrusive and demanding and to the "primitive" or raw quality of these patients' emotions that increases their interpersonal impact. Having accepted the feeling, it needs to be examined and understood. When treating patients, we need to be able to step back and reflect on what is happening both in terms of what the patient is doing and in terms of why we are reacting in a given way.

2. *Contain reactions*: Counter-transferences should be contained rather than revealed. They are the therapist's problem, not the patient's. Personal revelations about counter-transference reactions are a slope down which it is easy to slip but difficult to recover. Usually any disclosure feeds the need for more.

3. *Avoid taking patients' comments personally*: An important way to contain and reduce counter-transference reactions is to avoid personalizing patients' comments. This is an obvious point but it is noteworthy that many staff dealing with these patients get enraged or hurt by them because they interpret their comments as reflections on themselves rather than indications of the patient's problems and hence respond either angrily or defensively. This is often seen in institutional settings when a patient is angry, demanding, or hostile to a member of staff. If the staff person takes the patient's comments personally and responds in a similar fashion because he/she feels disrespected or controlled in some way, the situation escalates whereas a quieter limit-setting response usually allows things to settle down. This does not mean that abusive behaviour by patients should be tolerated; rather it should be dealt with in a way that focuses on changing psychopathology and not colluding with it. Nor does this approach mean that therapists do not need to examine whether they did something to evoke the anger or criticism. If this is the case, the therapist needs to discuss this with the patient and accept responsibility and apologize as the case may be.

4. *Use counter-transference reactions to understand the patient*: It is often easier to manage our personal reactions if we use them to understand the patient. If a patient evokes strong feelings in the therapist, they almost certainly evoke similar feelings in other people in everyday life so that the therapist can use his or her reactions to understand the patient's relationships with others and why their interpersonal life is so stressful. Engaging in such a cognitive exercise creates a little distance from immediate reactions that facilitates control.

5. *Use support and supervision sessions*: Working with patients with BPD can be stressful. Hence it is helpful to have opportunities to debrief and to discuss problems encountered in therapy with colleagues or supervisors. The availability of such sessions helps to maintain consistency and reduce the therapist's stress and burnout.

9.5 Concluding Comments

Consistency is largely a matter of managing the treatment relationship. Throughout therapy, the therapist needs to do minor, almost unnoticeable, things continually to keep things consistent and on track to prevent problems growing to the point where they threaten treatment. But these adjustments need to be done in a way that is consistent with the supportive, empathic, and validating stance that underpins therapy. This means that when acting to maintain consistency, therapists need to remind themselves of what was referred to in Chapter 1 as the second voice or tone of therapy. This tone features large in supportive limit setting, which requires therapists to be consistent but flexible, firm but supportive, and confrontational (in the sense of pointing out a problem) but empathic. It is the "tone" that often helps to meet these requirements and maintain consistency in a way that strengthens the relationship.

Notes

1. Critchfield and Benjamin (2006).

2. Livesley (2007).

3. Frank (1992).

4. Many experts stress the importance of the therapist being able to tolerate the patient's anger, criticisms, hostility, and devaluation without retaliating or withdrawing (see Gunderson, 1984; Waldinger, 1987).

Chapter 10

General Treatment Module 4: Validation
Promoting Validation

Most therapies concur that validation has a crucial role in treating borderline personality disorder (BPD)[1] and that it forms an essential ingredient of a supportive and empathic stance. Validation refers to the therapist's *recognition, acknowledgement,* and *affirmation of the legitimacy of the patient's experience.* Essentially, validating interventions affirm the therapist's empathic understanding and acceptance of the patient's mental state. The important feature for the patient is having one's subjective experiences understood, a process that creates feelings of safety and trust needed to explore, reflect, understand, and change.

Although validation may be applied to specific emotions, opinions and points of view, and behaviours, it also refers to something more general – the therapist's affirmation of the patient as a person. This includes affirming the patient's strengths and successes, something that is readily overlooked with a purely problem-focused approach.

10.1 Functions of Validation

Validation contributes to a treatment process that provides an ongoing corrective experience that helps to restructure maladaptive schemas. It is also an important first step in the change process. Patients need to feel validated before they can work on making changes. This is seen with deliberate self-harm. Many patients have been criticized previously for engaging in this behaviour and hence they need the therapist's non-judgemental approach to feel secure enough to make the effort to change. Indications of acceptance are liberating: they reduce rigidity and the need to spend time justifying actions.

Validation is also central to managing core self and interpersonal pathology. It helps to correct the empathic failures that compromised the development of the self as knower and counters self-invalidating thinking. Experience of a validating relationship contributes to building new expectations about relationships and correcting distorted perceptions and interpersonal distrust. Perhaps most importantly, consistent validation builds trust in oneself as an authentic and autonomous individual and confidence in one's ability to differentiate social communications that are genuine and trustworthy from those that are not.

Besides these more general functions, validation is also useful in managing emotional arousal. Research shows that validating responses reduces negative emotions and physiological responses to stress such as heart rate.[2]

10.2 Validating Interventions

Validation is as much an attitude as a set of interventions. As with the alliance, validation is built through the accumulative effects of multiple interventions, each having a small effect.

10.2.1 Non-Judgemental Recognition and Acceptance

Validation is based on the open, receptive, non-judgemental, and accepting stance discussed in Chapter 7, which is largely conveyed by the tone of voice, listening carefully, and empathic and respectful responding. Such actions indicate that the therapist is taking the person seriously and encourages him/her to accept his/her experiences without questioning or second-guessing them. The expressive component of verbal responses also contributes to validation. Comments that match the patient's tone and rate of speech contribute to feeling understood, provided that they are not delivered in a stereotyped manner.

Validation promotes self-acceptance. Patients spend considerable time and energy trying to suppress or deny painful feelings and memories or wishing that distressing events had not happened. The therapist's acceptance and validation of these thoughts, feelings, and experiences allow the patient to accept them as well as increasing self-awareness and opening up the possibility of change.

10.2.2 Provide Meaning and Understanding

Patients also feel validated when they are helped to understand their problems and the reasons for their difficulties. As one patient noted, "The problem is I don't understand why I am such a mess. I don't seem to be able to do anything right, nothing works out, all my relationships are a mess and yet there is no reason for it. It is not as if I was abused as a child. My parents really looked after me. I don't know why it is; there must be something really wrong with me. I must be flawed." This kind of self-invalidating sentiment not only adds to demoralization but also impedes therapy because it leads to patients blaming themselves rather than trying to understand themselves. A brief explanation of the origins of the patient's problems reduced self-blame and allowed her to focus on managing her chaotic emotional life.

With other patients the confusion is more specific. For example, some patients blame themselves for not coping better because they dissociate or because their thinking becomes confused at times of stress. Here simple explanations of the nature and causes of dissociation or how intense emotions make it difficult to think clearly help to reduce distress sufficiently for patients to focus on how to handle the problem. Similarly, abused patients who blame themselves for what happened and for not "getting over it" are helped by an explanation of why trauma has a lasting impact. Such problems need to be explained in ways that are not overwhelming without undermining personal responsibility for dealing with them.

Dialectical behaviour therapy emphasizes a specific form of validation – helping the patient to recognize that their problem behaviours are the best way that they have found to cope given his or her life experiences.[3] The idea that therapists search for the adaptive significance of maladaptive behaviour and then communicate this understanding to their patients differs from the usual approach of viewing such behaviours as purely pathological. While not all behaviour is explicable in this way, this is a useful form of validation for behaviours that make adaptive sense. For example, patients who engage in deliberate self-injury in emotional crises are often relieved to learn that these behaviours are the best way they have found to terminate the intolerable nature of the "distress without resolution" that characterizes crises (see Chapter 4).

10.2.3   Distinguish Experiences from Causes and Consequences

Validation does not mean that the therapist agrees with the reasons patients give for their experiences or how they respond to these experiences: therapists should not validate ideas and actions that are invalid.[4] Faced with situations in which the patient's feelings seem to be based on a misinterpretation or maladaptive thinking, the best approach is to acknowledge and thereby validate the feeling but not its origins and consequences. This requires helping the patients to differentiate between feelings and the reasons for, and the conclusions drawn from, these feelings. Validation of the feeling makes it possible to discuss any misinterpretation that caused the feeling and any actions that the feeling caused. Attempts to deal with misinterpretations directly without validation often evoke anger and defensive responses. This is illustrated by the following vignette.

A patient in twice-weekly therapy arrived for a session furious with the therapist because she had attended for a regular session two days earlier and found the therapist's office closed. She was disappointed because there had been a dreadful scene with her parents who eventually asked her to leave home. Although distraught, she was reassured because she had an appointment and needed to discuss the event with the therapist. It was devastating to find the therapist was not there. It made her realize that the therapist, like everyone else, did not really care about her. Consequently, she wanted to end therapy.

At this point, the therapist has to decide how to proceed. The difficulty was that the therapist had actually cancelled the session several weeks earlier and had regularly reminded the patient of this in subsequent sessions. One approach would be to remind the patient of the facts. However, the patient was intensely distressed, which influenced her ability to think clearly. She was also sensitive to being blamed for things that she did not consider her fault, which stemmed from feeling that she was the family scapegoat who was blamed for everything that went wrong. She also considered her parents hypercritical and uncaring.

Since this was relatively early in therapy, the therapist decided to use a less direct route because the alliance was still tentative largely due to distrust and beliefs that no one cared about her. The situation was also complicated by the failure of a previous therapy and the patient was convinced that her previous therapist thought the failure was her fault. Consequently, the therapist decided to validate her feelings by noting how upsetting it must have been to find that he was not there. This led to further talk about leaving therapy because the therapist obviously did care about her. These feelings were further validated by the therapist commenting that "No one would want to be in therapy if they felt that the therapist did not care about them." And, added that this "would be really unfortunate because last session you told me that you were beginning to feel better."

With this approach, the anger began to dissipate. It was replaced by talk about the hurt and disappointment she felt when she discovered the therapist was like everyone else and did not care about her. Exploration and reflection of these themes led to a further reduction in distress and a more thoughtful attitude that enabled the therapist to address the fact that the patient had forgotten the session was cancelled. He noted that "It sounds that what happened with your parents was dreadful upsetting and left you devastated and overwhelmed." The patient agreed and reiterated how dreadfully she felt. The therapist noted that "It sounds that it made you so upset and that you were so desperate to see me that you forgot I had cancelled the appointment."

The patient reacted with surprise – "Oh!! I remember now!! I totally forgot. How could I do that, it was stupid of me." The therapist quickly intervened, "It seems that what happened with your mum and dad so upsetting that you couldn't think of anything else." "But it was stupid. I should have remembered." The therapist responded, "But doesn't it tell us just how painful these feelings are – they block everything else out. Everyone has difficulty remembering things when they are that hurt and upset." This led the patient to talk more about how she longed for her mother to love her. Eventually, the therapist returned to the patient's earlier comment that she wanted to end therapy. "Something else happened when you came to the office and found I was not here – you got so upset and angry that you decided that you wanted to stop seeing me." The patient commented, "I was so upset and disappointed. I thought that you did not care about me. I got mad and decided to hell with you, I am not going to see you again." Further discussion led to the patient deciding to continue in treatment.

The vignette illustrates the importance of validation in the change process: intense emotions need to be validated before problems can be explored and restructured. It also illustrates the importance of avoiding validating things that are invalid (in this case, the assumption the therapist was absent because he did not care about her) and actions based on the emotion that are also invalid (deciding to end treatment when progress is being made). The example also illustrates the earlier point that validation is an effective way to reduce emotional arousal. When the therapist validated the anger and disappointment, distress settled sufficiently for the patient to begin reflecting on events rather than simply emoting. Of course, work on this event did not end here. The incident indicated the intensity of the schema "no one cares" and how it caused the patient to jump to conclusions and prevented her from seeing the event in other ways. For example, it did not seem to cross her mind that even if the therapist had missed an appointment this could have been for other reasons than her assumption that he did not care about her. But this was all work for later in treatment.

10.2.4 Acknowledge Areas of Competence

The affirmation aspect of validation involves recognizing and supporting the patient's strengths and competencies (see also Chapter 8). This is especially useful with patients who are self-critical, those who are exposed to hypercritical caregivers, and those who have felt criticized previously by health care professionals. This approach seems to be most effective if areas of successful coping are not examined or explored in detail but rather accepted as achievements to build on.

10.2.5 Recognize Painful and Traumatic Events

Most patients need more than the opportunity to talk about their distress: they also need someone to recognize the painful things that have happened to them. The escalating distress seen in crises leads to an urgent need for someone to understand how terrible they feel and how painful their lives have been, and to validate the conviction that life has been unfair. For example, one patient with a long history of abuse spent most of one session protesting about the unfairness of life with increasing fervour and distress. She regained control and began processing the material when her therapist simply commented that, "everyone would agree that what happened to you was absolutely dreadful." Clinicians are often reluctant to simply acknowledge their patient's pain lest it exacerbate their distress. They also seem to feel the need to do something about it. However, as the example illustrates, affirmation of the patient's pain has a settling effect that reduces the need to convince others that they have a problem or that things are unfair. This is often sufficient to allow them to move forward.

10.2.6 Counteract Self-Invalidation

Consistent use of validating interventions helps to change the self-invalidating mode of thinking that is common among individuals with BPD by continually affirming the authenticity of the patient's experiences. The value of validation in changing the tendency to question or second-guess basic experiences is enhanced by helping the patient to recognize and later challenge his/her tendency to think in self-invalidating ways. Behaviour patterns such as self-invalidating thinking can be managed by using a specific event to draw attention to the behaviour and then encouraging the patient to identify other examples of the same behaviour in therapy and everyday life. Thus, an event such as the patient saying that she was upset and then wondering if she was really upset and then asking painfully "How do I know I am really upset?" is used to draw attention to this way of thinking with a comment such as "Have you noticed that you seem to think in ways that confuse yourself?" If the patient recognizes the pattern, he/she is then encouraged to identify other examples of self-invalidation such as doubting feelings, second-guessing decisions, questioning the genuineness of wants and desires, dismissing his/her own opinions as having no merit, deferring to the opinions of others, self-criticism, and trivializing his/her distress. Recognizing a pattern in this way draws things together and connects actions that were previously not seen to be related. Once the pattern is recognized, attention can be given to how this way of thinking undermines self-confidence and makes it difficult to establish goals and decide on courses of action. Subsequently, the patient's attention can be drawn to how his or her tendency to doubt the authenticity of his or her feelings contrasts with the therapist's acceptance of the patients experiences.

10.2.7 Reduce Self-Derogation

Self-blame and self-criticism are common examples of self-invalidating thinking that contribute to distress and low self-esteem. Given the pervasiveness of this thinking style, it is useful for therapists to develop a repertoire of interventions to validate actions that usually evoke a self-critical response. For example, "Of course you behaved in that way; what choice did you have? It was the only way you could survive as a child"; "It is not surprising that you avoid showing your feelings because you were criticized if you did"; "It is not surprising that you get angry and full of rage in these situations. They remind you of what happened in the past and no one helped you to talk about it." Such interventions help the patient to see that the behaviour is understandable and adaptive in the circumstances in which it developed, while also holding open the possibility of change.

On other occasions, patients can be helped to recognize how self-blame hinders self-understanding. Contrasting their own responses with those of the therapist, who seeks to understand rather than blame, often gives patients sufficient perspective to recognize how they maintain a continual commentary of self-criticism. One patient was helped to recognize the automatic nature of self-critical thoughts when the therapist punctuated a seemingly unstoppable barrage of self-criticism by commenting that, "There are two people in this room but only one is on your side, and it's not you." The patient recalled this event long afterwards as a point of change that not only helped her to recognize her self-blaming style but also to see the therapist as supportive and understanding.

10.2.8 Avoiding Invalidating Interventions

In the intensity of therapy, it is easy not only to miss opportunities to validate but also to inadvertently do things that are experienced as invalidating.

1. Common Invalidating Interventions Common therapist behaviours that invalidate include not listening and decreased attention; focusing prematurely on the positive ("You are only focusing on the bad, what about the good things in your life?"); minimizing ("It may not be as bad as you think"), dismissing, and criticizing experiences and actions; failing to take problems and feelings seriously; insisting that an interpretation is correct when the patient disagrees; interpreting disagreement as resistance; communicating unreasonable expectations of change; blaming patients for the therapist's own mistakes; not acknowledging mistakes or lapses of concentration; not recognizing areas of competence; providing inappropriate reassurance, thereby trivializing patients' concerns; failing to provide support; and inadvertently failing to show empathy. When dealing with events the patient finds invalidating, it is important to recognize that messages sent are not always messages received. What matters is not what the therapist intended by any intervention but rather how the patient perceived it.

2. Interpreting Normality as Pathology A common source of invalidation is the tendency to interpret normal experiences and all problems as pathological. Because clinicians inevitably focus on pathology, it is easy to overlook that fact that frustration, ambivalence, rationalization, and so on are normal reactions that need not be maladaptive. Interpreting normal reactions as pathological is confusing for patients who have difficulty understanding what is normal and healthy. A related problem is interpreting all the patient's problems as arising from personality psychopathology or from a single cause. Therapists with strong ideological views or one-dimensional ideas about the origins of BPD sometimes fall into the trap of attributing everything to a single cause such as sexual abuse, trauma, or substance abuse, which can create the impression that the therapist does not understand.

Although some patients like the clarity of a one-dimensional perspective, others feel invalidated, especially when they believe that the therapist has preconceived ideas that prevent him/her from seeing the patient as an individual. For example, a patient in therapy for self-mutilation also attended an addiction group. He complained bitterly that the group did not take his problems seriously because everything was attributed to alcoholism and other problems were ignored. Even real-life situational problems unrelated to his addiction problems were often interpreted as being due to the fact he was an alcoholic. Thus, it is important to keep in mind that patients with BPD also have problems that are not related to their disorder. Even when practical problems are consequences of the condition, their practical significance needs to be recognized.

3. Premature Closure of Important Themes Therapists are often tempted to close off expression of painful experiences too quickly by moving to factual issues or focusing on more positive matters, partly out of concern for the patient and partly because it is often painful to listen to these things. A thoughtful balance is needed between appropriate ventilation and excessive exploration to avoid the danger of emotions spiralling out of control.

10.2.9 Managing Validation Ruptures

Invalidation occurs in most treatments because patients' hypersensitivity to invalidation makes it easy for therapists to invalidate inadvertently. As with the therapeutic alliance, it is the patient's view of these events that matters. Validation failures are common causes of alliance ruptures and should be dealt with in the same way: note the change in the alliance and the failure of validation; draw the patient's attention to what happened; explore the reasons for it and the patient's feelings about the failure; validate the patient's responses; and acknowledge your contribution to the event.

10.3 Concluding Comments

As with the alliance and consistency, validation is not achieved through complex interventions but through multiple simple interventions and a therapeutic approach based on acceptance and affirmation. In this sense, validation is woven into the fabric of treatment. The goal of validation is to affirm the legitimacy of the patient's experiences, especially those experiences linked to basic emotions and needs that are so important for self-development. However, validation is not confined to affirming important aspects of the person but also with affirming the integrity of the patient as an autonomous individual. Again this is not achieved through any complex intervention but rather through a listening and reflective stance that conveys acceptance and respect by taking the patient's concerns seriously.

Notes

1. Many therapies for BPD including dialectical behaviour therapy (Linehan, 1993), mentalizing-based therapy (Bateman and Fonagy, 2004, 2006), and self psychology (Kohut, 1971, 1977) concur that accurate and sustained validation of feelings and experiences is an essential component of treatment.

2. Shenk and Fruzzetti (2011).

3. Linehan (1993).

4. Linehan (1993)

General Treatment Module 5: Self-Reflection

Increasing Self-Knowledge and Self-Reflection

Therapists of most persuasions seek to deepen patients' knowledge about themselves and their ability to reflect on this knowledge. Although the idea of "increasing self-knowledge" seems self-evident, we need to be clear about what is involved because patients often claim to be well aware of their problems. In a sense, this is often true: most patients do indeed have some awareness of their difficulties. However, the self-knowledge that matters is more than simple awareness: it is also recognition of significance of the problem coupled with emotional acceptance of that problem. Patients often recognize this distinction – they talk about knowing something but not really feeling it. But it is the feeling part that matters. As many theorists that noted, emotion is critical to understanding and changing experience and behaviour.[1]

Most of us have experienced a sudden realization about ourselves that causes us to think about ourselves a little differently – as if we suddenly connect the dots even though we have always been aware of the dots. This happened with Anna who suddenly realized that her tendency to agree to even the most unreasonable demands made by her extended family caused her to feel used and exhausted. She noted: "I have always known I am like this but I thought it was the right thing to do. I hadn't realized how agreeing to do whatever people ask causes me to neglect my own family and makes me feel depressed and a loser." This is the kind of self-knowledge we want to generate in therapy – the kind that catalyses change by changing how people think about themselves.

However, awareness and acceptance are not sufficient. Patients also need to reflect on their actions and experience if they are to change. The term "self-reflection" refers to the cognitive and metacognitive processes involved in reflecting on inner experience and understanding the mental states of self and others. Self-reflection is the capacity to think about, appraise, and evaluate one's mental processes and products. An important feature of human thinking is the reflexive loop built into the way we think: we not only are aware of our experience but are also able to think about this experience and our awareness of it. This ability to think about thinking allows us to manipulate our experiences and change their impact on us, and hence to self-regulate. This is why therapy relies heavily on stimulating patients' curiosity about their own minds and how they work.

The richness of self-knowledge and self-understanding ultimately depends on how open we are to new inputs and ideas. Unfortunately, openness is limited in borderline personality disorder (BPD): adversity leads to inflexibility – the tendency to interpret and respond to events in fixed ways – and to difficulty seeing different perspectives. There is a tendency to cling to old ways of thinking and acting and to be closed to new experiences and hence to change. To increase the self-knowledge and self-reflection needed for change requires that we re-establish the natural openness of the personality system. This requires a collaborative alliance and a trusting relationship.

11.1 Self-Knowledge

Increased self-knowledge is a prerequisite for change: we can only change things that we recognize as problems. Self-knowledge increases when patients become aware of aspects of behaviour and experience that were not recognized, denied, or suppressed and when they understand the meaning and significance of this knowledge. This requires increased self-observation and self-monitoring.

11.1.1 Increasing Self-Knowledge and Self-Understanding

Self-knowledge is increased by (i) using open-ended questions, (ii) focusing on inner mental processes and states, (iii) decomposing global experiences, and (iv) integrating self-knowledge through the use of summary statements and narratives.

11.1.1.1 Open-Ended Questions

Self-understanding increases when therapists use questions that require more than "yes," "no," or simple concrete responses to build the therapeutic dialogue. Such questions also facilitate reflective thinking. At the same time, simple verbal and non-verbal interventions and indications of support such as nods of agreement and requests to "tell me more" are used to "grease" the process. To be effective, this process also requires increased self-acceptance. As one patient noted: "I only began to know myself when I accepted myself for who I am." Self-acceptance is rare with BPD: most patients are in conflict with themselves as they continually struggle to suppress important aspects of their experience, hence the importance of validation.

11.1.1.2 Focus on Mental Processes

Patients need encouragement to attend to what is going on in their minds so that they begin to recognize that many of their problems arise from inner mental processes. This is a crucial step in the change process. Patients with BPD readily attribute their problems to other people so that their efforts are to get other people to change rather than to change themselves. Anna, for example, was initially convinced everything would be fine if her partner and family were more supportive.

This tendency to externalize responsibility for one's problems reflects a general cognitive bias in how we explain behaviour. We usually attribute the actions of others to their inner characteristics and our own behaviour to situational factors. Thus, a partner's anger may be explained by seeing him or her as angry and aggressive, whereas we tend to explain our own anger as an understandable response to how we were treated. This natural bias is exacerbated in patients with BPD, creating a strong tendency for them to see the causes of their behaviour as external to themselves. To modulate this bias, we need to help patients to focus not just on events and other people's actions but also on their own thoughts and feelings at the time.

11.1.1.3 Decompose Experience by Pursuing Details

Patients with BPD often think in an impressionistic way that leads them to describe things in a global and diffuse way that lacks sharp details – a way of thinking that blurs the emotional significance of events.[2] This is an avoidant way of thinking that hinders an in-depth understanding of mental processes. To build self-knowledge, we need to help patients to focus on the specifics of events and emotional reactions to them by asking for details about exactly what happened, when it happened, what was going on at the time, what was said and done, and what were the feelings evoked. These details often reveal the emotional significance of events and the process reduces emotional avoidance.

11.1.1.4 Provide Integrative Statements and Summaries

The final component of the descriptive process is summary statements that draw things together by linking and connecting components of the patient's descriptions so as to clarify and extend what is being discussed. The experience of patients with BPD tends to be fragmented and poorly integrated. Helping them to see links and patterns makes experience meaningful and reduces the panicky feelings that occur when things do not make sense. Summary statements are also part of the process of promoting more integrative personality functioning. Summaries differ in breadth and scope. Some are brief statements linking events, feelings, thoughts, and actions. Others are broader narratives that draw together different aspects of experience and behaviour around a common theme.

1. Creating Links within Descriptions Self-knowledge is built by establishing the temporal chains that link events, experiences, actions, and consequences. Most patients have difficulty linking events in this way. For example, they are often unaware of what triggers the emotional distress that leads them to deliberate self-harm. Nor do they pay much attention to the longer-term consequences of such actions. Analysing the scenarios patients describe in therapy provides the therapist with a tool to help them make sense of their experience. Emphasis is also placed on connecting feelings, cognitions, and behaviours because many patients have difficulty understanding how thoughts and feelings are con-nected, leading to discontinuities in subjective experience and a tendency for emotional arousal to lead rapidly to action without attention to either the thoughts that preceded the feelings or the consequences of the action.

2. Identifying Patterns and Themes A different form of summary helps the patient to recognize behavioural patterns and themes. A simple example is helping the patient to recognize that overdosing, cutting, binge-eating, alcohol misuse, and impulsive and risky sexual behaviour may all be forms of self-harm that are used to cope with emotional pain. Other summary statements draw attention to broad patterns such as the self-invalidating thinking discussed in the previous chapter or patterns of interpersonal behaviour. Drawing things together in these ways helps to integrate experience in a way that facilitates change. This is where traits such as anxiousness, insecure attachment, and submissiveness discussed in Chapter 3 are helpful. They alert the therapist to broad patterns that patients need to recognize.

3. Descriptive Re-framing Self-knowledge is also increased by re-framing the meaning attributed to experience. Re-framing changes the way events are perceived and alters their significance for the self. It also stimulates further exploration. Re-framing statements can be unsettling because they offer a new perspective. They range from simple reinterpretations of simple behaviours or specific events to more complex interpretations resulting from a lengthy exploration.

4. Constructing Narratives We are story-telling beings[3] who need and enjoy narratives about ourselves and our lives. Besides increasing self-knowledge by decomposing experi-ence and connecting events with emotions, thoughts, and action, patients need stories to explain what has happened to them and help them to function more adaptively. The formulation begins the process of helping patients to construct more adaptive narratives, which continues throughout treatment.

11.1.2 Promoting Self-Observation and Self-Monitoring

A consequence of collaborative efforts to increase self-knowledge is an improvement in the patient's capacity to self-monitor. Self-monitoring differs from self-awareness. Self-awareness occurs when attention is focused on an aspect of the self.[4] Patients are often self-aware but poor at monitoring themselves. Self-monitoring combines awareness with an evaluation of the experience. This evaluation establishes the reflective loop needed for self-regulation.[5] Self-monitoring is promoted by encouraging patients to reflect on their experiences in therapy and through specific training in mindfulness or attention control (see Chapter 16).[6] This is facilitated with comments such as: "You seem to be recognizing how you react"; "You seem to be finding it easier to recognize your patterns"; and "You seem to be able to stand back more and take a look at what is going on." Keeping a journal of experiences associated with everyday events also promotes self-monitoring if it is used to reflect on experiences rather than simply emote.

11.1.3 Managing Avoidance

Avoidance is common in BPD: suppression, distraction, diverting attention, and acting out are among the many behaviours used to limit self-understanding and avoid the fear, guilt, shame, or pain that is believed will result from acknowledging, thinking about, and revealing what is being avoided. Thus it is common for patients to say, "I don't want to think about that" or "I don't want to talk about that." However, in many instances, the avoidance is more automatic. For example, one patient usually talked about someone in her life, usually her partner, whenever a painful emotion was aroused in therapy. The diversion always maintained the same theme, giving the appearance that she was engaged in therapeutic work when she was really avoiding affect. If her attention was drawn to the avoidance, she acknowledged what she was doing but moments later resumed discussing how her partner acted in this way. Usually, her attention had to be drawn to the avoidance repeatedly to get her to focus on the avoided issue.

As therapy progresses, a consistent focus on avoidant behaviour and exploration of avoided material is usually necessary because the greatest change occurs when patients are exposed to the things that they avoid.[7] Avoidance and self-deception can be managed using the two-step process used with self-invalidation. Attention is drawn to the avoidance and the reasons for it such as anxiety about losing control of painful feelings or the consequences of dealing with the avoided issue are discussed.[8] The patient is then encouraged to identify other examples of emotional avoidance in everyday life.

Before drawing the patient's attention to the avoidance, it is important to consider the likely consequences of exploring the avoided or warded-off material in terms of the level of emotional arousal that is likely to ensue and whether this is likely to be destabilizing. Generally, it is better to use an emotion-regulating approach that allows patients to deal with the warded-off experience in bearable amounts.[9] This is achieved by noting the avoidance and inviting the patient to join the therapist in observing his or her own behaviour. For example, Anna strenuously avoided her anger towards her mother by jumping to another topic. When her emotions became more stable and her ability to self-regulate distress increased, the therapist drew her attention to this pattern by asking, "Have you noticed that whenever we begin to discuss your anger with your mother, you quickly jump to talking about something else?" This kind of intervention invites collaborative self-observation. It is easy then to follow up by asking about the worse aspects of the patient's fears, guilt, shame, pain, or whatever. With this approach emotional arousal is managed by switching from exploration to simply reflecting the feelings.

11.2 Self-Reflection

The capacity to reflect on the mental states of self and others is essential for self-regulation, to change maladaptive thoughts and feelings, and to construct a coherent sense of self. We continually reflect on, organize, and reorganize our experience to enhance our understanding of self and others and to create new ideas and new meanings. Hence, integrated modular treatment (IMT) seeks to help patients to function as much as possible in the self-reflective mode. This mode of thinking is impaired by intense emotions regardless of their causes. Such impairment limits awareness of the details of inner experience and leads to attention being focused primarily on the moment, leading to difficulty seeing one's current mental state in a broader context.

A confusing variety of terms are used to describe the processes in self-reflection such as mindfulness, mentalization, metacognitive processes, psychological mindedness, and aspects of empathy. All refer to related if not identical processes. In IMT, self-reflection is used as a general term to encompass these constructs. However, to avoid confusion, it may be helpful to consider briefly how self-reflection relates to these other terms.

11.2.1 Self-Reflection and Related Concepts

Self-reflection is similar to the traditional concept of psychological mindedness and to more recent elaborations of this construct such as mentalization. "Psychological mindedness" refers to the capacity to relate actions and problems to intra-psychic factors such as thoughts and feelings.[10] "Mentalizing" extends this idea: it refers to the capacity to understand the mental processes of self and others and to see behaviour as linked to intentions.[11] The term is related to an older social psychological idea that adaptive social behaviour requires the ability to "take the role of another" and hence see things from the perspective of another – an idea that patients readily grasp. "Metacognitive," like mentalization, was coined more recently to refer to processes involved in "thinking about thinking." Here, self-reflection is used to encompass these ideas because it is straightforward, is readily understood, and lacks the theoretical connotations of other terms. It involves thinking about all mental processes and seeking to understand the nature and origins of these processes, the links among them, and the reasons behind them.

This broad conceptualization of self-reflection also captures some of the concepts used by dialectical behaviour therapy[12] such as "reasonable mind," "emotional mind," and "wise mind." The former involves mental processes dominated by cognitive factors. The emotional mind occurs when thoughts and actions are primarily controlled by feelings. The goal is a "wise mind" state that integrates rational thinking and feelings. This is also a goal of IMT.

Self-reflection depends on many abilities related to mindfulness. Traditionally mindfulness has at least five components: (i) observation of inner experience, (ii) description and labelling of experience, (iii) the ability to engage in activities with awareness without being distracted, (iv) non-judgemental acceptance of experience, and (v) the ability to avoid simply reacting to experience by reflecting on it.[13] Effective self-reflective thinking requires all these abilities but also stresses the importance of understanding how mental processes organize behaviour and experience.

11.2.2 Increasing Self-Reflection

The self-reflective mode is encouraged throughout treatment through the use of a therapeutic style that conveys an interest in the nature and reasons for the patient's actions and experiences. This provides a model that patients can use to increase their capacity for self-reflection.

11.2.2.1 Explain Self-Reflection

At some point relatively early in treatment, or even when discussing the treatment contract, it is useful to explain that one of the most useful things that patients can do to help themselves to feel better is to become curious about their own minds and how they work. Most patients are open to the idea of becoming interested in their own mental processes and why they think, feel, and act as they do and intuitively understand the need to become interested in their own minds in order to change. Others, however, are less introspective and rarely think about what goes on in their minds. Interestingly, this does not seem to be closely related to overall intelligence. Some highly articulate individuals find it hard to focus on inner experience.

The important thing about self-reflection that patients need to understand is that by thinking about our experience of events we can change the meaning and significance that we attach to them and hence change the impact they have on us. This idea is useful when patients protest that there is little point in discussing past events because they cannot be changed.

11.2.2.2 Adopt a Reflective Questioning Style

Questions like "Why do you think you did/thought/felt that?" "What were you feeling at the time?" or "What makes you want to hurt yourself?" encourage patients to go beyond simply describing what happened to begin to think about the reasons behind their feelings and actions. This questioning style should also be used to promote a focus on the mental states of others. Questions such as "why do you think they did that?" "What do you think they were feeling at the time?" or "Do you think they saw things differently from you?" divert attention from the details of what the other people did to thinking about why they did it, and what may have been going through the person's mind at the time.

11.2.2.3 Model Self-Reflection

Patients learn much from watching and imitating how therapists handle situations. For example, problem-solving skills are learned by noting how the therapist examines problems. Similarly, we can model the importance of reflecting on events. For example, if the patient reacts as if he/she thinks the therapist has not understood something, the therapist may comment that "I seem to have missed something" or "It seems that I have not understood what you were saying." Such comments indicate the therapist actively thinks about what the patient says. Or, the therapist may comment about a previous session by saying that "I was thinking about what you told me last week" and then explain these reflections. Such comments not only model reflective thinking but also show that the therapist takes the patient's comments seriously enough to think about them between sessions.

11.2.2.4 Generate Alternative Perspectives

Self-reflection is limited by the cognitive rigidity noted in Chapter 4. Patients tend to assume that their interpretations of events are the only possible interpretations and fail to recognize that their interpretation is one of many alternatives. Questions like "Is there another way to look at that?" or "Was there anything else you could have done?" (or, better still "Was there anything else *we* could have done?") open their minds to other possibilities and foster the capacity to generate multiple perspectives, a necessary ingredient of effective problem-solving.

Since patients tend to cling to their traditional ways of seeing things, the therapist's efforts to build greater flexibility are often experienced as threatening, leading to categorical statements that affirm that "There is no other way to see it." This tendency can sometimes be circumvented by encouraging the patient to "play" with the idea of alternatives.

11.3 Concluding Comments

Probably the most important thing we can do after building a good relationship with our patients is to encourage them to become more aware of themselves and to reflect on their mental states and behaviour. It is this process that catalyses change. Self-reflection is not usually something built quickly or easily and it usually requires persistent efforts to ensure that it becomes consolidated as the dominant mode of thought. In the early stages of therapy, intense emotions tend to hinder the self-reflective mode and it is only when distress begins to settle that it becomes more established. It also takes time to encourage patients to question their habitual ways of interpreting events and not to take things at face value but rather to question the way they and others do the things they do.

Notes

1. The importance of appropriate levels of emotional arousal for therapeutic change was initially described by Frank (1963) in his seminal work on persuasion and healing. Subsequently, the idea has been adopted and developed by many authors (see for example, Greenberg and Paivio, 1997).

2. Shapiro (1965).

3. Stanghellini and Rosfort (2013)

4. Wicklund and Duval (1971), Wicklund (1975).

5. Carver and Scheier (1998).

6. Linehan (1993), Teasdale et al. (1995).

7. Beutler and Harwood (2000).

8. This approach essentially makes use of classical psychodynamic interpretations of defences as described by Ezriel (1952) and Malan (1979) without adopting the underlying theoretical model.

9. McCullough Vaillant (1997).

10. Appelbaum (1973) defines "psychological mindedness" as the "ability to see relationships among thoughts, feelings, and actions, with the goal of learning the meanings and causes of ... experiences and behaviour" (p. 36). See also McCallum and Piper (1997).

11. Bateman and Fonagy (2006).

12. Linehan (1993).

13. Baer et al. (2006).

12

General Treatment Module 6: Motivation

Motivating for Change

Motivation for change predicts outcome. Unfortunately, motivation varies considerably in patients with borderline personality disorder (BPD), and many are not highly committed to therapeutic work at least in the early stages of therapy, which leads to poor compliance and high treatment dropout. Motivation is undermined by passivity and demoralization, expectations that someone or something will provide solutions, and a desire to use therapy only as a source of support. Motivation can also be impeded by external factors such as friendships and relationships. For example, significant others who have become accustomed to how the patient behaves may react adversely to attempts to behave differently, especially when these changes affect a status quo that they find comfortable.

Consequently, ambivalence about treatment is common: many patients want help but worry about the process, are doubtful about its potential benefits, and are concerned about the effort required. This means that motivation for change cannot be a prerequisite for treatment. Instead, therapists need to become skilled in building motivation: studies show that effective therapists are good at motivating their patients.[1] Readiness to change is not static: it fluctuates according to the effort involved and the level of distress that is anticipated to result from working on a problem. Motivation also depends of the focus of change: it is common for patients to be highly motivated to improve emotional stability but not to work on interpersonal problems or consequences of abuse because of the fears and shame involved. Although poor motivation is a serious problem, there is little research on how best to motivate patients with BPD, forcing us to draw on studies involving other disorders and the general literature on building motivation such as motivational interviewing[2] to identify useful methods.

12.1 Strategies for Building Motivation

Motivation is influenced by other generic interventions. It is closely related to the quality of patient–therapist bond and hence the alliance should be reviewed whenever motivational problems arise. Validation and empathy also help to create a context conducive to a commitment to change. As with other generic interventions, no single intervention dramatically increases motivation. Instead, a commitment to change is built through repeated use of diverse strategies.

12.1.1 Goal-Focused Approach

Outcome is better when treatment is based on goals.[3] The emphasis that cognitive therapies place on goal setting may explain why they have lower premature termination than psychodynamic therapy: patients are more motivated when their goals and concerns are addressed early in treatment. This is why treatment goals and what the patient wants from therapy should be discussed early in the assessment and contracting sessions.

Motivation is also increased by goal attainment. Ideally, we need successes early in treatment to build motivation and consolidate therapist and treatment credibility. Unfortunately, many patient goals are broad and require considerable work to achieve such as discontinuing self-injurious behaviour or establishing emotional stability. This is one reason why many patients find the prospect of change daunting. The solution is to decompose major goals into more easily achieved sub-goals.

12.1.1.1   Focus on Small Steps

Focusing on modest goals increases the probability of success. Implementation requires that the patient learns to analyse problems and decompose broad goals into specific tasks. For example, work towards the goal of stopping deliberate self-injury may begin by helping the patient to find ways to delay acting on the urge to self-injure for a short time and progressively increasing this interval until the patient manages to abort some episodes. Subsequently, the immediate goal would change to aborting some episodes, and so on.

A focus on small steps encourages therapists to view treatment as an incremental process. Treating BPD is not like pottery where a lump of clay is rapidly shaped into a pot or vase. Instead, the therapist is more like a sculptor, faced with a block of marble equipped with a small hammer and chisel. With each hammer blow, the flake that is chipped off is so small that progress is difficult to see. It is only over time that the sculptor is aware that the mound of chips has grown and the marble is beginning to take shape.

12.1.1.2   Reinforce Achievements and Support Self-Efficacy

Any progress towards attaining a sub-goal should be used to reinforce motivation, strengthen the alliance, and promote self-efficacy. Thus if a patient who is trying to delay self-injury manages to resist the urge for, say, five minutes, this is considered a success. The change is noted and used to promote the idea that change is possible.

With these small steps, the goal is to help patients to "own" the change process and to begin reinforcing themselves when their efforts are successful. The means that therapists should avoid being seen by the patient as a source of reinforcement or as acknowledging the patient's success in a way the patient considers condescending or patronizing. Consider this example. A clinician had been working with a patient on managing crises without deliberately injuring herself. Together, they agreed that she would try to go to the emergency room to talk to the clinician before she self-injured. On one occasion she managed to do this. Despite being very distressed, she arrived at the emergency room without harming herself. When discussing the event with the patient, the clinician said, "I am pleased you were able to come before you harmed yourself." He was surprised when she exploded in anger accusing him of being condescending and not understanding how dreadful she felt.

The clinician made several mistakes: he used language that seemed patronizing to the patient; he made himself the agent of reinforcement; and he used the personal pronoun "I," which emphasized that he was the source of reinforcement and made him, not the patient, the focus of his remarks. He also failed to validate the patient's distress. It would have been better if the clinician noted that "despite being very upset you were able to do what we talked about last session and come to see me before you hurt yourself." This could then be discussed in detail to understand how the patient was able to control the distress followed by a discussion of the event itself and the feelings involved. During this discussion, the patient could have been helped to recognize that "the feelings may not be as powerful as you thought" and that "there are things you can do to control them."

12.1.2 Maintain a Focus on Change

It is not sufficient to establish goals. Progress towards attaining them also needs to be monitored because a consistent focus on change predicts positive outcomes.[4]

12.1.2.1 Elicit a Commitment to Change

The change process begins by eliciting a commitment to work on making changes. It should not be assumed that patients necessarily want to change even if it involves obviously harmful behaviours such as deliberate self-injury. In fact, some patients are reluctant to stop hurting themselves because it reduces their distress. For them, the benefits of immediate distress relief outweigh the long-term consequences. Enquiring about whether the patient wants to change a specific behaviour involves the patient in the change process and makes change something the patient wants as opposed to something expected by the therapist. This builds motivation because people work harder to achieve goals they set for themselves. The process also makes the patient the author of any subsequent change.

12.1.2.2 Review Progress

Once elicited, this commitment needs to be monitored and progress reviewed regularly with the patient. These reviews remind patients of their goals and that therapy is about making changes. They also highlight the therapist's commitment to work on achieving the patient's goals. These reviews are essentially discussions about whether the patient thinks that the patient–therapist "team" is making progress. In effect, the therapist asks "How do you think we are doing in helping you get what you want out of therapy?" "Do you think we are making progress and is there anything else you think we should be doing?"

12.1.2.3 Balance Change, Support, and Validation

A focus on change with regular reviews of progress may appear inconsistent with the emphasis placed on validation.[5] A change-focus implies the patient has problems that need to be addressed whereas validation implies acceptance of the patient and recognition that the patient is doing his or her best. The apparent paradox is managed by embedding the focus on change within a non-judgemental, respectful, and affirming relationship. This means that a change-focus cannot afford to neglect the relationship and that progress reviews should be done in a collaborative way that enhances the alliance and avoids suggesting that any lack of progress is the patient's fault.

12.1.3 Encourage Talk about Change

Talking about change increases the likelihood of actual attempts to implement change.[6] Encouraging patients to "talk the walk" increases the chances that they will "walk the talk." We need to encourage talk about the changes they would like to make, and the effect these changes would have on themselves, their lives, and how they are treated by others. Also, any spontaneous comments about the need to change need to be reflected and reinforced.

Given patient ambivalence and high early dropout, talk about change should begin during assessment and continue throughout treatment. An encouraging sign is for change talk to increase during the early sessions. Talking about the desire or need to change is especially helpful when patients are ambivalent about change: it helps to tip the balance in the direction of change. It is less effective when there is more categorical resistance to change as when a patient refuses to stop an addiction or self-harming behaviour. Here change talk is incompatible with the patient's current position and any attempt by the therapist to discuss changing this behaviour puts the therapist in a polarized position, which is rarely helpful.

12.1.3.1 Characteristics of Effective Talk about Change

Talk about change is more likely to lead to actual change if directed towards specific problems. Patients often talk generally about the need to change – about how everything is wrong with their lives and that they need to change everything. Such general statements are not particularly helpful because they are difficult to translate into action. Patients who talk about change in this way need to be guided to focus on specific things they want to change such as structuring their day, improving sleep patterns, reducing deliberate self-injury, eating more healthily, managing their emotions better, and so on.

It also helps if talk about the need to change is in the present tense. Often, the need to change is projected into the future – "I will have to do this sometime," or "I hope to get round to dealing with it soon" – or into the past – "Cutting myself has caused a lot of problems in the past." Such statements distance the patient from the change process. They need to be rephrased to refer to the need to change now and extended to a discussion of how the behaviour in question causes problems in the present.

12.1.3.2 Preparatory and Mobilizing Talk

Developments in motivational interviewing[7] have identified two kinds of talk about change: (i) preparatory statements that indicate the patient is contemplating change and (ii) statements that indicate actual mobilization for change.

Preparatory statements include (i) desire to change ("I wish I could stop hurting myself" or "I want a better life"); (ii) ability and intent to change ("I think I can do this"); (iii) benefits of change ("My life would be much better if I did this," or "People wouldn't look down on me so much if I stopped this"); and (iv) need to change ("I can't keep doing this, it's getting serious"). Patients can be encouraged to elaborate on these statements by listing the reasons why change would be useful and how to begin making changes. Again this encourages patients to assume responsibility for change and to begin mobilizing the intent to change.

Preparatory statements are useful in building motivation. Therapists need to learn to spot them and reflect them in ways that encourage the patient to elaborate on their intent. However, they are not as useful as mobilizing statements that indicate an active intent to change, for example, "I am going to ..." and "I will do ... " Such statements need to be reinforced by eliciting details. For example, a patient commented that she was feeling lethargic and needed to exercise more and that she had decided to go to a gym. The therapist asked when she intended to go. She said later that day. The therapist expressed interest and asked what time she planned to go. This was followed up in the next session.

12.1.4 Increase Discontent, Build Hope

Discontent is a powerful motivator.[8] Most of us only contemplate making changes when we are discontented with ourselves or our situation. If we are contented with the way things are, there is little incentive to change. Discontent is often triggered by a specific incident that suddenly changes how we see ourselves and our situation. Such sudden shifts have been referred as the "crystallization of discontent."[9] These shifts galvanize us to take action especially when accompanied by emotional distress. For example, many years ago a woman told me she suddenly decided to end a relationship when at the end of a stressful day she decided to seek the comfort of a warm bath only to sit on fragments of toenail left when her partner cut his nails in the bathtub. Of course, the toenails did not cause her to end the relationship. They were simply the catalyst – the straw that broke the camel's back – that crystallized her growing discontent with the relationship.

The crystallization of discontent can be used in therapy when a specific incident causes the patient to stop and think about him-/herself and what he/she is doing. With one patient, this happened following a fight with her drug-abusing, video game-addicted boyfriend. As she stormed out of their apartment, she suddenly thought, "I have got to stop doing this – I've got to change my life." In the moment, she decided to stop socializing with people with addiction problems and to get help for her mood problems.

Such events have a radical impact when they occur. Unfortunately, they are relatively rare. However, we can "crystalize discontent" by exploring the discrepancy between the way the patient is and the way he or she would like to be.[10] For example, motivation to stop engaging in deliberate self-harm can sometimes be increased by discussing how other people react to this behaviour. Discontent needs to be increased sufficiently to mobilize a commitment to change but not to the extent that it causes despair or self-criticism. However, discontent alone is often not sufficient – it is also necessary to build the hope that change is possible. Without hope of success, there is little point in making the effort to change.

12.1.5 Create Options

The idea of change can be aversive when the patient cannot see that there are alternatives and that he or she is free to choose alternative paths – an aspect of the rigidity that characterizes BPD. Earlier, creating options was discussed as a way to increase self-knowledge. It also builds motivation. This requires teaching patients to examine problems from different perspectives.

12.1.6 Encourage Persistence

Maintenance of the commitment to change offer requires therapists to encourage patience and persistence. These are needed not because patients give up too easily but because they often believe that progress should be rapid and berate themselves for not progressing quickly enough once a problem is recognized. At this point, it is often useful to introduce information on the stability of personality and the way developmental experiences result in habitual ways of thinking and acting to help patients to accept that change takes time to implement.

12.1.7 Managing Motivation Problems

Obstacles to change range from outright opposition to treatment to avoidance of change and a desire to maintain the status quo. Attempts to maintain the status quo are commonly due to a fear of failing and fear that change may adversely affect relationships with significant others. For example, submissive individuals are often reluctant to be even modestly assertive lest others get angry with them.

12.1.7.1 Manage Resistance

Resistance to change may be passive or active. Passive opposition is usually linked to salient aspects of the patient's psychopathology. Strong oppositional tendencies, for example, can lead to poor compliance as part of a general tendency to reject ideas and suggestions emanating from others. This kind of resistance is often linked to the pseudo-compliant alliance discussed in Chapter 8 in which the patient readily agrees to various courses of action but somehow never manages to follow through. Narcissistic tendencies may also impede motivation if the patient feels that the therapist does not recognize how special the patient is or considers him-/herself to be so special that the therapist couldn't possibly understand him/her. More active resistance to treatment often occurs as a result of previous negative experiences in therapy or with other mental health professionals.

Motivation problems are best dealt with by offering support when patients feel stuck, recognizing and thereby validating both the difficulty of changing and fears about change, and by encouraging a discussion of options available. More confrontational methods do not work: little comes from directly challenging resistance to change. It is better to work on understanding the resistance and on talking about what patients really care about and what they want for their lives. One patient was feeling so stuck that she decided to end treatment. This changed when the therapist asked about what effect she thought this would have. This caused her to think about the impact her problems were having on her son. She was determined to ensure he had a better chance than she had and hence decided to stay in therapy for his sake. Gradually, this changed to wanting to stay in therapy because she also wanted a better life for herself.

12.1.7.2 Manage Personal Reactions to Motivation Problems

Motivation problems contribute to the difficulties many therapists experience when treating BPD. Ambivalence about therapy, low motivation, and relatively slow progress contribute to practitioner burnout. Hence an important part of managing motivation problems is managing the counter-transference problems they create. Several factors help with this process. Difficulties increase when clinicians begin to see patients as "not helping themselves" and as being almost wilfully unmotivated. Such perceptions negatively impact the therapeutic relationship and polarize the patient and the therapist. It is especially important to avoid getting into a polarized position in which the therapist directly or indirectly advocates for change and the patient adopts the opposite stance. Polarization is increased by the use of terms like "resistance" and "denial." Although these terms are part of the language of psychotherapy, they contribute to the therapist adopting a more challenging and confrontational stance that tends to shut things down further. A more open-minded and accepting approach is needed that assumes there are good reasons why the patient is not motivated and that these reasons need to be explored and understood. It also helps if therapists see motivation problems not primarily as hindrances that need to be removed but rather as expressions of borderline pathology or patient concerns that are important targets for change.

Finally, personal reactions to low motivation are also reduced by recalling that the therapist's function is to serve as a consultant who makes his or her expertise available to the patient and that the responsibility for change lies with the patient. Stress increases when therapists assume responsibility for change and then feel frustrated by lack of progress. These concerns are often projected onto the patient leading to a further deterioration in the alliance. The result is often a stalemate in which the patient resists the therapist's push for change.

12.1.7.3 Validate Difficulties in Making Changes

When patients feel frustrated by being stuck, they often blame themselves for lack of progress. This causes their focus to switch from struggling to make changes to berating themselves. At these times, it is important that therapists do not allow any frustration that they may feel about lack of progress to draw them into inadvertently colluding with the self-blame rather than validating just how difficult it is to change long-standing behaviours.

One of the things that clinicians often fail to take into account is just how exhausting it is to struggle to control intense emotions. Research suggests that the effort to exert self-control is tiring.[11] If you have to force yourself to do something, you are less likely to be able to exert self-control if another challenge comes along. The capacity to exert self-control gets depleted. Something like this must occur with BPD. Patients expend considerable resources attempting to control emotions and manage conflict, leaving few resources to be motivated to try anything else. Thus if the urge to self-harm occurs there are few resources left to resist. We need to recognize this phenomenon when treating these patients and use it to help them understand why motivation often fails and why they lack the ability to resist their urges. This sort of psychoeducation increases self-acceptance and self-compassion, which reduces time and energy spent on self-criticism and therefore helps to free up the resources needed to build motivation.

12.1.7.4 Identify Incentives for Not Changing

An important therapist task is to help patients understand reasons for being unable or not wanting to change.[12] This reduces the frustration and self-criticism that often accompany difficulties in implementing change and re-focuses attention to dealing with obstacles to change. Recognition of the incentives for not changing is also facilitated by encouraging patients to examine the costs and benefits of change versus not changing, something most patients rarely consider. Occasionally, the benefits of maladaptive actions such as self-injury are recognized because they reduce distress, but with other behaviours, the benefits derived from the action are rarely recognized. Instead, the behaviour may be viewed as unavoidable or inexplicable. However, many maladaptive behaviours benefit the patient in ways that are not always apparent. For example, deliberate self-injury not only reduces distress but also gratifies needs for care and attention and even for stimulation and excitement.

Encouraging patients to compile a list of benefits and costs of staying the same may tip the balance towards change. For example, one patient who adamantly maintained that she did not see the benefits of stopping cutting herself because it helped her to feel better and the cuts quickly healed changed her stance after a discussion of the costs involved forced her to recognize how her behaviour caused her friends to distance themselves from her, which made her feel ashamed. Another example is provided by the earlier discussion of the patient who suddenly recognized that she was a people pleaser who always gave in to the demands of others. Previously, she had thought of this as a desirable feature that made her feel needed and wanted. Suddenly, she realized it also made her feel exhausted and a loser because she had little time for her own family. Subsequently, this was used as the basis of a cost–benefit analysis that deepened her understanding of the costs involved that led her to conclude that the costs outweighed the benefits and that there were better ways to satisfy her need to care for others.

12.1.7.5 Manage Ambivalence

A common obstacle to treatment is the patient's ambivalence about change. Change is recognized as desirable but also evokes fear and even resentment, which occurs when patients feel that although their problems are caused by others they are the ones who have to change. Change therefore represents an approach-avoidance conflict.[13] Such conflicts are the most difficult to resolve. This is the same kind of conflict as the core interpersonal conflict of neediness versus fear of rejection. This conflict often contributes to ambivalence about change when the changes contemplated are interpersonal and hence activate the core conflict.

The first step in managing ambivalence is to help the patient understand it because patients usually have difficulty recognizing their concerns. They feel frustrated, irritable, uncertain about treatment, and stuck. The danger is they act out these frustrations in ways that threaten therapy. This danger is reduced by helping them to recognize the conflict. This can then be followed by an exploration of the costs and benefits of change. In the course of this discussion, opportunities usually arise to change the relative strengths of the positive and negative aspects of change. The strength of the positive side can be increased by reviewing the benefits of change and stimulating the patient's desire to relinquish old patterns. Similarly, the strength of the negative aspects of the conflict can be reduced by exploring the fear of change and restructuring these concerns. When these fears involve concerns about how significant others are likely to react, it may be helpful to arrange a few conjoint sessions to talk about the issue.

12.2 Concluding Comments

Motivating patients for therapy and change is one of the greatest challenges in treating BPD. Little seems to be achieved in treatment without a good relationship and a motivated patient. Unfortunately, the problem has received little research attention and it is largely neglected by contemporary therapies despite some outcome studies having dropouts of up to 50 per cent of patients who were intended to receive treatment. In this chapter, I have tried to draw together some ideas that are useful in promoting a commitment to change and retaining patients in therapy. However, it is also clear that we are still a long way from resolving the problem and many methods that seem to be effective with other disorders are less effective with BPD.

Notes

1. Meichenbaum and Turk (1987).

2. Miller and Rollnick (2002, 2013), Rosengren (2009)

3. See Critchfield and Benjamin (2006) for an overview of factors contributing to positive outcomes. Goal setting also tends to increase the treatment alliance (Persons and Bertagnolli, 1994).

4. Critchfield and Benjamin (2006).

5. See Linehan (1993) for a discussion on the importance of balancing validation with a focus on change. The latter implies that what the patient has been doing is inappropriate, which may be experienced as invalidating. Dialectical behaviour therapy addresses this problem by encouraging therapists to maintain a "dialectical balance" between validating the patient's experiences and teaching appropriate skills required for change.

6. See research on motivational interviewing: Amrhein et al. (2003, 2004), Rosengren (2009).

7. Amrhein et al. (2003, 2004), Rosengren (2009).

8. Baumeister (1991, 1994).

9. Baumeister (1991).

10. Miller and Rollnick (1991).

11. Research suggests the resources used for self-regulation can become depleted with successive attempts at self-regulation (see Baumeister and Heatherton, 1996; Kahneman, 2011; Muraven and Baumeister, 2000; Wagner and Heatherton, 2011). Given the self-control demands that patients with BPD experience in both the emotion and interpersonal realms, it seems very likely that the self-regulation resources are constantly being depleted, leaving little for other self-regulatory tasks.

12. Based on distinction made in motivational interviewing; see Miller and Rollnick (2002, 2013), Miller et al. (2006).

13. Miller and Rollnick (1991) suggested that conflicts between wanting to change and fear of change may be managed using Lewin's (1935) classic analysis of conflict. Lewin suggested that conflicts fall into three types. Approach-approach conflict occurs when the individual is faced with two desirable goals but only one can be achieved. For example, one could be faced with two pleasant options about how to spend the weekend. Such conflicts are usually easily resolved. Avoidance-avoidance conflicts present a slightly greater problem in that the individual is faced with two negative goals and is forced to choose between them. Approach-avoidance conflict occurs when the goal facing the individual has both positive and negative features. These conflicts are the most difficult to resolve and classically lead to ambivalence.

Introduction

Having described the core modules, we can now begin to consider their use in treating the different domains of impairment and how they can be supplemented with specific modules. Specific intervention modules will be described in the typical sequence that they are used when treatment starts with the patient in a crisis state and proceeds to longer-term therapy.

Previous chapters suggested that treatment progresses through five phases: safety, containment, regulation and modulation, exploration and change, and integration and synthesis. It is convenient to consider the safety and containment phases together because these are essentially components of crisis management. Treatment typically begins by evaluating suicidality followed by steps to ensure the patient's safety. This is quickly followed by interventions to settle and contain emotional distress and resolve the crisis. The primary treatment goals for this phase of treatment are as follows:

1. Ensure the safety of the patient and others.
2. Contain and settle emotional crises and reactivity.
3. Reduce the frequency of crises and the escalation of psychopathology.
4. Engage the patient in treatment and form the foundation for longer-term treatment.

It is useful to keep engagement in mind to ensure that all opportunities are used to promote the treatment relationship and build motivation.

Chapter 13

Managing Crises and Containing Emotions and Suicidality

Since most treatments begin with a crisis presentation and crises are common in the early stages of most treatments, therapists need to be skilled in managing crises and reducing their occurrence. This requires an understanding of crisis behaviour, the events that trigger crises, and how crises typically unfold.

13.1 Understanding Crises

13.1.1 Crisis Behaviour

Crises are characterized by emotional states that typically involve relatively undifferentiated emotional distress that escalates into a state of distress without resolution (see Chapter 4) which continues until it culminates in an urgent need to terminate the distress, which often results in deliberate self-injury. Escalation occurs because intense emotions overwhelm the cognitive mechanisms that regulate emotions and because maladaptive thoughts increase emotional arousal. Intense emotional arousal also impairs logical thinking, information processing, and problem-solving, making it difficult for patients to follow verbal interventions, instructions, or explanations. Consequently, interventions need to be kept simple and attempts should be made to align with the patient's distress and reflect an understanding of how the patient is feeling rather than attempting to confront the distress or address more complex matters. Unfortunately, the impact of intense emotions on thinking and information processing is not always recognized by those professionals who deal with these patients in crises.

As cognitive processes become more disorganized, other phenomena emerge such as transient psychotic symptoms and dissociative behaviour. Perceptual-cognitive symptoms occur in about 75 per cent of patients with borderline personality disorder (BPD). These usually take the form of quasi-psychotic symptoms such as pseudo-hallucinations, illusions, and ideas of reference, which include suspiciousness and mild paranoid ideation. Dissociative behaviour is also common, ranging from mild feelings of depersonalization and derealization to more pervasive dissociative episodes that may include decreased responsiveness. Impaired emotional control and thinking also contribute to behavioural disorganization. Besides the sense of urgency that leads to deliberate self-harm, coping skills become increasingly impaired, leading to regressive behaviour that sometimes progresses to the point that the individual cannot manage the routine tasks of everyday living. This occurred with Anna who sometimes took to her bed for several days because she felt overwhelmed and unable to cope.

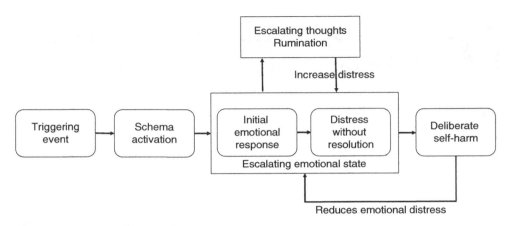

Figure 13.1 Sequence of Events in Crisis States

13.1.2 The Crisis Sequence

Crises are typically triggered by interpersonal events that evoke feelings of rejection and abandonment. These schemas initiate an escalating dysphoric state that leads to various emotional, cognitive, and behavioural consequences[1] (Figure 13.1). Although many triggering events occur outside therapy, they can result from within-therapy events such as the therapist cancelling appointments with inadequate notice, poorly timed discussion of trauma, or the patient feeling criticized or judged.

Healthy individuals who are distressed by negative events usually have a repertoire of coping strategies to manage their feelings. They may distract themselves, soothe themselves by doing something enjoyable, or try to solve the problem. Such options are not readily available to patients with BPD. Their emotional reactions are more intense and they lack self-soothing and self-regulating skills. To make matters worse, many patients also react to emotional distress in ways that make matters worse. They ruminate about what has happened or engage in self-talk that increases their distress: "This is not right, I should not have these feelings – there must be something wrong with me," "If these feelings don't stop I will have to kill myself," or "It's not fair that this is happening to me."

13.1.3 Crises, Deliberate Self-Harm, and Suicidality

Deliberate self-injury and suicidality are common with BPD: 60 to 80 per cent of patients report significant suicidality and between 40 and 90 per cent engage in deliberate self-injurious behaviour.[2] Deliberate self-harm is linked to severity of BPD and the occurrence of other disorders[3] such as eating, depressive, and schizotypal disorders. Those who self-harm are also likely to report more depersonalization and delusions and be more paranoid, hyper-vigilant, and resentful than those who do not.[4] They are also younger, make more suicidal threats and attempts, and have more serious suicidal ideation.[5] Although deliberate self-injury is associated with sexual abuse and dissociative behaviour,[6] deliberate self-harm and dissociation do not necessarily indicate a history of sexual abuse: they also occur in patients who have not been abused. Suicide risk is high in patients with BPD: about 10 per cent of patients take their own lives.[7] The average age of suicide is approximately

37 years although there is wide variation across cases[8] and there is some evidence that there is also a peak among patients in their early 20s. Risk is increased when treatment is terminated under difficult conditions and reduced when patients are in regular outpatient treatment and agree to follow up,[9] pointing to the value of long-term support.

13.2 Ensuring Safety: Strategies for Managing Acute Crises

The first step in managing any crisis is to ensure safety. This requires an evaluation of suicide risk and the patient's ability to manage self-harming impulses without external interventions.[10]

13.2.1.1 Assessing Suicidality

When assessing suicidality, it is helpful to distinguish between (i) deliberate self-injurious behaviour, (ii) chronic suicidal ideation, (iii) acute suicidal state, and (iv) acute-on-chronic suicidality. These states are often confused by patients, families, support groups, and even health care professionals. Although it is sometimes difficult to make these distinctions during a crisis, they are useful because these conditions are managed differently. Deliberate self-harm and chronic suicidal ideation are persistent features of BPD, which are managed as part of ongoing treatment. Acute suicidal states are different and may require additional interventions and possibly a brief hospital admission.

Most instances of deliberate self-injury are usually attempts to self-manage distress rather than suicide attempts. Patients usually understand this and many emphasize that their self-harm was not a suicide attempt but occurred because they felt desperate and could not think of another way to end their distress. Nevertheless, patients often use the word "suicide" to describe their actions to ensure that others take their distress seriously. Although most instances of deliberate self-injury are readily differentiated from suicidal behaviour, this does not mean that they should not be taken seriously. The risk of a fatal consequence from deliberate self-harm increases with the number of instances probably because these actions can have unintended consequences.

Chronic suicidal ideation is common: patients frequently think and talk about killing themselves and often say things like: "If things don't get better, I can always kill myself" or "If things are not better by the end of year (or some other date) I will end it all." This way of thinking becomes a way of life – an ingrained response to distress that reduces motivation and hinders treatment because the patient feels that there is little point in making the effort to change – "why bother, I am going to kill myself anyway." This needs to be addressed in therapy, and it is important that suicidality is not allowed to control the treatment. However, chronic suicidal ideation is remarkably persistent and often continues long after deliberate self-injurious behaviour has remitted.

The main difficulty in assessing suicide risk is in differentiating chronic suicidal ideation from acute suicidal intent. The frequency and chronicity of these thoughts can cause clinicians to overlook situations when acute stressors increase suicide risk in patients with chronic suicidal ideation. This is the acute-on-chronic situation.[11] Establishing acute risk is difficult because it is not possible to predict which patients are most at risk of suicide. Research suggests that risk is increased by a history of previous suicide attempts, past major depressive episodes, substance use disorders, antisocial behaviour, and history of sexual abuse. However, these factors are not very helpful when evaluating risk in a specific patient in a crisis situation. More useful are factors such as increased severity of a comorbid condition especially a major depressive episode and substance use disorder that increase acute-on-chronic risk. Other important risk factors are a recent discharge from a psychiatric inpatient service and recent negative life events such as loss of immediate family support, legal problems, or problems in the treatment relationship.[12]

Nevertheless, it is difficult to identify which patients are at greatest risk except in the most general terms. This means that the evaluation of current risk for a given patient is essentially a clinical judgement based on current level of intent and whether the intent has changed recently as indicated by the formation of a detailed plan and assessment of current level of impulse control. Risk is heightened when cognitive control is impaired by intense emotions, alcohol and drugs, impaired consciousness due to dissociative reactions or drugs, and a transient psychotic episode or quasi-psychotic symptoms.

13.2.1.2 Admission for Inpatient Treatment

When suicide risk is high, the usual course of action is admission to an inpatient unit. However, this should only be used when other options are not available or inappropriate because patients with BPD generally respond badly to general psychiatric care. Crisis behaviour usually settles fairly rapidly following admission, but if the patient is not discharged at this point, problems often recur due to the interaction between the patient's psychopathology and the dynamics of the inpatient service. The solution is to keep admissions brief – 24–48 hours.

Inpatient treatment may also undermine the patient's perception of his/her ability to manage problems, leading all too often to a repetitive cycle of crises and admissions. This is not surprising because hospital admission implicitly indicates that the clinician does not think that the patient can manage the current situation without external help. This inevitably undermines coping capacity. At the same time, the admission also gratifies dependency needs in ways that amplify these needs and encourages repeated crises. Although these untoward effects can usually be mitigated by working through them with the patient, this does not always occur, leading to more chronic problems.

There is also little evidence that long-term admission is effective in treating BPD or that medium-term admissions of several months produce better results than ambulatory care. Studies suggest that even after an extended admission to a unit designed to treat personality disorder, patients still show serious pathology.[13] There is also little evidence that inpatient treatment reduces deliberate self-harm.

The main indications for short-term admission are (i) high risk of suicide that cannot be managed in other ways, (ii) brief psychotic episode that cannot be managed with ambulatory care, and (iii) severe dissociative reaction with an amnesic or a non-responsive state.

These indications are not absolute and much depends on the patient's resources and support systems and the treatment options available. Chronic suicidal ideation and self-harm alone are not indications for admission nor are brief psychotic episodes unless the reaction is severe and the patient is unable to comply with treatment.

13.2.1.3 Alternatives to Inpatient Treatment

In most instances, crises can be managed through extra appointments and mobilizing family and social support systems. When patients are already in therapy, it is often possible to arrange extra sessions and telephone contact between sessions. For those who are not in treatment, short-term support from a crisis service can often be arranged until arrangements are made for longer-term treatment. In some settings, partial hospitalization or day treatment programmes are available. These are effective ways to treat BPD[14] but their value in managing crises is unclear although they are preferable to inpatient treatment.

When treating suicidal and chronically suicidal patients, some clinicians seek a verbal or written no-suicide contract in which patients agree to inform a relative or health care professional if they are suicidal rather than acting on the intent. Unfortunately these contracts are not effective.[15] Also the patient's acceptance of the contract may give the clinician a false sense of security so that necessary steps to ensure safety are not taken. This does not mean, however, that the clinician should not try to get a commitment from the patient to use resources available and to follow their crisis plan.

13.3 Containment: Settling Distress and Reactivity

Following actions to ensure safety, the next step is to return the patient to his/her previous level of functioning as soon as possible. This involves containing emotional reactivity, reducing symptoms, and helping the patient regain control. These objectives are usually achieved using containment interventions supplemented with medication as indicated. Containment interventions are based on the general treatment interventions modified for use in crises. The clinician's task is to make a connection with the patient, demonstrate non-judgemental acceptance, and convey understanding.

13.3.1.1 Basic Containment Strategy

The basic tenet of crisis management is that the patient's primary concern is to obtain relief from distress and that relief comes from contact with someone who communicates that they understand what the patient is experiencing.[16] The task is NOT to help the patient to understand his/her distress or the reasons for it. We are going to meet this basic principle repeatedly in various forms. Patients need to have their basic feelings and subjective experiences understood. This is critical to managing crises and later we will see that it is critical to improving emotion regulation generally.

13.3.1.2 Focus on Current Distress

Containment is best achieved by focusing on the emotional component of the patient's immediate concerns rather than factual details of what happened and why.[17] The current situation is only explored sufficiently to understand the patient's feelings and make informed decisions. The purpose of focusing on what the patient is feeling is to convey an empathic understanding of how the patient feels and not to encourage further ventilation. This is best avoided because it usually increases instability. Having someone recognize how dreadful they feel provides the support and help patients need to regain emotional control.

13.3.1.3 Reflect Rather Than Interpret

The most effective way to convey empathic understanding is to reflect rather than interpret what the patient has to say using simple, concrete statements that show that the therapist understands the patient's emotional state. Statements should be kept short and worded so that they have enough punch that they penetrate the distress. For example, with a patient in a self-harming crisis due to the break-up of a relationship, it may be more effective to simply note that "You're devastated" than engage in more long-winded statements about how you understand what happened and how it affected the patient.

More complex statements may exceed the patient's information-processing capacity and run the risk of being interpreted as an indication that the clinician does not really care or understand. Patients in a crisis are often hypersensitive and easily feel misunderstood, invalidated, or criticized. These risks are reduced by using statements that incorporate the patient's own language and by avoiding interpretations. Often it is not the words that are important but the way they are communicated. What matters is that the clinician presents a stable, consistent, caring, and non-punitive presence and demonstrates an ability to tolerate distress and anger while continuing to provide support and understanding.[18]

13.3.1.4 Avoid Interventions That Hinder Containment

Since containment is hindered by any intervention that conflicts with the patient's need for acceptance and understanding, containment is weakened by the failure to acknowledge distress, lengthy attempts to clarify feelings, discussion of coping strategies, and interpretations of the origins of thoughts, feelings, or impulses. It is also weakened by excessive sympathy as opposed to empathy.

Health care staff dealing with crises commonly make three mistakes. First, they ask too many questions and seek too much detail. Information is obviously needed to understand the situation and evaluate risk but this rarely requires detailed exploration of what happened. Too many questions especially when they are not balanced by the clinician demonstrating any understanding of the patient's distress increase frustration and emotional distress. Even questions intended to clarify the patient's feelings may cause frustration because the patient urgently wants understanding and acceptance.

Second, clinicians often attempt to reassure the patient that things are not as bad as the patient thinks by focusing on the positive things in the patient's life or offering the reassurance that things will look different in a short while. This rarely works. Such platitudes may actually make things worse if the patient feels the need to escalate his or her distress in order to convince the clinician that things are indeed desperate. It is best to simply acknowledge how the patient feels. However, clinicians often have difficulty simply reflecting the patient's pain as if this would reinforce or confirm the patient's perception of his/her situation.

Third, clinicians are often tempted to explain or interpret the reasons for the current crisis. Many get caught up in trying to reason with the patient as if a rational discussion would help the patient to see things differently and hence settle his/her distress. They forget that the intense emotions hinder thinking and problem-solving. Interpretations usually fail to contain distress because they do not match patients' ideas about what they need. At best, they decrease rapport because the patient considers them irrelevant or because they are too complex for the patient to process. At worst, they escalate the distress because they are viewed as critical, intrusive, or challenging or because they are taken as confirmation that the therapist does not understand.

13.3.1.5 Stabilize the Environment

Emotional crises are often triggered by problems in the patient's relationships with significant others, which can also help to maintain and even escalate the situation.

In these circumstances, it may be helpful to promote greater stability in the immediate social environment.[19] A brief inpatient admission, for example, can provide a respite that allows everyone to reflect on events as opposed to reacting to them. Stabilization can also be achieved by encouraging the patient to temporarily avoid the person or situation that triggers problems, by working with the patient and significant others to defuse the situation, or by calling a moratorium on any ongoing dispute. In an immediate crisis, it is often possible to help significant others to understand the patient's problems sufficiently to allow them to step back and be more supportive and less reactive.

13.3.1.6 Prevent an Escalation of Psychopathology

Crises need to be managed so as to minimize the risk of establishing a repetitive cycle of crises and an escalation of psychopathology. Short-term escalation is avoided by establishing a connection with the patient, using containment interventions to settle distress, and avoiding interventions that decrease containment and inadvertently reinforce maladaptive behaviour. Many patients with BPD are not helped by the health care system and some may even get worse.[20] Sometimes this is an unavoidable consequence of actions to ensure safety. For example, an inpatient admission needed to manage suicidality may also undermine coping behaviour and gratify the need for care, leading to repeated demands for inpatient care. In most cases, the risk of negative consequences of emergency care can be mitigated by discussing them later in therapy.

Perhaps the most common reason for an escalation of crisis behaviour is the failure to provide empathic emergency care. Many health care professionals with mistaken ideas about the reasons for crises and deliberate self-injury adopt a coercive and unsympathetic stance in the mistaken belief that this will reduce the chances of the patient engaging in further self-injury. This approach invariably fails because it assumes that self-injury is primarily attention-seeking behaviour. It also overlooks the fact that many self-harming patients are the victims of abuse and trauma and that this often leads them to seek out abusive situations unwittingly. Hence, rather than reducing the chances of future episodes, coerciveness actually increases the risk of future presentations.

13.3.1.7 Containment Interventions and the Management of Within-Session Emotional Arousal

Since intense emotions are destabilizing for patients with BPD, it is important to manage the patient's level of emotional arousal to keep it within tolerable limits. The first indications of adverse effects of heightened arousal are difficulty thinking, losing track of what is being discussed, feeling confused, and difficulty concentrating. These behaviours should not be managed as if they are purely defensive actions or indications of resistance but rather as indications of the need to intervene by discontinuing current interventions and switching to containment interventions to provide support until emotional control is regained. This approach uses the treatment relationship to regulate emotional arousal until the patient has developed the capacity to self-regulate emotions.

13.3.1.8 Medication

Since patients in a crisis are commonly prescribed medication, now is a useful time to consider the use of medication within integrated modular treatment (IMT). The position adopted by IMT based on reviews of treatment guidelines is that the primary treatment for BPD is psychotherapy and that if medication is used it should be considered as an adjunctive therapy. Nevertheless, medication is widely prescribed despite uncertainties and debates over its value[21] with studies showing that up to 80 per cent of patients take medication much of the time.[22] Polypharmacy is also common.

Since this book is primarily concerned with psychotherapy, medication is not reviewed in detail; instead the interested reader is referred to appropriate sources.[23] Reviews largely agree that medication does not improve borderline pathology in general. However, there is evidence that mood stabilizers reduce some features of emotional dysregulation and that second-generation neuroleptics are useful in treating cognitive perceptual symptoms and impairments. The evidence on the value of selective serotonin reuptake inhibitors (SSRIs) in treating emotional dysregulation is mixed. There is no evidence of medication effects on interpersonal problems although effects of medication on emotional dysregulation may have indirect effects on relationships. Evidence of the value of medications in crises is stronger than their longer-term use.

The use of medication in IMT is based on the following guidelines.[24] First, mediation is considered a specific treatment module, which means that like other specific modules it is used in the context of the general treatment modules. This means that the same attention is given to the alliance and motivation when prescribing medication as with other specific interventions. Second, medication is used in the targeted way to treat three symptom clusters: cognitive-perceptual symptoms, impulse-behavioural dyscontrol, and symptoms of emotional dysregulation. Third, the use of medication should be clearly explained to the patient, and if necessary significant others. Specifically, patients should understand that medication is not being used to treat the overall disorder but rather treat specific problems in order to avoid unrealistic expectations about the possible benefits of medication. It also helps to explain both the specific problems that medication is being used to treat and that many of the other problems associated with the disorder are unlikely to change to the same degree, for example, interpersonal problems. This is important to avoid patients seeking continual medication changes in search for a "cure" and to reduce the impact that taking medication may have on motivation. It is often useful to reinforce the idea that one of the benefits of medication is that it may help patients to work on their problems in therapy because they may feel less distressed.

Finally, it is helpful if patients clearly understand that the decision whether or not to use medication is theirs and that the therapist is merely making a recommendation. This helps to ensure compliance. However, it also avoids potential conflict arising from the polarization that can occur when the patient feels pressured by the clinician. Hence the value of medication is not something to be debated. Rather the clinician should state the case and leave it to the patient to decide. If medication is not being prescribed by the psychotherapist, it is important that the therapist and psychopharmacologist work collaboratively and that their respective roles are clearly understood by all parties.

It will be recalled that Anna was prescribed a low dose of the neuroleptic at the end of the assessment/treatment contact sessions to deal with acute distress and for cognitive-perceptual reasons. This was continued for about two years. She was also prescribed an SSRI to manage depressive symptoms and intense emotional lability. The treatment guidelines in widespread use at the time recommended SSRIs for this purpose.[25]

Subsequent studies called this into question although Anna subsequently improved. During the initial phase of treatment Madison was also prescribed quetiapine (25–50mg) for two weeks when experiencing some severe short-term symptoms. She was also prescribed an SSRI during the first year of treatment for severe anxiety symptoms.

13.4 Concluding Comments

Crisis management is an important aspect of treating BPD. Crises early in therapy provide the first opportunity for patients to see how the therapist copes with and manages their problems. In a sense, crises are a test that patients can use to evaluate the therapist and his/her commitment to the process. The outcome strongly influences the patient's perception of therapist credibility and his/her ability to provide the help the patient is seeking. The key to success is to keep things simple and not to try to achieve too much when the patient is in a decompensated state.

Notes

1. Swenson (1989).

2. Dulit et al. (1994), Friedman et al. (1983), Fyer et al. (1988), Mehlum et al. (1994), Shearer et al. (1988), Soloff et al. (1994).

3. Soloff et al. (1994).

4. Dulit et al. (1994), Soloff et al. (1994).

5. Soloff et al. (1994).

6. Zweig-Frank et al. (1994).

7. See Paris (2003) for a review. See also McGlashan (1986), Paris et al. (1987, 1989), Sansome (2004), Stone (1989, 1990, 1993, 2001).

8. Paris (2003).

9. Zanarini et al. (2006), Perry et al. (2009).

10. Kjelsberg et al. (1991).

11. Links and Kolla (2005), Zaheer et al. (2008), Links and Bergmans (2015), Sansome (2004).

12. Links and Kolla (2005), Gunderson and Links (2008).

13. McGlashan (1986).

14. Bateman and Fonagy (1999, 2000, 2001), Piper et al. (1993, 1996), Arnevik et al. (2009).

15. Stanford et al. (1994), Kroll (2000).

16. Joseph (1983), Livesley (2003), Steiner (1994).

17. Linehan (1993).

18. Buie and Adler (1982).

19. Vaillant (1992).

20. Frances (1992), Kroll (1988), Rockland (1992).

21. Silk and Friedel (2015).

22. Zanarini et al. (2004).

23. For more detailed reviews, see Binks et al. (2006), Duggan et al. (2008), Ingenhoven et al. (2010), Lieb et al. (2010), Markovitz (in press), Silk and Friedel (2015), Saunders and Silk (2009).

24. See Silk and Friedel (2015) for a detailed discussion of the use of medication in IMT.

25. American Psychiatric Association: Practice guideline for the treatment of patients with borderline personality disorder (2001). American Journal of Psychiatry, 158 (suppl.), 1–52.

Chapter 14
Managing the Early Sessions

The early stages of treatment set the stage for the rest of therapy and have a substantial bearing on outcome. Active attention needs to be given to engagement because relationship issues are easily neglected when faced with such urgent problems as intense distress, suicidality, and deliberate self-harm. In the early sessions, engagement is enhanced when the patient sees the therapist as open, realistically optimistic, attentive, sensitively attuned to his/her personal concerns, and flexible in responding to the issues raised.[1]

14.1 The First Session

The primary goal for the first session is to ensure that the patient has a positive experience because this session is the template for the rest of therapy and influences the ultimate depth of the therapist–patient relationship and the patient's expectations for treatment.[2] Ideally, the first session should end with the patient feeling a connection with the therapist and that the session was useful. This requires a flexible approach that combines efforts to engage the patient with a focus on immediate concerns and current mental state.

Most patients feel relief about starting therapy although this is often accompanied with anxiety about treatment and even wariness about the therapist. Hence patients need support throughout the session, especially at the beginning. When dealing with any anxiety about treatment, the patient's actual concerns should be discussed rather than just engage in chatting in an attempt to put the patient at ease. Apart from a little small talk at the beginning of a session that is part of normal social politeness, small talk is not helpful and sets a tone that is not conducive to therapeutic work. When patients are anxious about treatment, sufficient time will need to be given to these concerns to ensure that the patient is calmer by the end of the session.

The need to put patients at their ease and build rapport means that the therapist usually needs to be fairly active throughout the session. It is often useful to begin the session with an open-ended enquiry about how things have been since the assessment sessions or about the patient's reactions to what was discussed in those sessions. However, many patients have an agenda and often want to discuss a recent distressing event. This scenario is used to explore and reflect the feelings involved and to attempt to relate them to treatment goals such as self-harming behaviour. It can also be used to learn more about triggering events although, at this stage, exploration will be limited since the main goal is to convey understanding. Besides linking the theme of the session to treatment goals, it is also useful to summarize what is discussed in a way that extends patients' understanding of their difficulties because patients who see their therapists as understanding and knowledgeable and as providing insights into their problems in the first session are more likely return to the next session.[3]

At some point, during the session, the therapist should ask about how the patient feels about the session, whether it is what the patient expected, and how the patient feels about talking to the therapist about these matters.

14.1.1 Case Examples

Anna arrived for the first session very distressed due to a fight with her husband a few days earlier that led to him threatening to leave her. She felt overwhelmed by sadness and emptiness that made her feel as if everything hurt. She was so distressed that it was difficult for her to talk about what had happened or how she felt. Consistent with the treatment plan (see Chapter 6), most of the session was taken up by attempts to provide support and contain the distress by listening and reflecting Anna's feelings. Gradually, the distress settled sufficiently for Anna to describe more about the incident with her husband and her overwhelming fear that he would leave and how this aroused intense memories of her previous husband who had also abandoned her. She also talked of how she longed to be loved. The focus, however, continued to be placed on identifying and reflecting the feelings because her mood was still volatile. By the end of the session, Anna felt a little more in control.

The first session with Madison was equally stormy. She arrived in a distraught and furious state due to a fight with her mother. She had gone to see mother because she was very upset about something that had happened two days earlier and had been distressed since and had cut herself the previous evening. The first part of the session was concerned with settling the distress using containment interventions. This was effective and the distress settled quickly, allowing more detailed discussion of the event and the factors that triggered the initial crisis two days earlier. This led to a discussion of the specific events that triggered the distress both with mother and the earlier incident. Madison noted that in both cases she had felt let down. This discussion led to a further improvement in emotional control, which confirmed the impression formed during the assessment that Madison felt better when she talked about her emotional pain and began to understand it.

14.2 The Early Sessions: General Issues

The evolution of therapy during the early sessions differs widely across patients. Some settle quickly into therapy but typically, when therapy begins with the patient in a decompensated state, crises continue for some time. Throughout these sessions, emphasis is placed on both engagement and alliance building and containing emotional reactivity and suicidality.

14.2.1 Relationship Issues

Although intense emotions and suicidality demand attention, it is also important to monitor the relationship and focus on building the relationship because this is the best way to engage the patient in therapy and reduce crises because the patient's connection with the therapist provides an anchor that has a settling effect.

14.2.1.1 Pace of Therapy

An issue in the early sessions is how quickly to proceed. With severely decompensated and self-harming patients, therapists often feel intense pressure to deal with these problems immediately using relatively specific interventions. Patients also add to the pressure therapists experience because they often express a terrible urgency for someone or something to do something to change how they feel. Some demand action and suicide is often an ever-present threat. It is usually best to resist this temptation in favour of containment and engagement even if this seems counterintuitive. With severely decompensated patients, a slow pace is often best because intense treatment at this stage can be overwhelming, leading to further decompensation. If such caution proves unnecessary, no harm is done – it is easy to increase the tempo of therapy whereas the effects of further decompensation may be more difficult to resolve.

14.2.1.2 The Importance of Modelling

The therapist's response to crises is important because patients learn from how the therapist reacts to their panic and urgency. When the therapist reacts calmly and remains consistent and attentive, patients begin to recognize that even if they are panicking, the therapist is not. This happened with Anna. She found it helpful that the therapist was not panicked by her distress or self-harming behaviour. Initially, she was irritated by it and thought that the therapist should be doing more but over time it helped her to recognize that she did not need to be afraid of her apparently uncontrollable feelings and that they would settle and that they could be managed and understood.

14.2.1.3 Level of Therapist Activity

Level of therapist activity needs to be managed carefully during the early sessions. A relatively high level of activity is needed to provide the structure required to contain distress and avoid the rumination and preoccupation with inner experience that impairs cognitive functioning and increases anxiety and dissociation. However, it is also possible to be too active, which runs the danger of the patient concluding that the therapist is not interested in what the patient has to say or that the therapist has his/her own agenda.

14.2.1.4 The Therapist's Presence

A critical factor linked to the level of therapist activity is the presence of the therapist. This idea is difficult to describe succinctly. However, many patients, especially those with severe disorder who dissociate, comment later in therapy that the thing that helped them to settle into therapy and contain their distress was the presence of the therapist. One patient, who at the beginning of therapy spent most of her time at home sitting on her couch in a dissociated state oblivious to time, noted later that when therapy began she "felt all over the place" and that the therapist was the only stable thing in her life. She recalled that her life was chaotic and that "everything was blurry and ran together" and she had no sense of time. However, the therapist was always there and the same. The twice-weekly sessions provided an anchor and a safe harbour from a world that was bewildering, presumably because she was dissociating. She added that it seemed as if the therapist acted as her memory – she did not recall things from one session to the next and had little recall of what was going on in her life but the therapist seemed to remember and this made her feel as if she existed.

The important issue raised by these statements is the impact of the therapist early in therapy. Anna said something similar. During a session in the second year of treatment, she spontaneously noted that she was feeling better and that she had been thinking about why she had improved. This seemed to the therapist to be a good opportunity to deepen the alliance by reviewing progress and recalling a little of the history of therapy – two simple methods for alliance building discussed in Chapter 8 – because some difficult issues had been discussed in previous sessions. She described how she had learned to understand and control her feelings and mentioned that what helped was that the therapist "was there." When asked what she meant, she explained how, at the beginning of therapy, she felt distraught and overwhelmed, which caused her to panic. She constantly felt a desperate urge to do something to get out of this state because she cut herself frequently and always seemed to be fighting with her partner. She would arrive for her appointment in "a state" and the therapist "was just there and listened and talked about things and didn't get upset about what I had done to myself."

What seems to matter early in therapy with severely impaired patients is the presence of a therapist who is empathically attuned to the patient's inner world and communicates this understanding to the patient. An important part of this communication is non-verbal – the therapist is simply there. This is important because, in these states, the patient's capacity to process verbal information is limited. However, it is also important to communicate meaning and understanding so that the patient begins to make sense of inner experience. The settling effect of this combination of presence and understanding can be understood in terms of attachment concepts. With a good attachment relationship, the attachment figure helps soothe the child's distress until the child learns to self-soothe. Something similar occurs in therapy: the therapist acts as an external regulator to the patient's distress until the patient learns to self-soothe. One patient described how she learned to do this by listening to her therapist's voice mail. When she got upset she would telephone the therapist's office just to hear his voice even though she knew he was not there. This soothed her even though the message was a simple request to leave a message. It was as if the voice mail was a transitional object that helped her to self-soothe until she learned to do it without an external input.

14.2.2 Managing the Therapeutic Dialogue

Therapy may be thought of as a conversation with the patient who describes recent or past events that are then explored collaboratively. The scenarios presented change as different problems come into focus. They are also handled differently over time – typically they are explored in greater depth as treatment progresses and themes embedded in the scenarios that are explored change according to which domain of impairment is the focus of treatment.

The scenarios presented in the early sessions usually involve distressing recent events and their recounting often reactivates intense emotions. These scenarios are used to settle distress using containment interventions and to connect with the patient by listening to the scenario in a non-judgemental way and communicating an understanding of the feelings involved. Interventions that increase emotional arousal such as uncovering methods used in psychodynamic therapy and detailed exploration of trauma are avoided.

If the scenario presented by the patient deals with an emotionally charged event such as abuse, the therapist attends to these issues sufficiently to validate them without exploring them in ways that increase distress. For example, the patient may describe an argument with a partner that resulted in deliberate self-injury and mention that the fight activated memories of early childhood abuse. Since the concern at this phase of treatment is to contain distress and self-injury, the abuse is acknowledged and the impact of the memory is discussed without eliciting details of the abuse. This is left for later in therapy. If necessary, the therapist may note that this is an important issue that will need to be discussed when the patient feels more stable and able to manage his or her feelings better. Later in therapy, the same kind of scenario may be used to increase the capacity for self-regulation and later still to explore interpersonal problems including the abuse itself.

During this early phase of treatment, general interventions are used almost exclusively apart from simple behavioural interventions such as distraction and self-soothing. The patient's problems and concerns raised in the scenarios discussed are explored in a collaborative way to increase awareness of the thoughts and feelings associated with these problems. At the same time, these experiences are validated and the patient is encouraged to move beyond simply describing problems in increasing depth to reflecting on experiences and the reasons for them and to pay attention to the mental states of self and others.

14.3   Early Sessions: Interventions

With this broad overview of the early sessions in mind, we can now consider in more detail how to manage the early sessions to reduce crises and manage deliberate self-injury. Ultimately, a lasting decrease in crises requires increased emotional regulation. However, it takes time to acquire the requisite skills and a degree of stability is needed to learn them. For now the focus is on establishing stability through the continued use of the general intervention modules and containment interventions and on helping patients handle crises more effectively.

14.3.1   Increase Awareness of Crisis Behaviour

The behavioural sequence depicted in Figure 13.1 (see Chapter 13) provides a useful scheme to teach patients about crises. The first step is to help patients to see the connections between intense emotional states and self-harm and, possibly, to link distress to specific triggering events. The intent is to demonstrate that these crises are meaningful because this promotes stability. By linking crises to specific triggering events, we begin helping patients to construct a narrative about their crises, which draws together different behaviours and experiences. This is a process that occurs repeatedly throughout therapy as patients are helped to construct new narratives about their problems and concerns.

14.3.2   Teach How to Monitor Safety

At this stage, it is useful to teach patients (and significant others) how to monitor safety. This requires that they learn to (i) distinguish non-lethal suicidal behaviour and deliberate self-harm from "real" suicidal intent[4] and (ii) identify the early signs of distress before it escalates into a full-blown crisis. Previously it was noted that patients and others often confuse deliberate self-harm with suicidality. The realization that self-harm is often a way to self-manage emotions helps to reduce alarm sufficiently to allow significant others to be more supportive.

To control crises, patients need to learn to recognize early warning signs that something is wrong.[5] Most cannot do this because they are not aware of their emotions or else they actively avoid or suppress them in the hope that they will go away. As a result, many only attend to their feelings when they get out of control. Early recognition of warning signs allows them to deal with the problem while it is still manageable. However, patients often have difficulty pinpointing when things began to go wrong. Simple enquiries about what was the first thing they noticed that was wrong are often difficult to answer. Nevertheless, these queries may help to "prime" the patient by suggesting that the next time the patient gets upset he/she should try to identify signs that indicate that his or her sense of safety is changing. These early signs differ substantially across patients. Sometimes, the earliest sign may be feeling irritable, feeling tense, or developing a headache. In other cases, the signs may be less obvious indicators that something is wrong – feeling sleepy, drowsy, or more cut off from the world. Some signs are cognitive such as thoughts about being worthless. Behavioural signs include staying in bed or feeling an intense desire to curl up in bed or even just to curl up in a fetal position regardless of the situation. It is useful to draw up a list of these signs with the patient – the task engages the patient in treatment and models collaboration. This also indicates that the therapist is confident that the patient can learn to recognize early indications of impending problems and has the ability to manage things differently.

Some patients also find it helpful to have a personal scale to describe their level of emotional distress. This helps them to communicate with others more effectively and it often gives them a little "distance" over their emotional reactions. The scale should run from safe to very unsafe or calm and in control to out of control with steps in between. As the patients learn to recognize their own reactions, the scale often becomes more refined and more steps are added with labels for each step. For each step in the scale, the patient is encouraged to identify his/her main feelings and what he/she can do to settle things down and reduce his/her distress. It is helpful to include the names of people to contact for help and, in some cases, information about whom not to contact. This is helpful when patients are extremely distressed because they often turn to people who are either unable to help or do things that exacerbate the problem.

For example, Madison usually contacted her parents when she felt out of control. However, they always became very anxious because they felt helpless, which caused them to get angry and critical, which led to an acrimonious exchange that made things worse. Having discussed this with her therapist, Madison decided that she would only contact her parents when mildly distressed. At these times, her parents did not feel pressured and were able to act supportively by suggesting a variety of activities that usually helped to settle things down. She also realized that when extremely distressed she needed to seek help from other source. The value of developing this scale and list of actions to take at each level is that it provides patients with a toolkit that they can refer to when their emotions overwhelm their ability to think about what to do.

14.3.3 Teach Distraction and Self-Soothing

The purpose of recognizing the early signs of emotional distress is to allow the patient to take appropriate action before things spiral out of control. The action taken will vary according to the situation and the progress the patient has made in treatment. Early in treatment, simple distracting and self-soothing activities are helpful. As treatment progresses, these can be supplemented with other methods to self-manage emotions (self-soothing and other emotion-regulating strategies are discussed in Chapter 16).

Distraction and self-soothing are easier to use if patients compile lists of distracting and self-soothing activities that they refer to as soon as a problem is recognized rather having to think about what to do at a time when it is often difficult to think clearly. Distraction is also useful in dealing with minor problems or when alternatives are not readily available. Problems arise when it is used persistently as a way to avoid intense feelings with limited awareness that it is being used in this way. Most of us also have a variety of methods we use to soothe ourselves. We listen to music, read a book, go for a walk, have a drink, or talk to a friend. If the problem is more persistent we may argue with ourselves about whether our distress is appropriate or try to solve the problem. Attachment trauma can lead to difficulty self-soothing because patients feel undeserving of pleasure, which makes self-soothing a source of guilt rather than comfort. The therapist's participation in compiling a list of self-soothing activities along with the therapist's empathy and compassion for the patient's distress is often an important factor in helping patients to acquire and use this skill.

14.3.4 Foster Self-Efficacy

During a crisis, patients usually feel there is nothing that they can do to change how dreadful they feel. This perceived lack of self-efficacy and self-agency exacerbates their distress. These are similar concepts. Broadly speaking, both refer to a person's belief in his/her ability to produce desired outcomes and results including responses from others. Hence, they are used interchangeably in this volume.[6] Limited self-efficacy adds to suicidal and self-harming behaviour; faced with overwhelming distress, the patient feels that there is nothing that he/she can do to change the way he/she feels and that the only solution is either suicide or self-injury. Hence it is desirable to begin working on building self-efficacy as early as possible by helping patients to understand that there are things they can do to manage their emotions and to recognize occasions when they have been able to control their feelings and the urge to self-harm. Attainment of these modest goals can then be used to challenge beliefs that change is not possible and thus begin the long process of building a sense of competency and self-efficacy.

14.3.5 Teach Appropriate Help-Seeking Behaviour

In a crisis, patients often seek help in ways that alienate those they turn to for help.[7] Most patients do not realize how they talk to other people and how their sense of urgency and desperation can lead to an angry, demanding manner that is off-putting to even the most well-intentioned person. Instead of asking for help, they demand it, often in a challenging and accusatory way. Consequently, attempts to seek help from friends and family or from emergency and crisis services are often unrewarding and lead to increased distress and more frequent crises.

Although it takes time to develop the reflective attitude needed to see things from the other person's perspective, patients can be encouraged to develop better communication skills early in therapy to allow them get the help needed and reduce the escalation that often occurs when requests for help are unsuccessful. More effective ways to communicate distress and the need for help include the following:

1. *Ask rather than demand.* For example, "I am having problems (dreadfully upset, or feeling like harming myself), could you help me?" rather than, "You have got to help me," or "You must do ... "
2. *Request rather than accuse.* Ask for help and support rather than accuse the other person of not helping, for example, "You never listen to me," or "you're never there for me," or "you don't care about me." Such statements are often used to initiate a request for help from significant others and patients do not realize how such statements alienate people. Even if feeling uncared for or unloved is part of the crisis, it is more effective to say something like: "I get very hurt when I think that you are not listening to me (or when I feel you don't care) about me. It would help me just now if you could listen and be supportive." It also helps if the patient could add a rider that explains what he/she needs because often family members are frustrated because they do not know what to do. For example, "I don't need you to do anything, just listen and support me."
3. *Use an appropriate tone of voice: do not shout but also do not speak in a meek or hesitant way.* Some patients speak with a great intensity when upset that comes across as aggressive and confrontational. Others talk in a quiet or meek way that fails to engage the other person.
4. *Approach as quietly as possible, don't just barge in.* When distressed, patients often rush to contact people for help without paying attention to what the other person is doing, which can be seen as intrusive and dramatic, causing the other person to step back just when the patient wants him/her to step forward.
5. *Talk in the first person.* For example, "I am very upset and it would help if I could talk to you about it" rather than "you need to listen to me" or "you have to do ... "

One reason why family and significant others have difficulty being supportive in crises is that they do not know what to do, which causes them to feel both frustrated and guilty. Hence when faced with an angry, demanding, accusing, and in-your-face attitude, they respond in similar fashion. Consequently, besides helping patients to communicate their needs more effectively, it is also useful to teach family members how to respond to crises. However, before discussing this, there is another component to patients' communications when they are in a crisis to consider – how they communicate to emergency room staff.

Patients who use accident and emergency resources often need help in making more effective use of these services.[8] It helps if patients understand the pressures placed on emergency department staff and hence the importance of quickly providing staff with the information needed to decide what to do. Since it is usually difficult to organize thoughts and communicate effectively when emotionally distressed, it is useful for patients to prepare an information sheet to take with them when they next visit the emergency department, which provides details of medications, physicians' contact information, important personal supports, and even their crisis plan.

Another way to think about teaching more appropriate help-seeking behaviour is that the therapist is helping the patient to construct a new script and narrative for how to act in crises. Their previous script was to demand help as if people would only help if coerced. This needs to be replaced with a more effective script for how and when to approach people and how to ask for help without being demanding or blaming.

14.3.6 Incorporate Significant Others

Living with someone with borderline personality disorder (BPD) can be stressful. A session with significant others explaining crises and offering guidance about helpful responses can help to reduce their stress and enable them to help the patient to self-manage distress. People are action-oriented and want information on specific things they can do to help their loved ones. Hence, it is important to spend some time stressing that the most important thing to do is to provide support and that this simply involves listening and communicating that they understand what the patient is telling them.

Case Example

The value of incorporating family is illustrated in the treatment of Madison. Early in therapy, it became apparent that many crises were triggered and exacerbated by family issues. A conjoint session with Madison's parents indicated the level of family stress. Throughout the session, Madison was overtly hostile about her parents' apparent inability to provide support. Her parents were similarly angry and frustrated. However, it was also apparent that the parents were concerned but did not know what to do. Mother was upset about her inability to help, and father, who seemed very solution-focused, was frustrated at being unable to find a solution. The therapist decided that the most effective strategy was to meet the parents alone. Madison agreed with this suggestion.

The meeting with the parents revealed the intensity of their distress and frustration. Mother felt guilty about being unable to help and blamed herself. Father was also angry with himself because he thought of himself as a problem-solver but here was a problem he could not solve. He was also angry with Madison because, as he saw things, he offered her good advice that she ignored. The parents were also a little afraid of Madison. She would turn up suddenly filled with rage and demand help. They lived on eggshells not knowing when this would happen. Nevertheless, they cared deeply about their daughter and wanted to help her but did not know how.

The therapist provided some basic information about crises and what it was like to have one and explained how it was difficult to think in a crisis, which made it difficult to process information. The parents seemed to accept this but father still had trouble understanding why Madison could not see things that seemed to him to be very clear. He wanted to know what they could do.

The therapist explained that the most important thing was to be supportive and that this meant listening to Madison and making sure that she felt that they had heard her and understood what she was going through. However, father said that they did all that and there must be something else they could do. The therapist said that was probably not the case. On these occasions, Madison was not in a state to listen to advice no matter how thoughtful. What she needed was to feel that they cared and understood. Mother suddenly got it. She exclaimed, "You think I should do what I did when she was little and was upset or hurt herself. I would pick her up and dust her off, sit her on my knee and comfort her." The therapist nodded and added "Yes, she just needs to feel understood and loved." Mother turned to her husband saying, "Darling, it's just like me! I've told you when I get stressed out that all I need is for you to listen to me while I go on about everything. I don't need you to fix it. You're Mr Fix-it but you can't fix everything." The therapist commented. "No, that's Madison job but it is what you have both been trying to do and beating yourselves up because you couldn't." A few more sessions occurred with the parents to help them manage their relationship with Madison differently and to deal with the guilt they continued to feel. Family stress gradually decreased and Madison became more stable. Some weeks after the meeting with her parents, Madison arrived for a session looking happy – a rare occurrence.

MADISON: Things are much better with my mum.

THERAPIST: Oh yes!

M: Yes, much.

T: That sounds great. What happened?

M: I had some problems with Tim (her boyfriend) that hurt me and I was getting upset. But it wasn't too bad so I thought I should talk to mum before it got worse like we said. So I asked if I could come round. She was OK with it. I was proud of myself.

T: Yes! You did what we'd talked about.

M: Yea and I walked in quietly and asked if I could talk to her. She said "of course." I told her I was really upset about something that happened with Tim and that I really needed to talk to her. I also told her that I didn't need her to do anything just listen. She gave me a hug and made us a coffee and I talked to her. She didn't say much, she just listened. Then we didn't talk much we just sat and drank coffee together. It felt good.

In the initial interview with the parents, the therapist responded to the parents' request for advice by stressing support because of a concern that the father's eagerness for action would distract him from listening and reflecting. However, in subsequent sessions, further information was provided about early-warning signs so that they could help Madison to monitor her emotions and use distraction and self-soothing when her emotions were becoming more intense. Later, they were encouraged to help her to react differently during a crisis by encouraging her to breathe normally and use relaxation, distraction, and self-soothing. Father in particular seemed comfortable with this combination of providing support and actually doing something and managed to stop trying to find a rational solution for the immediate problem and giving advice.

14.3.7 Building Structure into Everyday Life

The lives of many severely disordered patients are disorganized and unstructured. The normal rhythms of life do not apply. Even the diurnal pattern of sleep and wakefulness is disrupted. Patients sleep much of the day and then complain of being unable to sleep at night. These patients need to be helped to introduce some structure to their day, although this is often remarkably difficult. Simply being in therapy helps. Regular appointments begin to structure the patient's week. At some point during the first phase of treatment, the issue of daily routine needs to be raised, especially with patients who complain of insomnia. The first step is often to re-establish a set routine for sleeping and waking and perhaps to have a discussion about how exercise helps to improve both sleep and mood. These discussions probably have little immediate impact but they set the stage for future discussions about self-care and self-neglect and the idea of structuring the day by having a regular schedule and later by possibly getting a part-time job or volunteering.

14.3.8 Specific Interventions to Reduce Deliberate Self-Harm

Many of the interventions discussed thus far help in managing deliberate self-harm. This section draws these ideas together into an overall treatment approach that is based on the assumption that deliberate self-injurious behaviour is a self-regulatory action used to reduce negative emotions.[9] This suggests that treatment should seek to identify alternatives to self-harming behaviour and reduce the negative emotions that self-harm is intended to reduce. Although improving emotion regulation is ultimately the definitive way to reduce deliberate self-harm, this usually takes time to accomplish. In the meantime, attention can be given to finding alternatives to self-harm that can begin to reduce its incidence.

As with all problems, treatment begins by eliciting a commitment to change because patients do not necessarily see the need to change behaviours that make them feel better. If necessary, the benefits and costs or consequences of these behaviours can be discussed to establish such a commitment. Subsequently, immediate goals are agreed to. Earlier it was suggested that the immediate goal should be to delay such behaviours or even abort an episode when the urge arises because this is readily attainable. Some successes are needed at this phase of treatment to build the alliance, promote hope, and help patients to develop confidence in their ability to control these behaviours and to change.

At this stage of treatment, interventions usually need to be simple, especially with patients like Anna and Madison who are acutely symptomatic. Usually simple behavioural interventions that are easy to use such as distraction, self-soothing, substitution, and avoidance are usually sufficient to achieve the delay that we are looking for. In the case of distraction, it is usually a matter of working with the patient to identify activities that they think are likely to help them and then encouraging their consistent use. When the self-harm involves cutting, hitting, or burning, it is sometime possible to find substitutes that also reduce negative emotions. One method commonly referred to is to squeeze an ice cube tightly but the only time I have found this effective was when the patient coloured the ice with red food-colouring, which made it look as if she had actually cut herself. Avoidance is also useful when the patient self-harms in specific situations or with a specific weapon. Some patients who carry knives or razor blades or keep a stock at home so that they can cut themselves if the urge arises can be discouraged to stop having these instruments so readily available. Or, patients who have the urge to jump off a bridge if they cross one when distressed can be encouraged to take a different route. When working with patients to identify things that are likely to be useful, the point made earlier should be borne in mind that the goal is to delay or avoid some incidents of self-harm using these methods until they have learned other ways to deal with their emotions.

14.4 Re-Formulation during the First Phase of Treatment

The first opportunity to elaborate the initial formulation based on new information occurs when the patient is engaged in treatment and working on reducing crises and deliberate self-harm. The purpose is to give the patient a road map that makes sense of crisis behaviour. Any earlier discussion of the behavioural sequence leading to crises can now be extended to cover the overall sequence, beginning with a triggering event and culminating in deliberate self-harm.[10] This sequence is readily understood and makes crises more understandable, which helps to reduce their intensity. This is what happened with Madison.

Case Example

For the first few months, sessions were dominated by the most recent crisis but, gradually, within-session distress settled, the alliance increased, and Madison started to discuss events in more detail. In one session, she said that two days earlier in the early hours of the morning she had been taken by the police and paramedics to the hospital. The event had woken her neighbours and she was very embarrassed about what happened. Her distress had progressed during the day until it became intolerable in the evening. She went to bed hoping to escape the pain by falling asleep. However, she became so upset and lonely that she could not stand it. In desperation, she telephoned a crisis line. She had been telling the counsellor for some time about being depressed and how she had thought about harming herself and that she had cut herself when suddenly the police and paramedics arrived at her apartment.

After reviewing the details of the visit to the emergency room and her current state, the therapist asked about what had happened during the day. Madison said that she had been feeling upset and angry for most of the previous day and things got worse as the day progressed. At one point, she contacted a friend who was too busy to join her and her mood got worse. When the therapist asked about when she first noticed feeling upset, Madison said she had felt like that all day. When the therapist asked whether she woke up that way, she initially thought that she did but further inquiry revealed that it seemed to start in mid-morning. When asked about what she was doing at the time, Madison insisted nothing happened, she just got upset. Further discussion led Madison to say that the only thing she could remember doing was telephoning her mother but that was all. The therapist asked whether the call had upset her. Madison thought not. The therapist asked what the call was about. She had called her mother to ask if she would go shopping with her, that was all. When asked what mother said, she said that mother was too busy. The therapist asked how she felt about this. She said she was absolutely fine with it. When the therapist reflected this, she got into a rant saying that she was mad at the way mother did not care and how she favoured her brother and that it was all unfair.

Let us pause here and look at what has happened. This vignette illustrates the impressionistic way of thinking adopted by patients with BPD who prefer to talk in generalities. This is dealt with by pursuing details as illustrated by the therapist's persistent search for the specifics of what happened. This needs to be done in a casual and conversational way to avoid appearing to be conducting an interrogation. The vignette also illustrates how this style of thinking is also an effective avoidance strategy. Madison sought to avoid the anger with mother by maintaining that her distress simply happened and nothing caused it probably because the feelings activated the painful schemas that mother did not care and jealousy about her brother, and also because she felt ashamed of these thoughts and feelings.

Apparently, Madison ruminated about the unfairness of it all and how hurt she was for the rest of the day becoming increasingly upset. The phone call to a friend asking her if they could get together added to her feelings of rejection and hence to her rage. The therapist then summarized what had happened using the behavioural sequence of event-escalating emotional state response (see Figure 14.1). It was noted that Madison had often said that she did not know what caused her to get so upset but on this occasion it seemed that it was the phone call to mother and especially mother declining Madison's invitation to go shopping. The therapist noted that this seemed to suggest that an important trigger to her crises was feeling hurt and rejected and wondered what Madison thought. Madison agreed and added that these feelings seemed to occur whenever she felt rejected and unloved. She went on to give examples of similar incidents.

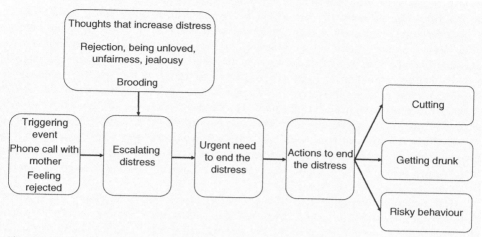

Figure 14.1 Diagram of Madison's Crisis Behaviour

Having established the trigger for many crises, the feelings aroused by these events and their associated thoughts were explored. Attention was drawn to the way ruminative thoughts of rejection, how unfair things were, jealousy, and being unloved increased the distress until it became intolerable. This led to a discussion of the things that Madison did to reduce distress. On this occasion, she cut herself. On other occasions, she abused alcohol, engaged in risky sexual behaviour, or binged on ice cream. These actions were explained as the best way she could think of to end how terrible she felt.

While exploring the crisis and the flow of feelings and thoughts, the therapist drew a diagram of what happened and then showed it to Madison (see Figure 14.1) for her comments. The therapist recalled how when they first discussed Madison's treatment goals she had said that she wanted to learn how to deal with her intense emotions, which seem to arise from no one reason and that it seemed that there was a reason and that this was something that could be dealt with. Madison noted that "it all makes sense."

This incident had a substantial impact on treatment because it helped Madison to make sense of what had seemed to her to be chaotic and meaningless episodes by drawing together a variety of experiences and behaviours. The subsequent change was not dramatic. Emotional crises and self-harming behaviour continued for some months but these incidents progressively became less intense and shorter in duration. More importantly, Madison began to work more determinedly on learning to control her feelings and reducing self-harm. The incident illustrates how a successful formulation has a settling effect that reduces distress and demoralization and facilitates engagement.[11] It also illustrates how patients need to make sense of their experience before they can learn to regulate it.

14.5 Case Example: The Early Sessions in Therapy with Anna

For the first few months, Anna's treatment followed a similar course to that of Madison but within-session distress was more intense and in some sessions she dissociated and had difficulty thinking and even recalling what she had been discussing. Life continued to be chaotic and stormy and visits to emergency departments continued to be an almost weekly occurrence that occasionally led to brief hospital admissions. Since Anna travelled a considerable distance for therapy and lived in a different health region, the therapist often did not learn of these events until the next session and there was little that could be done to influence what happened during these occasions. Under other circumstances, twice-weekly sessions would have been offered from the onset of therapy with someone so decompensated; however, this was not practical because of the distance involved. Another alternative would have been day hospital treatment but this was not available. Attempts were made to arrange additional support from a community care team in the town in which she lived but this did not work out. Part of the difficulty was that Anna's frequent crises involved intense inconsolable distress (distress without resolution described in Chapter 4), intense rage, fear of abandonment, and dissociative features. This led to angry demanding behaviour that was difficult to manage.

Most sessions were concerned with providing support and containing the reactivity. This pattern continued for about thirty sessions spread over the first year of treatment. However, sessions were not uniformly the same. During some sessions she was distressed and dissociated. On other occasions, she was angry about her life and the way she was treated by her husband and siblings and the demands they made of her, demands that she sought to meet despite the anger she felt. On one occasion, she became enraged with the therapist because she wanted additional medication, benzodiazepines and another medication that was inappropriate. The therapist explained this but Anna could not listen. She was filled with rage and her attention was focused totally on what she wanted and she did not seem to either listen to or think about anything else. She was relentless in her demands that the therapist quietly but firmly resisted. When the session ended, Anna stormed out but an hour later during the long trip home she telephoned to leave a message saying she was sorry for the way she behaved. During the next session she was fearful that the therapist would end treatment.

It seems that the first year was a test of the therapist not in a deliberate conscious way but rather in the sense that Anna needed to be confident that the therapist would be there to help her and would not abandon her. Given her history, this pattern is not surprising. Anna had never felt loved or cared for. The only person she felt cared about her was her father and he was often not around. As a result she did not trust anyone. Moreover, earlier therapies had failed. So all the therapist had to do was to be there, survive, and accept the intense feelings without being overwhelmed by them, judging Anna for having them, or retaliating (see also the section of Chapter 13 dealing with the presence of the therapist). This also required consistent limit setting to contain the demands and neediness in a way that was accepting and non-judgemental, something that was sometimes a challenge given Anna's angry, demanding, in-your-face behaviour.

Interspersed with the emotionally intense sessions were occasional sessions or, more often, short periods in a session in which Anna was more settled and reflective. On those occasions, she showed remarkable insights into her problems. She talked about her neediness and her longing to be loved and cared for and linked this to childhood events. However, the therapist simply validated and reflected these insights by noting both their importance and Anna's understanding of her difficulties without exploring them because it was not clear that she could tolerate further emotional distress that might result from discussing the neglect. In responding, the therapist also indicated that these were important issues and that Anna's understanding of them would stand her in good stead as therapy progressed (see later discussion of treatment of these problems in Chapter 20). These situations were, however, also used to introduce simple behavioural methods to control self-harm and reduce distress such as distraction and self-soothing and to do a little work on changing Anna's help-seeking behaviour. She also learned to disengage from fights with her husband.

Given the need to manage emotions, cognitive dysregulation, and dissociation in most sessions and Anna's overall mental state, there was no opportunity during this phase to reformulate Anna's problems as was done with Madison. This phase also took much longer to navigate. Whereas with Madison, therapy rapidly moved to the control and regulation phase, the transition took much longer with Anna, partly because of the severity of her problems and partly because of situational problems. Anna's personal life circumstances were chaotic and unstable. Her husband's problems increased substantially for reasons unrelated to Anna's difficulties, and conjoint sessions did not prove helpful because her husband needed help himself, which he refused to get. As a result, problems and crises continued for the first eighteen months of therapy. However, despite these issues the alliance increased steadily and during sessions there was little doubt about the level of engagement or commitment to therapy even when she was angry with the therapist.

14.6 Transition to the Regulation and Modulation Phase

The length of the safety, containment, and engagement phases varies substantially from weeks to a year or more, depending on the severity and whether the patient has had previous treatment. With most patients, the frequency of crises gradually decreases in the first few months of treatment although incidents continue to occur and thoughts of self-harm continue even if they are not acted upon. Throughout therapy, a critical decision is when to move to the next phase of treatment and the next domain of impairment. This is not an issue with the safety and containment phases because they are so closely intertwined that it is never necessary to decide when to move from safety to containment. The first time that the therapist faces the question of when to move to the next phase of treatment occurs when considering the transition from containment to the regulation and modulation phase and hence when to begin systematic work on building emotion-regulation capacity. There are no real guidelines for when to make this transition: it is usually a matter of clinical judgement. What usually happens is that within-session distress gradually settles and the alliance flourishes, creating the conditions needed to begin incorporating more specific interventions. The transition is usually smooth because relevant interventions are fairly simple and highly structured such as the distraction and self-soothing methods discussed earlier along with attempts to identify and label emotions, and a brief discussion of sequence of events leading to crises. Although these methods hardly qualify as specific interventions, they pave the way for introducing skill building and related modules to increase emotional control and reduce deliberate self-harm, interventions that require a little more of the patient in terms of commitment and effort.

14.7 Concluding Comments

Although crises and self-harm gradually decrease, problems usually continue to occur for some time albeit in muted form. When such events occur, they need to be taken seriously without overreacting. As with addictions, it is best to concentrate on the occasions when an intense emotional state or deliberate self-harm has been delayed or aborted and on the days in which these events did not occur so that relapses are seen within this broader context rather than viewing each incident as a failure.

Notes

1. Sexton et al. (2005). This study investigated the impact of the psychotherapy process in the first session and the alliance. Although not conducted on personality disordered patients, there is little reason to assume that patients with personality disorder would differ.

2. Sexton et al. (2005).

3. Tyron (1988).

4. Links and Bergmans (2015).

5. See Links and Bergmans (2015) for a thoughtful discussion of crisis management and methods to help patients monitor safety within an integrated treatment approach.

6. See Layden et al. (1993) for a helpful discussion of ways to help patients communicate more effectively in crises. The methods proposed were guided by their recommendations.

7. "Self-efficacy" refers to an individual's belief in his or her capacity to be effective in producing desired results (see Bandura, 1977, 1986), whereas "self-agency" has been defined as the belief that we can influence our environment and produce a response from others (Knox, 2011). These terms are used interchangeably in this volume although it could be argued that self-agency as used by Knox is a somewhat broader conception. However, these terms are used in the narrower way as defined in the text.

8. Links and Bergmans (2015).

9. Klonsky (2007), Kemperman et al. (1997), Suyemoto (1998).

10. Swenson (1989).

11. Davidson (2008) makes the point that formulation as she conceptualizes it within a cognitive therapy model is very useful in containing suicidality, self-harm, and emotionality and in helping the patient to settle into treatment.

Introduction

The three chapters in this section present an eclectic array of strategies and interventions for improving the capacity to regulate, organize, and modulate emotional experience. Until now, efforts to reduce emotionality have relied largely on generic interventions to provide structure, support, and containment. Treatment now makes greater use of specific interventions drawn from diverse treatment models. Nevertheless, expansion of the therapeutic focus and treatment methods occurs within the structure established by the general modules. Generic interventions continue to be important but they now take second stage to specific methods unless the alliance, motivation, or self-reflection falters, when they again assume priority.

The first chapter, Chapter 15, sets the stage for treating emotional dysregulation by considering the part emotion plays in adaptive functioning and how emotional regulation develops. This information is used to establish the general goals for this phase of therapy and the interventions needed to achieve them. Interventions are organized into four modules: (i) patient education, (ii) building emotional awareness, (iii) developing emotion-regulating skills and strategies, and (iv) enhancing emotion-processing capacity. Chapter 16 describes the first three modules and Chapter 17 describes methods to enhance emotional processing capacity, an important issue that is often neglected.

Chapter 15

General Principles for Improving Emotional Stability

Unstable emotions dominate patients' thoughts, behaviour, and experience. A more regulated and nuanced expression of emotion is necessary to provide the stability needed to treat other aspects of borderline personality disorder (BPD) and provide long-term stability. Thus success in increasing emotional regulation is a crucial change that governs overall rate of progress and determines ultimate outcome.

Emotion regulation is the ability to control the occurrence, intensity, experience, and expression of emotions.[1] This requires skills in monitoring, appraising, and modulating emotional responses.[2] This phase of treatment seeks to develop these abilities. However, in order to divide this broad goal into specific therapeutic tasks and identify suitable interventions, we need to understand the purpose of emotions, their role in adaptive behaviour, and how emotions are regulated.

15.1 What Do Emotions Do?

Emotions are crucial to organizing our experience of reality, regulating behaviour, guiding social interaction, and constructing an understanding of ourselves. Emotions are a rich source of information: they give meaning to experience by telling us what is important and what is not, what should be feared and avoided, and what is desirable and should be sought. Without them, the world would appear bland and nothing would stand out. The informational function of emotion was illustrated by the earlier discussion of anxiousness (Chapter 3) where it was noted that the anxiety aroused by the threat system tells us that something is wrong that needs our attention. With BPD, the constant heightened state of emotional arousal means that much of the informational value of emotions is lost. Since the same intense and diffuse emotions are aroused in many situations, they provide little useful information other than to indicate that something is wrong.

Emotions also direct our behaviour and help us to deal with situations: they tell us what to do, set priorities, and organize our actions. Worry or stress, for example, influence our thoughts and actions in various ways. We ponder on the problem, seek comfort from a loved one, turn to a friend for advice, or even withdraw within ourselves.

Emotions are also used to establish long-term goals such as pursuing an interest or deciding on a career. Such goals are not established using a rational process. Rather, the idea often springs to mind fully formed. Only then does rational thinking take over to evaluate the goal, establish an action plan, and appraise subsequent progress towards goal attainment. However, emotion initiates and guides the process. In a sense, emotions establish the problems, goals, and tasks for rational thinking to solve.[3] This means that we need to be aware of our emotions and not allow them to overwhelm our thinking capacity. The clearer we are about our emotions, the more accessible they are, and the more they are integrated with the rest of our experience, the clearer we will be about our wants, goals, and personal concerns. This is why patients with BPD have difficulty setting goals. Uncertainty and distrust of basic emotions and the sheer intensity of emotions reduce their information value. At the same time, the energy needed to deal with intense feelings leaves few resources for goal setting and even less for sustaining goal-directed activity. And, even if goals are set, they often change with fluctuations in emotional state and are rarely attained.

If we are healthy and adapted, emotion, thought, and action work together seamlessly. Emotions are integrated into our experience of ourselves and our lives and become part of who we are. This does not occur to the same degree for people with BPD. Intense and fragmented emotions are difficult to integrate with the rest of the personality. Instead of informing the sense of self, emotion dominates self-experience, contributing to its fragmentation. Therapy seeks to correct this situation by integrating emotions with reason and into an overall understanding of self.

15.2 How Emotional Regulation Develops

If our emotions are to provide useful information about ourselves and our world and guide our action, we need to self-regulate emotion so that it is not overwhelming. From early infancy onwards, we learn multiple ways to do this. Philosophical treaties often distinguish between *feelings* and *emotions*.[4] This distinction is useful in understanding how emotions are regulated and what we need to do in treatment. Feelings are the physiological sensations associated with emotions whereas emotions are the cognitive understanding of these sensations. The cognitive elaboration of feelings gives meaning and structure to experience and changes feelings into emotions. This is what we do in therapy. We help patients to understand and thereby organize their emotional experiences.

The gradual process of transforming feelings into emotions begins with the actions of caregivers who intuitively know why the infant is upset and respond appropriately by feeding, changing, or soothing the infant as needed (see Figure 15.1). Here, the caregiver acts as an external regulator of the infant's emotional state. As the infant matures and cognitive functions develop, the soothing actions and qualities of caregivers are internalized so that the child learns to self-soothe, a development that supplements other

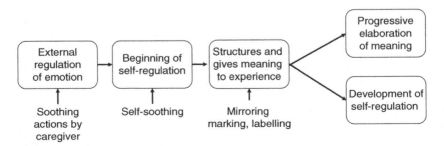

Figure 15.1 Development of Self-Regulation on Emotions

self-soothing actions such as thumb-sucking and crying to gain care and attention. Something similar happens in therapy: the therapist uses containment interventions to settle and soothe distress, which are gradually internalized to create self-soothing skills.

The next step in the process is for the caregiver to help the infant to organize experience by identifying and labelling feelings. This is done by mirroring and marking the infant's feelings in a slightly exaggerated way. Sensitive caregivers constantly say things like: "Who's a happy boy?" "Why are you so angry, Didi?" "Isn't this fun, Saleh?" "Did something scare my little darling?" Such comments help to transform what William James characterized as the "big booming confusion" that he assumed was the infant's experience into a coherent pattern of emotions such as anger or joy. Labelling develops the child's awareness and supplies meaning to experience. It also conveys understanding and acceptance of the feelings involved. This is also internalized, leading to the self-acceptance needed for self-regulation.

As cognitive functions mature, emotional schemas are formed, which progressively organize experience and enable emotions to be used in organizing interactions with the world. Like all schemas, emotional schemas consist of beliefs, expectations, rules, and values and associated memories and sensations that form an acquired body of *knowledge* about the emotion and its effects. Schemas also contain an *appraisal* component that evaluates the emotion and its value and effects along with the individual's capacity to manage the emotion and the situation that evoked it. These developments give additional meaning to emotional experiences, which forms an additional level of self-regulation. The process continues throughout development as cognitive functions mature and self-reflective capacity develops. Links are established among schemas, leading to the final stage of self-regulation – the formation of complex schemas and narratives that regulate emotional experience and integrate it with other aspects of adaptive functioning, an issue that will be considered further in Chapter 17.

The cognitive elaboration of emotion is paralleled with the acquisition of emotion-regulating skills and behaviours that extend self-soothing capacity. These include distraction; avoidance; refocusing of attention away from emotions and emotional events or memories; social behaviours for seeking help, soothing, and support; and communication of emotional distress.

Most aspects of emotional regulation are impaired in BPD. There are problems identifying and labelling feelings. Certainty about basic feelings and emotions is undermined by self-invalidating thinking, leading to patients treating their own experiences as invalid. Maladaptive emotional schemas are formed that fail to organize emotional experiences adaptively and may increase distress. The appraisal component of emotional schemas is invariably negative, consisting of beliefs about adverse consequences of emotions and the patient's inability to manage them, and assumptions that negative emotions are best avoided. These schemas escalate emotional distress and encourage maladaptive emotional expression. Consequently, most patients are anxious to "get rid" of their emotions rather than learn to understand and use them. Finally, emotions are not effectively integrated with other aspects of behaviour, and the higher-order meaning systems and narratives constructed around emotions often hinder adaptive functioning. Effective treatment of emotional dysregulation requires a broad range of interventions to address these diverse problems.

15.3 General Plan for Treating Emotional Dysregulation

In Chapter 3, it was suggested that unstable emotions are linked to anxiousness and emotional lability – a distinction that is useful in helping patients to identify their feelings accurately and selecting interventions. It was also noted that patients tend to "fuse" with intense emotions, so these feelings come to define the self, and that dysregulated emotions lead to an intense self-focus, narrowing of attention, and limited awareness of both the specific emotions involved and the situational factors that contribute to them. These ideas, along with an understanding of the functions of emotion and how emotion regulation develops, are the basis for an overall treatment strategy.

15.3.1 Structure and Sequence of Treatment

The natural progression in the acquisition of emotion regulation in therapy is represented schematically in Figure 15.2. First, the intense and disorganized nature of emotions needs to be reduced by containment by the therapist and then by self-soothing. Second, feelings are identified and labelled. Third, increased awareness of emotional experiences is developed through the cognitive elaboration of the emotion within a relationship that facilitates emotional acceptance and tolerance. In the process, schemas associated with each emotion are explored and restructured. These factors add an additional dimension to emotion regulation that generally contributes to a further settling of distress. Identification and awareness are not independent but rather interwoven because labelling is not possible without awareness.

The fourth step is to learn emotion-regulating skills and strategies. This requires a modest level of within-session stability because it is difficult to give attention and time to learning specific tasks when threatened by overwhelming emotions. This step leads to greater emotional control that makes it possible to focus on the final step of enhancing the way emotions are processed. This involves creating more flexibility in the arousal and expression of emotions, encouraging greater experience of positive emotions, integrating emotions and thinking, and developing higher-order meaning systems and narratives to organize emotional experiences and integrate them with other aspects of adaptive behaviour. This sequence represents the continuous cognitive elaboration of emotions, a process that underlies the acquisition of emotional self-regulation.

This sequence suggests that the broad goal of enhancing emotion regulation devolves into four specific goals: (i) increase knowledge about emotions and emotional dysregulation, (ii) increase awareness of emotional experience, (iii) learn emotion-regulating skills and strategies, and (iv) increase emotional processing capacity. Each goal is associated with a specific module and hence a specific set of sub-modules and interventions. The complexity of these goals requires a multifaceted approach that may include the use of medication to help settle emotional reactivity and facilitate psychotherapeutic interventions.

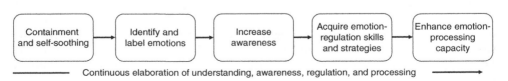

Figure 15.2 Steps in the Treatment of Emotional Dysregulation

15.3.2 Specific Treatment Modules

Four specific modules are proposed to treat the various facets of emotion dysregulation:[5]

1. Patient education: This module provides information about the nature of emotional dysregulation and emotions, the adaptive origins of emotions, the way emotions affect thought and action, and the role of emotions in everyday behaviour and normal personality functioning.
2. Awareness: The module seeks to increase awareness, recognition, and acceptance of emotions by identifying and labelling emotions, developing the ability to track the flow of emotional experience, and increasing awareness by recognizing and modulating emotional avoidance.
3. Self-regulation: This module focuses on learning emotion-regulating skills and strategies to self-manage the intensity and consequences of emotional arousal.
4. Emotion-processing module: The intent is to develop an understanding of the way emotions are processed and enhance the capacity to reflect on emotions and their consequences. The module is also concerned with developing higher-order meaning systems and narratives that provide an additional level to the self-management of emotions and allow emotions to serve an adaptive function.

A practical issue is whether modules should be delivered as discrete packages using a predetermined number of sessions or whether the interventions should be incorporated into the therapeutic process as the opportunity presents. Both methods are used in treating personality disorder although my preference is to integrate these modules into the overall process.

15.3.3 Role of General Treatment Modules

The progressive incorporation of specific interventions into treatment does not mean that the general treatment modules no longer have a role. They continue to be important in maintaining the therapeutic process needed to implement specific intervention modules because specific modules are used only when there is a satisfactory alliance and a motivated patient. Improvements in emotional self-regulation are also dependent on reflecting on the nature, origins, and consequences of emotional arousal. Validation also tends to increase emotional control and it can be used throughout treatment to manage emotional arousal.[6]

Throughout therapy, the general and specific components of treatment operate in parallel. The general modules form the matrix into which specific interventions are woven. Successful implementation of a specific intervention is then used to enhance the alliance and motivation. Hence general and specific treatment modules support and reinforce each other. It is this combination and the interplay between them that make therapy effective.

15.4 Concluding Comments

The treatment of emotional dysregulation illustrates the value of a trans-theoretical approach. The wide-ranging problems associated with unstable emotions suggest that comprehensive treatment requires the use of an eclectic set of interventions. It also suggests the important point that it is not sufficient to focus exclusively on building emotion-regulation skills. Attention also has to be given to building emotion-processing capacity to enable patients to express emotions in a modulated and nuanced way rather that gushing out in ways that are unhelpful and overwhelming – a development that restores the adaptive value of emotions.

The general approach proposed involves an approximate sequence for facilitating the development of emotion-regulating abilities. Although there is a general progression based on the way emotion regulation normally develops, the sequence is largely intended to be a heuristic for thinking about the therapeutic tasks of this phase. Most interventions address several issues and the process of therapy moves fluidly between promoting awareness and developing regulatory skills.

Notes

1. Gross and Thompson (2007).

2. Nolen-Hoeksema (2012).

3. Greenberg and Paivio (1997), Damasio (1994).

4. Stanghellini and Rosfort (2013).

5. For more details of the rationale for a modular approach to treating unstable emotions, see Livesley (2015).

6. Research shows that individuals who receive validating responses while completing stressor tasks experience significantly less emotional reactivity than individuals who did not (Shenk and Fruzzetti, 2011).

Chapter 16

Building Emotional Stability
Patient Education, Awareness, and Emotion-Regulation Modules

The previous chapter outlined the overall strategy of treating emotional dysregulation using four specific treatment modules. This chapter describes the first three modules: patient education, awareness, and increasing self-regulatory skills.

16.1 Patient Education Module

Providing information about the disorder is important because most patients are poorly informed about their condition.[1] Some general information is provided when establishing the treatment contract (see Chapter 6) and managing crises (Chapter 13) but more information is now required about emotions and emotional dysregulation. The following topics outline what needs to be explained and discussed during this phase.

   1. Emotions are adaptive: Many patients consider emotions as threatening or dangerous and hence they do not realize that emotions are an inherent part of human nature rather than harmful things that they need to "get rid of" or that emotions play a crucial role in responding adaptively to events. Examples that can be provided are how anxiety and anger alert us to important events that we need to deal with.

   2. Emotions have a genetic basis: An understanding that emotions are adaptive and have a genetic basis helps to build tolerance and acceptance and reduce self-criticism.

   3. Emotions provide information about the world and organize our experience of reality: Emotions tell us what is frightening and to be avoided, what is pleasant and should be sought out, and what is interesting and should be pursued. It is useful for patients to understand how intense and persistent emotions undermine the informational value of emotions and that an important treatment task is to reinstate the informational value of emotions by enhancing the ability to self-regulate emotions.

   4. Emotions are important in setting goals and regulating behaviour: Since emotions tell us what is interesting and valuable, they help us to set goals and direct our efforts to attain them. Without this information it is difficult to establish major goals and long-term interests.

   5. Emotions are crucial to effective social interaction: Our feelings are important sources of information about other people and guide our interaction with them.

   6. Emotions are integral to our sense of self: Our feelings are part of who we are: they organize an understanding of ourselves and our place in the world.

   Besides information about the value and function of emotions and the part they play in adaption, patients also need information on the following aspects of emotional dysregulation. Although much of this information was probably discussed at various times earlier in treatment, it is useful at this time to work through this information again to ensure the patient understands the following points: (i) the nature of emotional dysregulation, especially how a complex mixture of feelings contribute to their emotional states and the value of unpacking these states to identify specific emotions involved; (ii) impact of intense emotions on thinking and information processing and the way strong emotions undermine cognitive control over feeling; and (iii) the sequence of emotional arousal involving the sequence of triggering event → emotion → responses to emotion.

The module is not intended to be delivered within a fixed time period or through a designated number of sessions. Rather, information is imparted gradually as different aspects of the patient's emotional life become the focus of treatment to avoid overwhelming patients who are vulnerable to information overload.

16.2 Awareness Module

The awareness module has four sub-modules: (i) recognizing and labelling emotions, (ii) tracking emotions and responses to them, (iii) developing moment-by-moment awareness of emotions, and (iv) promoting emotion acceptance. The goal is to help the patient to progress along the sequence of an intense self-focus→self-awareness→self-reflection.

16.2.1 Recognizing Emotions

Undifferentiated emotions are difficult to control. We need to be able to recognize, identify, and label emotions before we can control them. When we put a label on something, we feel that we understand it better, which gives us a sense of being in control. Thus, labelling helps to structure emotional experiences and to distance the person from his or her emotions. This promotes self-observation and self-reflection and reduces the tendency to "fuse" with emotions.

16.2.1.1 Decomposing Global Emotional Experiences

Identification of emotions requires the decomposition of global states into specific components. Most patients are not aware of the complexity of their emotional states and often simplify their experiences by focusing on the most obvious or least painful feelings present. Although identification of emotions is sometimes taught as a specific exercise with a set workbook, it is often best to make it part of the general flow of therapy because this allows the therapist to deal with emotion avoidance, provide support and containment if feelings threaten to be overwhelming, and validate feelings as they are recognized, which has the added benefit of strengthening the aspect of the self described earlier as the self as knower.

16.2.1.2 Specific Emotions and Emotion Regulation

Decomposing global states is also useful because different emotions are often managed somewhat differently.[2] For example, differentiating anxiety from general emotional distress is helpful because general distress is best managed initially through self-soothing whereas with anxiety it is also useful to modify fear arousal by changing the way threatening situations are perceived, by building confidence in the ability to manage threats, and by teaching specific anxiety management skills. A recent crisis often provides an opportunity to help patients to differentiate feelings of anxiety and threat from more global distress. This distinction is useful because many patients (and clinicians) focus on emotional lability and neglect the intense panicky fearfulness that also contributes to dysphoric states.

With emotions such as shame, sadness, and hurt, the main task is to access them rather than regulate them because they are often suppressed and masked by more reactive emotions such as anger. This is often the case with those who have been abused. Bringing these emotions into awareness helps the patient to process them rather than suppress them and to work through the issues involved. The experience of positive emotions such as joy, interest, enthusiasm, love, and contentment often results from regulating and resolving intense negative emotions. Whenever positive emotions occur, they need to be nurtured and strengthened so that they become an increasing part of the patient's emotional life because most patients do not know how to play or to experience joy and contentment.

16.2.2 Observing and Tracking the Flow of Emotions and Their Consequences

Having begun to identify emotions accurately, the next step is to learn to observe the flow of emotions and their consequences: the antecedents (triggering events)–responses (thoughts, emotions, behaviours)–consequences structure discussed earlier. The first step is to identify the emotional trigger. Since many patients maintain that their feelings occur for no apparent reason, identification of triggers changes this belief and enables patients to use self-regulation techniques such as self-soothing before their emotions become overwhelming. Subsequently, patients are helped to track the effect of the emotions aroused on subsequent thoughts, other emotions besides the initial emotion, and actions.

Attention is also drawn to thoughts and actions that increase distress without the patient realizing it. Many engage in negative self-talk: they criticise themselves, ruminate, or catastrophize, which increases emotional arousal. For example, one patient talked to herself when in a rage. Although she did not say anything aloud her lips moved as if she was engaged in an intense exchange. When the therapist drew her attention to it, she was surprised because she was not aware of what she was doing or how it fed her anger. The incident illustrates the intensity of the focus on inner experience during these states and the almost total lack of awareness of anything else.

The emotions activated by an initial trigger often arouse other emotions such as fearfulness and anxiety not only about the event but also about the feelings it aroused. Many patients are almost phobic about their negative emotions. These "secondary emotions" create a vicious cycle that adds to the urgency to terminate the distress, which leads to self-injury. Finally, it is useful to explore the short-term and long-term effects of emotions and responses to them. Most patients recognize the short-term benefits of actions such as deliberate self-injury that are self-reinforcing because they reduce distress or how their rage gives a temporary sense of being in control. However, they often fail to recognize the long-term impact of these behaviours on their well-being and on how other people treat them.

Tracking the flow of emotions and their effects in this way helps to organize emotional experiences by making them part of a chain of events that may not have been fully recognized. It begins to give meaning and structure to experiences that often seem to the person to be chaotic and disorganized.

16.2.3 Promoting Present-Focused Non-Judgemental Awareness

To be adaptive, emotions need to be integrated into awareness. Problems arise when emotions are suppressed or avoided. Increased emotional control depends on the development of moment-to-moment awareness of emotional experiences.[3] The core skill is to observe emotional reactions in a non-judgemental way. This is not something most patients do. They focus on how distressed they are but not on the nuances of their experience, and they are extremely judgemental about the experience, criticizing themselves for being this way and ruminating about how unfair it is to have such problems.

Present-focused awareness is helpful because initial emotional responses to events are often useful, for example, feeling fear in response to a threat,[4] but subsequent reactions are often more judgemental and self-critical. Hence it is important to distinguish the initial emotion from the subsequent cascade of other emotions and reactions. Recognition of the usefulness of initial emotional reactions reinforces earlier information on the adaptive functions of emotions and begins to build tolerance and self-compassion. The task is to help patients to attend to these reactions and observe the flow of inner experience without evaluating it.

Since it is difficult for patients to tease out the different emotional, cognitive, and behavioural responses to emotional triggers, it helps to explore specific scenarios that evoked strong emotions. Talking about the event and the feelings it activated encourages a more detached way of observing what happened rather than simply reliving the event. This can be promoted with the open-ended questions used to encourage the self-reflective mode discussed in Chapter 11. For example, "What was it about the event that caused you to react in this way?" "What was your initial reaction?" and so on.

Many therapies stress the value of mindfulness exercises in promoting present-focused awareness and it may be useful to include these interventions as a sub-module at this point[5] both to promote this ability and to help control ruminative tendencies. Many patients with borderline personality disorder (BPD) brood about the wrongs, humiliations, and rejections they have suffered at the hands of others both in the immediate and in the distant past. These ruminations strongly influence emotional arousal and reactions. The evidence suggests that mindfulness-based interventions are helpful in treating these problems and building present-focused awareness. As with identification of emotions, mindfulness is often taught as a separate exercise with a fixed number of sessions. While this is often useful, it is also often helpful to incorporate mindfulness into the treatment process. When treating BPD, the collaborative process involved in teaching and learning skills is often as helpful as the skills themselves. Since, a present-focused awareness depends in part on being able to identify and track emotions, mindfulness is best introduced when the patient has made progress in these areas.

16.2.4 Increasing Acceptance

Awareness of emotional experiences is hindered by the difficulty many patients have in accepting their emotions without self-criticism and in tolerating even modest levels of negative feelings. Acceptance and tolerance are important because the activation of emotions is automatic and outside our control. What we can control is what happens next: we can self-regulate the intensity of our emotional responses and how we respond to them. This requires that we accept our emotions rather than trying to avoid or suppress them and that we learn to tolerate distress long enough to begin to implement self-regulation skills and strategies.

Tolerance and acceptance are promoted by encouraging patients to examine and hold negative emotions as they occur in therapy. Although patients often seek to avoid such feelings and promptly suppress them when they occur, they often reveal their feelings fleetingly by changes in facial expression and other non-verbal responses that can be used to focus the patient's attention on these transient states. Monitoring the eyes is a particularly useful way to pick up signs of fleeting emotions. The treatment relationships can then be used to help the patient to tolerate these feelings. Tolerance is also built by the patient internalizing and modelling the therapist's empathic and non-judgemental response to his/her emotions. It is also increased by the therapist's capacity to handle intense feelings. A calm response tells the patient that the therapist is not alarmed by the patient's feelings. This occurred with Anna. As described in Chapter 14, Anna found that the therapist's calm acceptance and preparedness to discuss her distress helped her to manage her feelings better so that she gradually came to accept that she too need not be alarmed by these feelings.

16.2.5 Managing Avoidance

Emotional awareness is also hindered by cognitive and behavioural strategies to suppress feelings and avoid situations that activate them. As with self-talk, patients are often unaware of these behaviours. The problem can be managed by drawing the patient's attention to an event in therapy in which he/she avoided dealing with painful feelings. Patients vary in their awareness of avoidant behaviour. Some clearly recognize that they act in this way although they may not always recognize all instances but others are almost totally oblivious. Identification of the broad pattern helps the patient to see links among behaviours that may seem to be unrelated. Recognition may be facilitated by discussing how emotions are suppressed or avoided so that an educational component is integrated into the process.

Subsequently, the patient is encouraged to identify other examples both in therapy and in everyday situations. Some patients find it helpful to construct a list of avoidance behaviours such as rapidly changing topic when emotions begin to emerge, distracting behaviours, or avoiding eye contact, and specific cognitive avoidance strategies such as deliberate suppression of feelings, self-reassurance, or focusing on positive things. In most instances, it is sufficient simply to draw the patient's attention to his/her avoidant response. At other times, however, it is also necessary to address fears and concerns that motivate avoidance, a process akin to the defence interpretations of psychodynamic therapy in which attention is drawn to an avoidant response and anxieties that motivated the avoidance such as fear of losing control or guilt.

Patients also need information on the long-term consequences of avoidance, most notably how it limits self-understanding and perpetuates distress by hindering self-regulation – it is only possible to control feelings effectively if they are fully recognized and accepted. Their preparedness to reduce avoidance may also be increased by noting that suppression and avoidance do not work in the long term: suppressed and avoided feelings do not go away and often emerge more powerful than before.

16.3 Emotional Regulation Module

This module focuses on developing specific skills needed to self-regulate emotions. Multiple interventions are available for this purpose. A major accomplishment in developing treatments for BPD is the development of effective ways to increase emotion regulation. With integrated modular treatment (IMT), therapists are free to select any method that is congenial to their style of working. Here a limited array of relatively straightforward and commonly used methods are discussed. Although a wide range of methods are available that differ in complexity, with most patients, using a few methods judiciously in combination with the general strategies is often all that is needed.

16.3.1 Self-Soothing and Distraction

The use of self-soothing and distraction was briefly considered as a useful way to deal with acute distress and deliberate self-injury until other methods are acquired. Both self-soothing and distraction are useful first steps towards improving emotion regulation because they are probably used routinely by most patients and hence they are easily understood and applied. Any success in reducing distress can then be used to promote self-efficacy by showing that these feelings can be controlled. Both are only effective if used in the early stages of emotional arousal which is why it is important to help patients identify emotional triggers and be more aware of their emotions so that they recognize the early signs that something is wrong and take steps to manage emotions before they escalate.

An extension of encouraging self-soothing is to promote self-nurturance generally. Patients with BPD are often remarkably self-neglectful and show little respect or compassion towards themselves. They neglect themselves in many ways including nutrition, exercise, sleep, and relaxation and they often do not allow themselves to do things they enjoy. An active discussion of these matters with regular follow-up and review is a practical way to model concern and an interest in the patient's well-being.

16.3.2 Encouraging Incompatible Emotions

Negative emotions and moods can also be regulated especially in the early phases of arousal by deliberately inducing incompatible emotions and moods.[6] To take an extreme example, laughter is incompatible with feeling sad so that activities that promote laughter such as watching a funny movie may help to control mild feelings of sadness. Moods may be induced in different ways. Many of the activities used to self-soothe can be used for this purpose such as listening to pleasant music. However, it is often necessary to do something that involves more intense emotional stimulation such as watching an intense movie or spending time with people who are intensely engaged in a task. Looking after someone or helping another person also tends to engender different feelings, which is perhaps another reason why so many patients with BPD like looking after others or caring for animals. This method is only modestly effective and then in the early stages of emotional arousal. Nevertheless, it is another activity that patients can keep in mind.

16.3.3 Reducing Escalating Thoughts

Previously reference has been made to the tendency to think in ways that exacerbate distress so that a useful way to manage is to restructure these thoughts. Sometimes the problem is simply that the labels and interpretations that are applied to emotions add to distress. Thus one patient told herself that she was "falling apart" whenever she felt even a modest level of any negative emotion. She acted on this belief by assuming a fetal posture and hugged herself as if she were holding herself together. Things began to improve when she abandoned the "falling apart" label in favour of labelling the actual emotions she was experiencing and began to rate their intensity. It is common for patients to tell themselves their feelings are intolerable, that they cannot stand them any longer, or that if the feelings continue they will have to kill themselves. Simply drawing attention to this kind of self-talk and the way it increases negative feelings often helps to modulate its effects. Patients should also be taught to challenge and dispute these thoughts.

Many of these thoughts are linked to the tendency to expect the worst with catastrophic expectations that centre on fears of rejection or loss of significant others. As a result, minor interpersonal disagreements are rapidly assumed to be likely to result in the end of the relationship or someone who is a little late returning home is assumed to have been involved in a serious accident. It is useful to help patients to recognize catastrophizing as a general thinking style and then teach them to argue with themselves about their beliefs and to examine the evidence for and against a given belief. Disputing with oneself is one of the most useful cognitive techniques for patients to learn. Most readily adopt the idea although most patients initially forget to use the techniques so that frequent reminders and within-session practices are needed before it becomes an established way to deal with catastrophic thinking. Cognitive techniques are discussed further in Chapter 20, which deals with methods to change maladaptive schemas.

16.3.4 Relaxation

Although relaxation exercises are useful in managing a variety of negative emotions, they are particularly useful in treating the anxious element of emotional instability. However, it is best to use a simple method such as breath training. Other methods such as systematic relaxation are too complex for treating BPD especially when patients are unstable because these methods require too much effort and energy to learn and use. As noted when discussing motivation (Chapter 12), the effort to control intense emotions depletes the resources needed to learn and use complex exercises.

Breath training involves sitting or lying in a quiet place and taking a deep breath through the nose and allowing the abdomen to expand fully and then breathing out. When breathing out, patients can be instructed to say simple word like calm or relax and to let themselves go loose. Over time, the word becomes a conditioned stimulus that initiates relaxation. The method is easily learned and usually produces immediate benefits. It is also useful because breathing patterns can be disrupted by intense emotion, leading patients to hold their breath or hyperventilate. Since attention to breathing focuses attention on current sensations, it disrupts rumination and a preoccupation with inner experience and hence it is often useful to combine relaxation with grounding exercises. Breath training also tends not to evoke fear of losing control that can occur with other relaxation methods. When teaching the exercise in-session, relaxation can be introduced as a way to counter anxiety and that like all skills practice leads to improvement.

An advantage of this form of relaxation is that it can be used in everyday situations to manage feelings such as anxiety, fear, assumed slights, and anger without other people realizing that the person is practising relaxation. Anna used this method to control her anger with her husband without him knowing. Like grounding, it can also be taught to significant others who can then help the patient to use the exercise when they notice that he/she is becoming distressed. This also involves significant others in the patient's treatment, which often makes them more supportive.

16.3.5 Grounding

Patients who dissociate when intensely distressed or experience depersonalization or derealization are often helped by interventions that force them to attend to external stimuli rather than to painful thoughts, feelings, and memories. In these states, intense anxiety causes a preoccupation with inner experience that leads to further distress. This escalating sequence can be disrupted by getting the patient to focus on external stimuli and their surroundings.

In therapy, simple methods such as getting the patient to focus on the therapist may be sufficient to limit dissociation in its early stages. However, other techniques are often needed that increase the focus on current sensations. Simple acts such as placing one's feet firmly on the ground, feeling a solid object such as the arms of the chair, concentrating on specific objects in the immediate surroundings, and increasing diaphragmatic breathing by placing one's arms around the back of the chair substantially increase sensory input that counters the focus on inner experience.

This simple intervention works well with most patients. However, those with severe dissociative tendencies may require additional steps to increase external stimulation. For example, with one patient who sometimes dissociated when driving due to flashbacks, the most effective method was for her to stop her car in a safe place and stand on one leg on the passenger side with a hand just touching the top of the car. Being forced to concentrate on balancing in this way and hence on proprioceptive stimuli countered the pull of traumatic memories. With severe episodes, it also helped to say aloud the colours of the cars that went by. This exercise gave her some control over the dissociation until other methods were used to deal with the trauma. Initially, it was necessary for the therapist to talk her through the exercise over the phone but later she was able to do it without assistance.

The exercise is best introduced in a session when the patient begins to dissociate or describes a recent dissociative experience. Used in this way the exercise is a useful way to promote collaboration and any success is readily used to build the alliance and self-agency by showing in-session that these feelings can be controlled. Since success depends on a good alliance, the exercise should not be introduced when rapport is impaired.

Grounding is also something that can be taught to significant others or friends who can remind the patient of what to do when he or she feels overwhelmed. Significant others usually do not know what to do when the patient dissociates and hence tend to get caught up in the patient's panic.

16.3.6 Attention Training and Desensitizing Emotional Stimuli

An important aspect of emotion regulation is the ability to shift attention from emotionally arousing thoughts and images. Most patients cannot do this and hence they ruminate over wrongs that they have suffered and mistakes that they have made, which increases their distress. At the same time, the inability to shift attention reinforces beliefs about being unable to control their feelings. A simple extension of breath training is to ask the patient to also focus on a pleasant thought or scene. Once this skill is established, patients can be encouraged to use this to divert attention from ruminative thoughts. This is best done initially in-session so that the therapist can talk the patient through the exercise and help him/her to switch attention from the intrusive thought to the pleasant stimulus.

This technique is also useful in desensitizing specific emotional triggers such as intrusive images or memories associated with trauma experiences. For example, one of Anna's abusers had an unusual physical feature. Seeing someone with a similar feature caused her to panic and dissociate. With other patients, the trigger may be a traumatic memory, words or phrases used by an abuser, or a specific event. Anna had previously learned to practise relaxation while focusing on a pleasant scene that involved lying on a beach, feeling the warmth of the sun, and listening to the waves. In-session, she was asked to relax and visualize the pleasant scene. When relaxed, she was asked to imagine a man with this feature. The therapist observed her reactions and, when she began to experience anxiety, she was asked to shift her attention back to the pleasant scene. Initially, the therapist asked her to shift attention as soon as she became anxious to ensure that she was successful and talked her through the relaxation and visualization. When relaxation occurs, the cycle is repeated. When the exercise is first introduced, it is useful to complete three or four switches. On subsequent occasions, the time Anna was asked to tolerate anxiety was gradually increased until she was able to imagine someone with this feature without reacting to it.

The exercise is a version of systematic desensitization.[7] Systematic desensitization seeks to extinguish the fear evoked by a specific stimulus by presenting a low level of intensity of the stimulus while encouraging relaxation. More typical desensitization may be needed with more complex emotional triggers. For example, one patient was recurrently troubled by memories of a sexual assault that occurred in her mid-teens. The incident occurred when dusk was falling one winter evening when she was home alone. The doorbell rang and looking through the window she could see it was a neighbour. He tried to force his way in and she recalled his arm coming around the door. Later, at times of emotional instability she experienced anxiety at dusk and for a while she did not leave home at dusk, and while at home, memories of the incident caused her to dissociate. A hierarchy of stimuli was constructed as with systematic desensitization consisting of dusk, the doorbell ringing, and the arm coming around the door. Each was desensitized using this procedure.

An important feature of these kinds of exercises is that they have multiple effects. Besides desensitizing specific emotional stimuli, this exercise also enhances attention control, increases distress tolerance, and builds self-efficacy by demonstrating that emotions can be controlled.

16.3.7 Managing Hypersensitivity

Discussion of borderline traits in Chapter 3 noted that hypersensitivity to all kinds of stimulation increases emotional and interpersonal problems. The trait may be managed with low doses of a neuroleptic, for example, 0.25–0.5 mg of risperidone or 25 mg of quetiapine, as was prescribed for Anna. If a low dose is not effective, it is probably best to use other strategies to manage this problem because higher doses of neuroleptics can be sedating, which interferes with the cognitive processes needed to achieve emotional control.[8]

Regardless of the effects of medication, it is also useful to teach patients how to modulate their hypersensitivity using behavioural methods. It usually helps patients to understand how they are more sensitive to stimulation than other people. Sometimes the metaphor of not having a skin so that comments, criticisms, and barbs get through to them helps them to understand the problem.

No single intervention seems especially effective but it is usually possible to find a combination of simple things that can reduce sensitivity. When relaxation skills are well developed, it may be possible to respond to interpersonal barbs by practising relaxation. At the same time, the personal impact of such comments can be reduced by asking what could be happening in the mind or life of the other person to cause him/her to behave in this way. This diverts attention away from the self and makes the hurtful comment into a problem that the other person has, which may reduce the patient's tendency to take the comment personally. Together such simple techniques slow down the patient's reactions, which is often sufficient to avoid further escalation.

Another simple technique is to use the metaphor of not having a skin and of putting on an additional skin in the form of a rainproof or sou'wester so that comments run off like water off a duck's back. Patients who use a lot of visual imagery find this useful. They literally visualize themselves putting on a waterproof garment when someone is critical and imagining the comment running off. For example, one hypersensitive patient living in an institutional setting frequently got into angry exchanges with others, which precipitated suicidal crises triggered by a simple comment or jab. She learned to deal with the problem by first using relaxation to reduce her anxiety before leaving her room, which reduced her hypersensitivity, and then imagined putting on a bright yellow rainproof and walking out and things simply running off her.

16.4 Incorporating a Trauma Module

This phase of therapy is an appropriate time to consider incorporating a trauma module for patients with BPD and post-traumatic stress disorder (PTSD) because these patients have poorer outcomes than those without.[9] However, there has been some debate in the literature as to the optimal time to introduce treatment of co-occurring PTSD because of concerns that a direct focus on past trauma could be destabilizing and precipitate crises and suicidal or self-harming behaviour.[10] Clinical observations also suggest that early exploration of trauma, especially childhood sexual abuse, can be destabilizing especially for patients with severe BPD and hence that this work should be deferred until a measure of stability has been achieved. However, evidence of the decreased effectiveness of some therapies and a small study which suggested that trauma treatment could be combined with dialectical behaviour therapy (DBT) without adverse consequences[11] suggest that this guideline may need to be reconsidered. The issue is especially pertinent to DBT, which did not incorporate a trauma component in the first stage of therapy which is primarily concerned with teaching emotion-regulating skills. The small pilot study suggests that trauma treatment could in fact be combined with first-stage DBT. However, the authors suggested this should only occur when the patient had not shown serious suicidal or self-harming behaviour for two months. This implies that a reasonable level of stability had been achieved.

Although studies of the timing of trauma interventions have only been based on DBT, the recommendations are consistent with the basic emotion-regulating strategy of IMT, which seeks to regulate the level of emotional arousal within sessions and hence makes minimal use of emotion-activating interventions at least until emotion regulation improves. Hence a trauma module or specific trauma interventions are only used if the patient has been stable for several months as evidenced by more stable emotions and cessation of deliberate self-injury, and when the ability to self-manage emotions has increased. The issues that matter are whether the patient has acquired the capacity to tolerate that additional stress that is likely to be evoked without significant impairment of cognitive functions and a re-occurrence of suicidal and self-harming behaviour.

When the patient has trauma symptoms but does not meet the full criteria for PTSD, it is often sufficient to manage the trauma in the same way as other adverse events are handled, with perhaps the addition of some specific interventions to deal with specific symptoms. What typically happens is that as greater stability is achieved and as emotion-regulation skills develop, work on emotion regulation inevitably touches on trauma and abuse issues that are handled differently than in the containment phase. Rather than simply reflecting and validating these issues, they are now discussed in more depth and the feelings aroused are processed. At the same time, specific emotion-regulating interventions are used to manage level of arousal. Gradually, this work becomes more focused and the depth of discussion increases as the patient's capacity to manage distress develops. This is largely how sexual trauma was managed in the treatment of both Anna and Madison. Although both experienced disruptive memories, they settled with a combination of relaxation, attention-training, limited exploration, and the construction of new narratives about these events. In both cases, work on abuse- and trauma-associated emotions was integrated with the general focus on building emotion regulation.

For patients with the full range of PTSD symptoms, it would seem appropriate to incorporate a specific treatment module to the IMT framework. This would mean that the module would be used within the context provided by the general treatment modules and the general therapeutic stance.

16.5 Concluding Comments

This chapter has discussed a diverse set of interventions drawn from a wide range of therapies that are used to build emotion regulation. The methods described are not intended to be a set protocol to be used with all patients. They are merely suggestions of methods in common use. Therapists should be creative in selecting methods that fit their style of doing therapy and the personality and needs of the patient.

Throughout the chapter I have emphasized that these interventions should not be viewed merely as ways to build a specific aspect of emotional control but also as interventions that have the potential to serve multiple functions. Hence the successful use of any methods should be discussed with patients in ways that ensure that all potential benefits are fully exploited. Successful implementation is used to strengthen generic change mechanisms, especially the alliance, commitment to change, and self-reflection. They should also be used to deal with more specific aspects of borderline pathology including emotional awareness, tolerance, and regulation and to build self-efficacy and self-esteem.

Notes

1. Psychoeducation has not played a large role in the treatment of borderline personality disorder as it has with other disorders; see Ruiz-Sancho et al. (2001), Ridolfi and Gunderson (in press).

2. Greenberg and Paivio (1997).

3. Barlow et al. (2011), Kabat-Zinn (2005a).

4. Barlow et al. (2011).

5. Kabat-Zinn (2005a, 2005b). See Ottavi et al. (2015) for discussion on how to apply mindfulness to the treatment of personality disorder.

6. Davidson (2008), Linehan (1993).

7. Wolpe (1958).

8. See Soloff (2000) for a discussion of a medication strategy that targets specific symptoms of BPD rather than the global disorder. Silk and Friedel (2015) discuss the use of medication within an integrated treatment model.

9. Evidence of a poorer outcome for patients with BPD and post-traumatic stress has only been investigated in patients receiving one year of treatment with DBT (Barnicot and Priebe, 2013).

10. Foa et al. (2009). See also Linehan (1993) who suggested that extensive work on trauma should not occur until self-harming behaviour was under control and patients had been taught emotion-regulating skills.

11. A study with only a small number of subjects suggested that DBT could be combined with trauma therapy without adverse effects earlier than originally recommended (see Harned et al., 2014). See also Robins et al. (in press) for a discussion of this issue in the context of DBT.

Improving Emotional Processing

The previous modules sought to improve emotion-regulating skills and strategies. However, skill building alone is not sufficient. It needs to be supplemented by interventions that enhance emotional processing capacity, restore the informational value of emotions, and integrate emotions with other aspects of personality functioning.[1]

The term "enhance emotional processing" requires explanation. What we need to build is a more nuanced activation and expression of emotions by: (i) developing greater flexibility in how emotional events are interpreted and managed; (ii) integrating emotions with other mental processes so that behaviour is more coherent; and (iii) constructing higher-order meaning systems and narratives that integrate emotions with other personality processes and coordinate and regulate the way emotions are expressed.

Work on enhancing emotional processing begins to change therapy in subtle but important ways. First, less-structured interventions are needed both to restructure emotional schemas that are well-established and central parts of belief systems and to help patients to construct new narratives. Consequently, this chapter deals more with principles than specific interventions. Second, since interpersonal factors loom large in triggering emotion and influencing subsequent action, the focus of treatment becomes increasingly interpersonal and the regulation and modulation phase progressively merges with the exploration and change phase, which is primarily concerned with the interpersonal domain.

17.1 Enhancing Flexibility in Emotional Responses

The rigidity that is a prominent feature of borderline personality disorder (BPD) extends to the expression and processing of emotions. Emotional expression tends to lack flexibility and subtly is partly due to the intensity of emotions – it is difficult to be flexible when feelings are overwhelming – and partly due to the impact of maladaptive schemas that give rise to fixed ways of thinking about and responding to emotional events.

17.1.1 Promoting the Idea of Emotion as a Process

Rigid emotional reactions are also linked to assumptions that emotions are enduring states as opposed to processes that wax and wane. This assumption is not surprising given the intensity and persistency of emotional states in BPD and patients' tendency to "fuse" with their emotions and define themselves largely in terms of their current emotional state. It is also maintained by the limited time perspectives of patients who have difficulty integrating events across time and recalling how feelings change with fluctuations in mental state. Recognition that feelings are transient and that even painful feelings come and go is promoted by education about emotions and their dysregulation and by helping patients to track the flow of emotional changes during specific sessions. It is interesting how surprised patients are when their attention is drawn to the fact that although they talk about their feelings as if they never change, they actually change all the time.

17.1.2 Developing Flexibility in Interpreting Emotional Triggers

Emotional flexibility is impaired by the rigid ways emotional events are interpreted. Patients tend to see things in fixed ways and assume that their interpretation is correct and indeed the only conceivable way to interpret things.[2] Essentially, patients tend to treat an event and their interpretation of the event as identical. Consequently, the idea that events can be interpreted from different perspectives is not considered a possibility.

Earlier exploration of events that trigger intense emotions can now be extended to develop a greater understanding of how these events activate schemas that determine how the event is interpreted and dealt with. This allows patients to begin to accept the idea that their interpretation of an event is not a fixed property of the event but rather a result of the beliefs it activates, and hence to recognize that if they change their beliefs, their interpretation of the event and the way they react to it will change as well. This refocuses the patient's attention from the event and the details of what happened to thinking about the way the event is perceived. This change of focus helps patients to recognize that emotions are not simply evoked by external events but are also closely related to internal processes such as beliefs about abandonment and rejection. This realization opens up the possibility of seeing things differently and that other responses are possible. It also does something else: it contributes to feelings of personal agency and self-efficacy because it allows patients to recognize that their actions are not determined by other people but rather by internal processes, which means that they have options in how they react to events.

These changes are achieved by handling differently the scenarios patients present. This is illustrated by the case of Madison. It will be recalled that Madison described a self-harming scenario triggered by mother declining a request to go shopping with her. The scenario was used to explore the sequence of events leading to self-harm because treatment was focused primarily on containing distress and reducing self-harm. Later in therapy, Madison described a similar event. On this occasion, her response was more muted because she controlled her emotional reactions by self-soothing (listening to a favourite piece of music) and by distracting herself with a task that required concentration. She also argued with herself about the way she was catastrophizing. Nevertheless, the event caused distress, intense rumination, and thoughts of self-harm that she did not act on.

The therapist noted the similarity between this event and the one that occurred some months earlier. Madison agreed and added that mother was unfair. The therapist initially drew attention to how differently Madison had reacted and used the opportunity to review progress but then raised the possibility that other interpretations of the event were possible by asking "Why do you think mother did that?" and later by asking "What do you think was going on in her mind?" The questions surprised Madison and initially she maintained that mother did not care about her. However, the therapist's persistent query about whether there could be other reasons helped her to become more reflective (see Chapter 11 on questions that activate the reflective mode).

Further discussion revealed that mother had explained that she could not just drop everything whenever Madison wanted. This led the therapist to enquire further about what Madison thought mother meant and what she might have been thinking at the time. Encouragement to put herself in mother's shoes helped her generate several alternative interpretations of mother's behaviour and eventually to accept that mother did not react in this way because she did not care but because she had a prior commitment related to her work. In fact, Madison knew about this commitment but activation of the schema "mother does not care about me (or love me)" and the strong feelings it aroused led to her discounting this information and limited her ability to reflect on what happened.

As this scenario was worked through, Madison's ability to see things from the other's perspective gradually increased. At the same time, the possibility that Madison's schemas, especially sensitivity to rejection, may lead her to misinterpret some events was introduced and explored. At this stage of therapy, the mentalizing interventions used by mentalizing-based therapy are readily combined with the standard methods of cognitive therapy to help the patient to challenge and restructure interpretations based on maladaptive schemas and the misperceptions they generate.[3]

17.1.3 Creating Options in Emotional Responses

Flexibility in emotional expression also means being able to choose when and how emotions are expressed. This is something patients have difficulty recognizing. Since their emotions are intense and difficult to control, they tend to assume that their only option is to respond to them. The task is to help them to understand that emotions are experiences not actions and that they can be experienced but not necessarily expressed.[4] This means understanding that it is possible to be angry without acting in an angry way. This is usually what happens with most people. We experience a gamut of feelings each day but only express a few of them. In fact, normal social discourse would be impossible if we did not express our emotions selectively.

Flexibility in emotional responding also involves understanding that even if intense emotions are expressed, they need not be expressed in their full-blown state. Individuals with BPD tend to react in an all-or-nothing fashion. Hence, emotions are expressed with full intensity or not at all. They need to recognize that more nuanced expression is not only possible but also desirable.

17.1.4 Tolerating Ambivalence

Since patients with BPD tend to see things as either black or white, they have difficulty managing ambivalent emotions. The experience of some degree of contradictory feelings about significant others is an almost ubiquitous feature of human experience. However, when emotional processing is compromised, people find it difficult to recognize and accept that they may feel both love and resentment about the same person, leading them to worry over which is their "real" feeling, a concern that also reflects doubts about the authenticity of basic experiences that is part of self pathology. Tolerance and acceptance of ambivalence are needed in order to reconcile these feelings by integrating them by creating higher-order meaning structures that include a conception of the other person and their relationship with them. However, tolerance is often hindered by attempts to avoid the negative emotions involved as illustrated by the following vignette.

One patient, who talked throughout therapy of love for her long-standing partner in a way that suggested idealization and romanticization of the relationship, mentioned that they had quarrelled a few days earlier. With some prompting, she recounted being furious with him although she now realized that she was angry because she was tired and stressed. She insisted that he was a wonderful person and did not deserve her anger. The therapist noted how difficult it can be to be angry with someone you love. The patient acknowledged this but insisted she was not angry. The therapist asked about what had happened. Initially, the patient maintained that it was nothing and she was over it now. Further queries revealed that she had asked for her partner's help with a household chore that required both their efforts and he had refused. Queries about how she reacted to his refusal at the time revealed that it enraged her. However, this acknowledgement was accompanied by her insistence that the anger was not justified.

As the anger was acknowledged and processed in subsequent sessions, it became easier for her to tolerate having mixed feelings about her partner and to accept that this did not mean she loved him any the less. The process was aided by the therapist's affirmation and acceptance of both emotions as experienced in therapy. At the same time, the significance of both feelings was explored and understood especially in terms of the way the anger resonated with feelings she had as a teenager towards her mother for being unable to show love and caring. This led to an improvement in the relationship with her partner because she felt that she was more genuine and less pressured in the relationship and held back far less. These changes allowed the patient to talk not only about the anger but also about her disappointment with him over his inability to provide the support she needed.

Further work revealed that behind of the anger and disappointment lay intense feelings of hurt linked to feeling unloved and uncared for by him. Again, these feelings resonated with earlier feelings that mother did not love her. Over time, the patient was able to access the sadness she felt about her partner's and mother's inability to express love and affection. Gradually, she came to accept that difficulty showing caring was part of who they were and not a reflection on herself – previously she assumed it was because she was too needy, and even a bad person.

This vignette illustrates more than the value of promoting tolerance of ambivalent emotions. It also illustrates how significant emotions get masked by other more accessible and tolerable emotions and that improving emotional processing involves accessing suppressed or avoided feelings. In this case, the anger masked disappointment, hurt, and sadness. It was only when the ambivalence about, and fear of, the anger was recognized and tolerated that other feelings became accessible.

17.1.5 Promoting Positive Emotions

Emotional dysregulation predominantly affects negative emotions such as anxiety, anger, depression, distress, sadness, guilt, and shame. These emotions impact most aspects of a person's life. They cause people to hunker down and limit their activities and way of living. Horizons shrink and life becomes constricted. In contrast, positive emotions such as joy, interest, love, and happiness stimulate engagement with the world and communion with others. They are motivators that drive a range of adaptive behaviour. Without them, we are at a loss about what to do. The paucity of positive emotions in patients with BPD contributes to their constricted lifestyles and comparative lack of motivation and purpose. As the intensity of negative emotions decreases with therapy, there is often a void: despite increased emotional control, patients often feel disengaged from life, emotionally flat, and unenthusiastic.

Part of the difficulty is that patients with BPD experience less positive emotion than healthy individuals.[5] Unfortunately positive emotions are not easily stimulated. They seem to arise largely as a consequence of therapeutic improvement. Actual attempts to stimulate them are usually unsuccessful and may even cause patients to feel inadequate or to be self-critical because they are unable to feel more positive despite feeling better. An exception is the emotion of interest. With an improved sense of well-being, patients often begin to talk spontaneously about things that interest them often in response to accidental events. When this happens, the interest needs to be acknowledged and nurtured.

As Madison improved due to increased ability to manage her emotions, she suddenly became interested again in a sport in which she excelled but had given up when she was severely symptomatic. This was an important turning point in her recovery because the renewed interest suddenly changed her life and made her more engaged and enthusiastic. Sometimes, these opportunities may be more mundane. For example, another patient commented that she was interested in making minor renovations to her apartment, which led to discussion of her plans for wall colours and flooring materials, which was discussed in several sessions with the therapist taking an active interest in her plans. A few weeks later, she said that she was "very much enjoying" her apartment now the renovations were finished. This was a new comment. Although the emotional lability that had dominated her life had settled, she remained fearful lest it return and lived a constricted and socially isolated life. The new feelings of enjoyment were reflected and affirmed by enquiring about the changes and their effect. This led to the patient noting that she was thinking about inviting neighbours over for coffee, something that she would not normally do. The idea illustrates how positive emotions activate thoughts of social contact and bonding. The therapist enquired when she was planning to do this to strengthen the feelings and consolidate the implied commitment to change. This encouraged her to talk about specific plans to socialize (see Chapter 12 on the importance of "change-talk").

Within therapy, the treatment relationship itself is a source of positive emotions.[6] As therapy progresses, patients often comment on how they value and appreciate being understood, respected, and treated in a compassionate way. These aspects of the relationship can be nurtured to promote positive feelings about therapy that can be used to support the emergence of these feelings about other aspects of the patient's life.

17.2 Constructing More Adaptive Narratives

Discussion of the role of emotions in Chapter 15 noted how they shape higher-order meaning systems and personal narratives. Humans are meaning-seeking, interpretative beings who seek to understand their experiences, emotions, moods, and personal qualities by constructing and reconstructing interpretative narratives.[7] Once formed, these narratives help to regulate behaviour including the emotions that influenced their development.

The cognitive elaboration of emotions through the development of emotional schemas consisting of beliefs about the nature and value of emotions, the factors that trigger specific emotions, and personal capacity to manage feelings gives meaning to experience and influences the way that emotions are expressed When schemas are largely positive, they help to regulate emotional reactions, but when negative, they amplify emotional distress. Some schemas are used to construct narratives that ultimately become part of a broader self-narrative. These narratives constitute an additional level of meaning and regulation by providing a broad perspective that allows patients to see their emotions within the overall context of their lives. This perspective often helps to modulate distress. During the latter part of the regulation and modulation phase, treatment seeks to help individuals to restructure any negative narrative that is impeding self-regulation and develop new narratives to modulate emotional expression and promote adaptive functioning. The influence of narratives on emotions is illustrated by the case of Madison.

When Madison started therapy, she described her emotions as overwhelming and intolerable and she thought of herself as a weak, vulnerable, and dirty person who needed to be loved. She also thought of herself as something of a sham because she had been forced to withdraw from her university course and could not keep a relationship. Although she had difficulty articulating the different qualities she attributed to herself, she was aware of a pervasive negative self-image and sense of failure. This image was continually reinforced by events. Her life was unstructured and disorganized so that every day was a reminder of her failures. At the same time, the image of being a failure perpetuated the distress.

Once Madison began to understand her problems more as a result of the reformulation of her crises (Chapter 14), the emotional instability began to settle. This allowed her to acknowledge that her emotions were more intense and more difficult to manage than those of other people but whereas in the past she thought of this as a weakness – as an indication that she was a loser – she now began to draw on the competitive side of her nature and saw it as a challenge to be overcome. She decided that she needed to learn the skills needed to manage her anxiety and moods and keep them within tolerable limits. Over time, she also began to think about her emotions differently and recognized that they were not things to be feared but rather parts of herself that she could use constructively. She learned to draw on her feelings to motivate herself in competitive situations and came to recognize that modest levels of anxiety actually helped her to study more effectively. As a result of these changes, Madison, in effect, constructed a new narrative about her emotional life that helped to dampen the distress, making it possible for her to pursue new interests and establish positive goals that gave her a sense of purpose.

This vignette reveals the importance of a broad approach to treating emotion dysregulation within the context of the personality system and that effective treatment requires an emphasis on both the acquisition of appropriate skills and the construction of narratives capable of regulating emotions and integrating them with other personality processes. Narrative construction is not something that happens over a few sessions. Rather it begins towards the later part of the regulation and modulation phase with the construction of a new narrative about emotions, which is subsequently elaborated to incorporate changes resulting from work on interpersonal themes and finally into an overall self-narrative in the final phase of treatment.

17.3 Concluding Comments

The modular structure of IMT does not mean that treatment is assumed to follow a rigid and predictable sequence. In practice, most sessions will incorporate elements of multiple modules to match the flow of the therapeutic dialogue. Nevertheless, most treatments show a consistent pattern – treatment methods become less structured with progress and the scope of therapy and hence interventions progressively broaden. With progress, therapy gradually progresses from a focus on the patient's capacity to self-manage emotions to viewing emotions more broadly within the context of the overall personality. As this occurs, interventions become more dependent on using "chance" events to further the aims of treatment. This means that the therapist has to be alert to the importance of such things as comments about interests and other positive emotions and the narratives that guide the patient's reactions to events and then seize them as opportunities to move therapy along.

With these developments, an interpersonal focus is increasingly incorporated into treatment because emotions are essentially interpersonal in nature. As this occurs, attention begins to move from emotion regulation to the treatment of interpersonal problems. Emotions, however, are an intimate part of personality functioning and hence even though the primary focus changes, it will be necessary to work on most aspects of emotion regulation, especially emotional processing, throughout therapy.

Notes

1. Livesley (2015).

2. Dimaggio et al. (2015).

3. This scenario illustrates the importance of self-reflection and the ability to "take the role of the other" in emotional processing. This is the phase of treatment in which the interventions stressed by metacognitive approaches to treatment (see Dimaggio et al., 2015; Dimaggio et al., 2007) and mentalizing interventions (Bateman and Fonagy, 2004, 2006, 2015) become important in building on progress brought about by more skill building and cognitive restructuring interventions.

4. Note the similarity to the way self-harming behaviour was managed. Part of this process required patients to accept that ideas of self-harm need not be acted on. This required increasing tolerance of ideas of self-harm and separating thoughts of self-harm from self-harming behaviour.

5. Stepp et al. (2009), Sadikaj et al. (2010).

6. Greenberg and Paivio (1997).

7. Ricoeur (1981), Stanghellini and Rosfort (2013).

Introduction

With improved emotion regulation, treatment gradually shifts to treating interpersonal problems, becoming more complex in the process. The previous focus on the single impairment of emotional dysregulation now broadens to cover the multiple interpersonal problems that characterize borderline personality disorder (BPD). Treatment also becomes less structured in order to deal with the broader array of problems covered in most sessions. Although the use of generic interventions, cognitive-behavioural methods, and narrative construction continues, interpersonal and psychodynamic strategies and methods are added to the mix.

The scenarios patients present in the latter part of treatment tend to differ from earlier ones. They are less concerned with crises and unstable emotions and more with interpersonal problems. They are also handled differently. The interpersonal component is explored in more detail to identify and change maladaptive interpersonal schemas and interpersonal behaviour.

This phase of treatment makes more demands of the therapist than previous phases because it is less structured and much "messier." Previously, it was possible to focus on specific problems using well-defined interventions. The challenge for therapists was to manage intense emotions and suicidality, not what strategies and interventions to use – in many situations this was rather obvious. In contrast, interpersonal problems are complex and they interact in complex ways. This means that treatment becomes less predictable because the issues and scenarios patients present vary considerably across sessions. These challenges are addressed in two ways. First, a general framework is proposed for changing the maladaptive schemas, ways of thinking, and interpersonal problems that characterize individual patients, which is discussed in the next chapter. Second, this general framework is used to treat submissive behaviour (Chapter 19) and intense dependency needs and the core conflict of neediness versus fear of rejection (Chapter 20).

18 Principles for Treating Maladaptive Schemas and Interpersonal Patterns

This chapter begins by discussing the part schemas play in establishing and maintaining maladaptive interpersonal patterns and then proceeds to describe a general method for changing maladaptive schemas, interpersonal behaviours, and habitual ways of thinking. Repetitive interpersonal behaviours will be referred to as "patterns" because they involve the interplay of habitual ways of thinking, feeling, and acting. This term is useful because it is readily accepted by patients and because it implies order and meaning to their actions.

18.1 Schemas and Interpersonal Patterns

Since schemas influence what we notice, what we ignore, and how we respond to events, the treatment of interpersonal problems begins by helping patients to recognize their interpersonal schemas and their impact on interpersonal behaviour.

18.1.1 Teaching about Schemas

At some point in therapy, patients need to learn about schemas and how they function. It is difficult to be precise about when this should happen – much depends on the severity of the disorder and progress. The idea may be introduced when discussing beliefs that exacerbate emotional arousal. Or, the concept may be introduced when discussing alternative interpretations of the interpersonal events that trigger crises, as occurred with Madison. If not introduced previously, it should be discussed early in the interpersonal phase because it is central to interpersonal change. It is helpful to explain: (i) that a schema is a set of beliefs, ideas, feelings, and memories linked by a common theme; (ii) that people are often unaware of their schemas even though they influence their thoughts, feelings, and actions; (iii) why schemas are stable and self-perpetuating; and (iv) how they influence interpersonal behaviour.

18.1.1.1 Schema Stability

Schemas are stable because we tend to notice things that are consistent with our beliefs and ignore things that are not. Thus individuals who believe that people are hostile notice and ruminate over incidents when they were treated in a hostile way but tend to not notice the times when people were kind or friendly. They also tend to be hypersensitive to hostility, which causes them to see hostility when others would not and to be more likely to interpret ambiguous behaviour as hostile. Schemas are also stable because they give rise to actions that cause others to behave in ways that confirm the schema. Thus the tendency to see others

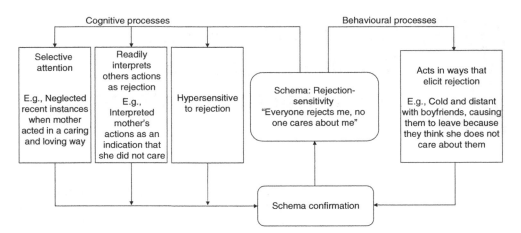

Figure 18.1 Schema Diagram: Cognitive and Behavioural Processes That Maintain Schemas

as hostile may lead to an unfriendly demeanour that evokes similar responses from others, which are taken as confirmation of the belief that people are hostile.

Many schemas are also maintained by avoiding actions and situations that may lead to experiences that are inconsistent with the schema. As a result, schema-based fears are rarely tested. For example, fear of social disapproval and social embarrassment may lead to avoidance of social events. As a result, there is no opportunity to learn that these outcomes are not inevitable. Thus one patient who was afraid of embarrassing herself because she thought that she was boring would accept invitations to social events but only stay a short time lest others get tired of her which prevented her from learning that her friends actually enjoyed her company.

The cognitive and behavioural processes that promote schema stability are seen in patients with rejection sensitivity who expect to be rejected and are hyper-vigilant to rejection but fail to notice behaviours that are inconsistent with this belief. Madison illustrated this perceptual bias when she interpreted mother's refusal to help as rejection and an indication that mother did not care. Other actions showing that mother was deeply concerned about Madison's well-being were ignored. Madison also behaved in ways that confirmed her expectations. She was distant, cautious, and uncaring towards boyfriends, which led them to withdraw because they thought that she was not really interested. Hence her actions led to the outcome she desperately sought to avoid.

Schema functioning is readily explained by a diagram showing how behavioural and cognitive processes contribute to schema stability (see Figure 18.1). Diagrams capture the essential details of a schema and its behavioural effects in a way that is readily understood and remembered. Patients can also be invited to contribute to the diagram and provide further details of maladaptive patterns so that the diagram becomes a collaborative project. A diagram also allows patients to view their actions more objectively.

18.1.2 Schema Change

Schemas can be changed either by replacing maladaptive schemas with more adaptive alternatives or, as is usually the case when treating BPD, by modifying schemas so that they are more adaptive.[1] Schema modification largely involves promoting more flexible application. For example, patients with pervasive mistrust may become more discriminating initially by developing trust in the therapist and later by incorporating the idea that some people can be trusted on some occasions. Perhaps later still, the schema may be restructured to accommodate the belief that some people are trustworthy. In many cases, this restructuring occurs as a result of new experiences in therapy. This is an important point: schema change is more often achieved through the provision of new experiences than by using the traditional cognitive therapy focus on schema restructuring.

18.2 Stage of Change Approach to Treating Schemas and Maladaptive Patterns

Changes to interpersonal patterns such as submissiveness and insecure attachment, cognitive modes such as self invalidation, and interpersonal and self schemas may be achieved using a general model that assumes that change occurs in four stages:[2]

1. Problem recognition, which involves identifying and accepting a problematic schema or pattern and affirming a commitment to change;
2. Exploration of the way a schema or behaviour pattern is expressed and its effects;
3. Change that is achieved by restructuring schemas, modifying interpersonal patterns, generating alternative responses, or acquiring new behaviours;
4. Consolidation and generalization, which involve strengthening new learning and applying it to situations outside therapy.

The stage approach to behavioural change implies that interventions should be relevant to the stage of change that the patient is at with regard to a given problem. There is little point in trying to help patients to behave differently such as being more assertive until they recognize the problem and are committed to change.

The stage approach may be used to change any behaviour or mode of thinking. In fact, the approach underlies early discussion of the treatment of deliberate self-harm and emotional dysregulation. In subsequent chapters, the approach will be used to organize the treatment of submissiveness, dependency needs, insecure attachment, and the core interpersonal conflict. Note that the stages of change model should not be confused with the *phases* of change model that refers to the overall process of treatment, not specific behaviour.

18.3 Stage 1: Recognition and Commitment to Change

Because patients usually have limited awareness of their habitual patterns, change begins, as it did with unstable emotions, by identifying and labelling problems. This may take considerable time because many schemas and problem behaviours are used automatically without the patient realizing it. Also problematic experiences tend to get warded off or avoided. Consequently, it is often necessary to draw attention to these problems repeatedly and work has to be done on avoidance before they are fully recognized.

Schema and pattern recognition follows the two-step process described earlier that first involves drawing the patient's attention to a particular problem such as submissiveness and the associated schema "I must do what others expect of me" and, second, encouraging the patient to identify the different ways the schema or behaviour is expressed. This process often leads naturally to establishing a commitment to change, which may be as simple as asking "Is this something you would like to change?" However, with some patients it may involve a lengthy discussion of the costs and benefits of continuing to act in this way as opposed to changing.

18.4 Stage 2: Schema Exploration

Schema exploration involves establishing the different ways it is used and how it influences experience and action. The following sections illustrate the kinds of methods that may be used.

18.4.1 Creating Links and Connecting Components

Identification of different ways a schema or pattern is expressed organizes diverse feelings, cognitions, and behaviours into a common theme that allows patients to see patterns to their behaviour and experiences. For example, helping a patient to recognize that worries about a romantic partner leaving, concerns about being criticized, worries that a parent may not be supportive, not expressing opinions lest others disagree are part of a generalized sensitivity to rejection changes the meaning of these experiences and draws them together in an integrative way. It also helps the patient to recognize and accept that the causes of these behaviours lie in themselves and not in the actions of others. Subsequently, it is also important to link schemas to the symptoms and problems that brought the patient to therapy – this seems to be a crucial part of the change process – and to establish the kinds of interpersonal events that trigger a particular schema or pattern.

18.4.2 Exploring the Origins of Schemas and Maladaptive Patterns

An issue to consider when exploring schemas and patterns is whether to focus exclusively on how they are expressed in the present or whether to also explore their developmental origins. Integrated modular treatment (IMT), like most therapies for BPD, assumes that change results primarily from modifying maladaptive processes as they occur in the present rather than through insight into their origins. Nevertheless, many patients need to understand the origins of their problems. We are going to encounter this repeatedly in the next few chapters and the fact that discussion of specific events that happened earlier in life can make a substantial contribution to understanding how these events and the maladaptive schemas that they generate influence current behaviour. A developmental account provides a perspective on problems that many patients find useful in constructing an adaptive self-narrative.

18.4.3 Exploring Relationships among Schemas

It was noted in Chapter 2 that schemas are organized into hierarchical systems. This structure creates a chain effect because the activation of one schema tends to activate others, both at the same level and higher in the hierarchy. A key task in changing interpersonal behaviour is to help patients to track the flow of schema arousal and its impact on emotions and action. This is illustrated by the way Madison's interpretation of mother's refusal to help as indicating that "mother does not care about me" subsequently activated the jealousy schema "mother prefers my brother," which led to the activation of the higher-order schema "mother does not love me." Later in therapy, this schema was found to activate the even higher-order and more distressing schema "I am unlovable."

18.4.4 Managing Non-Verbal Schemas

Some patients with severe BPD have difficulty describing some common states and ways of experiencing the world. When this is persistent, the possibility should be considered that these states involve non-verbal schemas that began to emerge before verbal skills were well established. Anna experienced a state of this type, which took some time to identify because it was a quiet, almost numb state characterized by silent withdrawal. When the state became apparent, Anna had difficulty describing how she felt or what she was thinking. To the therapist, it seemed as if she was trapped in a state of silent despair – a void that she found difficult to describe. Later in therapy, she recalled being told by a family member that they remembered that she used whimper in her cot for hours at a time and that the family used to joke about how she sounded like a motorcycle ticking over and they called her "little Harley." Perhaps most significantly no one tried to comfort her. When discussing these incidents, Anna realized that the feelings aroused when recounting these events were the same as those experienced in the recurrent state, which she had difficulty describing.

Exploration of non-verbal schemas is similar to that of other schemas. The first step is to find a label to represent these states and identify triggers. With Anna this took time and progress only occurred when she recalled the family story. This allowed her to describe how she felt and labelled the state "little Harley." This gave sufficient structure to the experience to enable further exploration. Previously, Anna had insisted that these feelings occurred spontaneously. The events triggering non-verbal schemas may also be non-verbal such as a physical stimulus associated with abuse, for example, someone getting physically too close, being touched, a non-responsive facial expression, or even a particular smell. With Anna, one trigger was being alone and feeling isolated and sad.

Within-therapy events are often especially useful in identifying these schemas and identifying triggers because therapist behaviour may inadvertently trigger them. With one patient, they occurred when she thought that the therapist was not listening. This evoked painful feelings of despair that were eventually related to abandonment and unlovable schemas and memories of a distant non-responsive depressed mother who rarely responded to her young daughter. With Anna, it was sometimes the approaching end to a session, which evoked the feelings that she had when left in her room for long periods.

18.4.5 Identifying Maintenance Factors

A key part of exploration is to identify factors that help to maintain problems. It was noted that cyclical maladaptive interpersonal patterns are maintained by internal factors such as selective attention to information and external factors such as other people's reactions that confirm these patterns. Patients do not always recognize, however, how other people reinforce their behaviour. Change requires that these reinforcing factors are identified and modified.

18.4.6 Managing Obstacles to Exploration

Schema exploration is often blocked by self-deception and schema avoidance. Avoidance is sometimes straightforward such as patients stating that they do not want to think about or talk about something. However, in most instances, patients are unaware of the avoidance. Madison, for example, rarely thought about the schema "I am unlovable" because of painful feelings it generated, and when she did, the thought was quickly suppressed. It was only when she began to talk about the anger she felt towards her mother and later about the sadness that lay beneath the anger that the schema became more accessible.

Increasing awareness of avoided thoughts or feelings is a critical therapeutic step: substantial change tends to occur when patients are exposed to the things that they avoid behaviourally or emotionally.[3] Suppression, avoidance, and distraction are among the many ways used to avoid the fear, pain, guilt, or shame that is believed will result from acknowledging, thinking about, and revealing what is being avoided. Awareness is often increased by inviting the patient to join the therapist in observing his or her own behaviour. For example, "I have noticed that whenever we begin to discuss your anger with your mother, you quickly start talking about something else. Have you noticed this?" Such interventions invite collaborative self-observation that is easily extended by enquiring about the worst possible consequences of talking about the fear, shame, or pain.

Other personality characteristics may also obstruct exploration. For example, intense emotional states are not conducive to exploration and reflection so that improvement in emotional self-management is often a prerequisite for schema exploration. Also the global, diffuse, and impressionistic thinking style common with BPD also makes it difficult to focus on the details of experience. Similarly, self-invalidation hinders exploration because it causes the person to doubt his/her experience.

18.5 Stage 3: Schema and Pattern Change

Exploration of a schema or pattern gradually evolves into steps to implement change. The cognitive therapies offer an impressive array of cognitive, interpersonal, behavioural, and emotional methods to change maladaptive schemas and patterns[4] some of which will be discussed in the following sections. First, however, we need to return to the ever important issue of motivation.

18.5.1 Maintaining Motivation to Change

Translating understanding into actual change is often difficult because understanding does not automatically bring about change. Considerable effort is needed to implement changes because old ways of thinking and acting are well entrenched and predictable. In contrast, change creates uncertainty by threatening to take patients into unknown terrain or requires that they relinquish cherished beliefs about self and others on which they have based their lives. Moreover, the patient's relationships often reinforce these patterns and undermine efforts to change. Hence motivation needs to be monitored closely and prompt intervention is needed when motivation declines and frustration mounts. Feeling stuck decreases self-esteem, increases self-blame, and often re-activates maladaptive patterns. Fear and frustration about change need to be validated and managed. Evidence suggests that successful outcomes require the therapist to be flexible and creative in managing the patient's difficulty in implementing change.[5] Direct and confrontational methods do not work and usually make matters worse. Empathy for the patient's predicament and continued encouragement and support are more effective.

Sometimes, a direct problem-solving focus on identifying new ways of behaving needs to be supplemented by a lighter touch by encouraging patients to "play" with the idea of doing things differently. When we play, we tell ourselves that what we are doing is not real. This often reduces anxiety about attempting to act differently. It also allows us to experiment without the worry that occurs when actions are really meant. The idea of play is also useful because many patients find it difficult to play and few have any sense of fun or pleasure. Hence this stage is an opportunity to encourage spontaneity, to try things out, and to explore the idea of doing things differently. Therapist support is an integral component. As attachment theory shows, young children only play and explore their environment when they feel secure. Therapy is similar: patients only make full use of the opportunity to explore problems and contemplate alternatives when they feel safe and supported.

Motivation is often easier to maintain and change is more likely when patients feel that they can change gradually rather than all at once. The gradual substitution of progressively more adaptive behaviours used earlier to modify self-harming behaviour acts (see Chapter 14) can now be extended to gradually modifying maladaptive patterns. The application of this strategy to modulating submissiveness is discussed in the next chapter.

18.5.2 Cognitive Strategies

Standard cognitive interventions that are the cornerstone of traditional cognitive-behavioural therapy are not as effective when treating BPD as with other disorders.[6] Early in treatment the struggle to manage distress depletes the resources needed to work on cognitive tasks. Also maladaptive thoughts often seem trivial compared to acute distress, suicidality, and conflicted relationships so that patients do not always understand the benefit of working on changing them. Nevertheless, as discussed in Chapter 16, simple interventions such as disputing dysfunctional thoughts, examining the evidence supporting a belief, and promoting greater flexibility in schema application are three simple techniques that should be introduced early in treatment and used extensively throughout. Often more complex cognitive interventions are not required.

Patients readily see the value of disputing and examining the evidence for and against catastrophic thoughts and other beliefs. With core schemas, this method is also useful but the examination of the evidence may extend over long periods of treatment because the evidence used to justify the belief is extensive. For example, the evidence Anna used to maintain the core schema "I am bad" included being sexually abused as a child, not being loved by mother, mother telling her that she was bad and everything was her fault, her siblings' anger towards her, engaging in self-injurious behaviour, and being abused by her partner. Over time, many of these pieces of "evidence" needed to be discussed and re-framed. For example, Anna thought that the fact that several people had abused her was evidence that "I must deserve it and I must be bad for everyone to treat me in this way." This kind of "evidence" was repeatedly re-framed by noting how she was raised by a physically abusive mother and abused by men when still a child and unable to protect herself and that as a result she had learned to pick abusive men. Over time, this allowed her to restructure the schema gradually until eventually, following a discussion of how abusive experiences affected her choice of men, she noted, "I hadn't thought of it that way. That means that I may not be bad, I simply made bad choices."

Discussions of core schema can also be used to re-frame childhood experiences and their effects. Work on changing the schema "I am bad" helped Anna to see how her family was dysfunctional and that this led to maladaptive ideas about herself and how the family continued to reinforce these ideas. This allows her to see the ideas and schema as the results of family dysfunction, not as the result of her being a bad person.

Disputing a schema also involves helping patients to recognize how they ignore or discount contradictory information. Madison's belief that "mother does not love me" was modulated substantially by drawing her attention to acts of caring that mother regularly showed. With Anna's "I am bad" schema, change also involved drawing attention to how she acted in ways that she considered good and caring while pointing out how these acts were inconsistent with her all-or-none belief that she was bad. Over time, she began to note how people regularly sought her help that she went out of her way to be helpful, how people confided in her, and how she was the only person to help a family member with severe personal problems.

The third cognitive method that is useful is to promote flexibility in the way core schemas are used. The significance of promoting alternative ways of interpreting events was first discussed in connection with Madison's difficulty interpreting her mother's behaviour more flexibly (Chapter 16). This strategy is central to building greater flexibility into information processing and to changing maladaptive interpersonal behaviour. Consequently, it is essential that we help patients to recognize the difficulty they have in understanding that perceptions are merely points of view and that they can change if viewed from a different perspective.[7] They also need to develop cognitive skills to promote the ability to see things from other perspectives by asking themselves consistently whether there are alternative ways to see or interpret events. This way of thinking is important because core schemas such as rejection sensitivity are almost imperialistic in their application: they are assumed to be widely applicable and hence become the person's favourite ways of interpreting events. The situation is like the old adage – when you have a hammer everything looks like a nail. When you feel threatened, everything looks like a threat, and when you are terrified of rejection, the possibility seems everywhere. Although patients usually recognize how these schemas are used frequently, it is often difficult to help them become more discriminating because they tend to assume that there is only one way to look at many events. Considerable work is usually done during this phase in promoting greater flexibility by exploring and re-framing specific scenarios aided by the use of interventions that encourage self-reflective modes of thought (Chapter 11).

18.5.3 Behavioural Strategies

Behavioural interventions include (i) reducing behavioural avoidance, (ii) changing habitual behaviours that contribute to schema stability, (iii) reducing schema avoidance, (iv) acting against schema-based rules to test the reality of fears and negative expectations using behavioural experiments, (v) behavioural rehearsal and developing new behaviours that support more adaptive schemas, and (vi) making environmental changes.[8]

18.5.3.1 Graded Tasks and Reducing Behavioural Avoidance

Schemas that are maintained by avoidance are changed by encouraging gradual exposure to avoided situations to test the validity of fears and negative expectations. As the treatment of trauma shows, this is a potent way to change schemas. Submissive individuals who avoid acting assertively lest they make people angry may be encouraged to act more assertively and note the effects on other people and feelings about the self. This was used to reduce Anna's subservience as described in the next chapter. Or, social avoidant individuals who have difficulty talking to others due to a fear of ridicule may be encouraged to talk to another person for a few moments in a no-risk situation and note how the other person responds. Over time, the range of situations may be extended and the duration of conversation increased.

18.5.3.2 Changing Schema-Maintaining Behaviour

Many schemas are maintained by acting in ways that elicit confirming responses from others. Change is more likely if the patient learns to recognize what he or she does to elicit such reactions with the aid of schema diagrams discussed earlier. Nevertheless, changing courses of action that maintain a schema is often difficult especially for patients who blame others for their problems. The idea should be introduced gradually by the therapist explicitly recognizing and acknowledging the terrible things that have happened to avoid inadvertently being invalidating and the patient dismissing the therapist's comments as indications the therapist does not understand.

18.5.3.3 Acting against Schema-Based Rules

Many schemas incorporate rules and beliefs that are adopted without question. These rules can be challenged through simple behavioural experiments. For example, Anna was encouraged to break the rule that she "should always agree to help people when asked" by occasionally saying "no." Similarly another patient who thought that she should never confront someone no matter what the other did was encouraged to express her concern when someone she worked with acted inappropriately. The therapist worked with her to identify a time and a way to do this which was likely to be effective. A successful outcome to this behavioural experiment allowed her to feel more comfortable about acting in this way. It also made her realize that she was not as incompetent as she thought – a development that initiated long-term changes.

18.5.3.4 Rehearsal and the Development of New Behaviours

Patient confidence in trying out new behaviours is often increased by rehearsing the behaviour in therapy by role playing or rehearsing in imagination and by working with them to work out what they would like to say and to find an appropriate way to say it. Sometimes it is even necessary for the patient to actually write down what she or he would like to say and discuss it with the therapist. This not only reduces anxiety but also gives an opportunity to discuss the kinds of words and phrasing that are likely to be successful. These kinds of changes often require the use of skills that are poorly developed or that the individual is uncomfortable using. Hence it may be necessary to do some preliminary work on developing new skills or strengthen old ones such as social, assertiveness, communication, and problem-solving skills.

18.5.3.5 Environmental Changes

Change to some schemas may also be achieved by encouraging the patient to deliberately seek out situations that are likely to generate information that challenges cherished schemas. For example, one patient who considered herself to be incompetent, a belief that had a pervasive effect on her life that was also resistant to change, was asked to describe any activity she thought she was good at or any situation in which she felt competent. With difficulty, she eventually acknowledged being good with animals. Dogs and cats seemed to like her and she felt confident handling them. A discussion of how she could use this ability led to her saying she would like to work with animals and hence to the decision to volunteer at an animal rescue centre. This worked out well because part of the rehabilitation planned for this phase was to get a part-time job. At the centre, her ability to handle difficult animals was quickly recognized and she was invited to assist the veterinarian with minor procedures. Again, she managed extremely well. The compliments she received and the thanks for donating her time helped to soften the incompetency schema sufficiently to allow the use of other interventions that helped her to extend and consolidate the changes. Sometimes it takes some kind of event in everyday life to kick-start changes to schemas that are rigidly held.

18.5.4 Interpersonal Strategies

The treatment of interpersonal problems makes extensive use of the therapeutic relationship as the major vehicle for changing core schemas and maladaptive interpersonal patterns.[9] This is achieved in two general ways. First, as discussed in Chapter 4, IMT provides a continuous corrective experience that challenges core schemas and ways of relating. Briefly, a treatment process based on collaboration, consistency, and validation modulates distrust, abandonment and rejection, neglect, defectiveness (being flawed or unlovable), cooperation/control, predictability, and reliability schemas while an emphasis on building motivation and competency modulates passivity, powerlessness, and incompetency schemas. This process occurs throughout therapy and continues to be important during the exploration and change phase.

Second, core schemas and patterns are invariably enacted in the treatment relationship where they can be explored and restructured in the here-and-now of therapy. It is not that this kind of work was not done at earlier phases. Rather, the frequency and depth of this work increase significantly because exploration of interpersonal issues leads to frequent activation of core schemas originating in childhood adversity that colour the treatment relationship. This creates an opportunity to rework these issues by examining the schemas involved in the context of the treatment relationship. Issues related to trust and intimacy in particular come to the fore as therapy focuses increasingly on the interpersonal aspects of trauma and adversity. These issues will be discussed in more detail in the next two chapters.

18.5.5 Emotional Strategies

Core schemas are usually highly emotion-laden. Cognitive therapies have developed emotional methods to address this aspect of schema change such as role playing and psychodrama. However, as noted previously, emotional arousal is potentially problematic with treating BPD due to the destabilizing effects on intense emotions. Although emotive techniques are likely to be used later rather than earlier in treatment, they still need to be used cautiously. The occurrence of high levels of cognitive dysregulation, regressive and dissociative behaviour, a history of severe abuse and deprivation leading to primitive object relationships, poor affect tolerance, and limited psychological mindedness are reasons for minimizing the use of these techniques.

Nevertheless, change in core schemas invariably evokes painful emotions and an important therapeutic task is to defuse some emotional intensity evoked by these schemas and associated memories of painful events. This seems to be best achieved using a graduated approach in which the therapist manages the intensity of emotional arousal with a strong emphasis on affect tolerance and regulation, especially when dealing with anger, rage, and shame associated with early trauma and deprivation. With this graduated approach, the goal is not to promote an intense cathartic reaction but rather to help the patient to assess and express painful feelings in tolerable doses to drain some of the intensity of emotions attached to core schemas while maintaining emotion regulation. Specific methods such as imaginative recall and role playing may be useful with some patients but often all that is needed is a simple psychodynamic approach that focuses attention on the feelings associated with schema arousal and the memories evoked and deals with any avoidant or defensive behaviour.

18.6   Stage 4: Consolidation and Generalization

Sustained change requires that new behaviours are consolidated and their use generalized to everyday situations. This requires that the patient is consistently encouraged to apply the things learned in therapy to specific everyday events and that the results are reviewed in therapy. This is something that occurs automatically with behavioural experiments, which needs to be applied to all new learning. If necessary, patients should be helped to identify situations in which they can apply what they have learned with an opportunity to rehearse these behaviours in therapy if they are hesitant about them.

Consolidation and generalization of change often require the inhibition or blocking of old ways of behaving.[10] The old ways were learned for a reason and these reasons often continue after the patient has begun to learn alternative behaviours. Hence, besides learning new behaviours, it is also necessary to help patients to block old ones so that they have the time to deploy the new one. This happened with Anna. Although she accepted that her tendency to be acquiescent made her feel a loser and her family to feel neglected, she was unable to say no despite being motivated to change. She also tended to respond to such requests automatically without thinking. As will be discussed in the next chapter, Anna's ability to implement the changes she wanted to make was aided by helping her to learn a new kind of self-talk in which she continually reminded herself that she could say no and that she did not want to be a doormat any more. These techniques helped her to block her automatic response. Progress also came from encouraging Anna to identify which requests she would find it easier to decline.

Successful change often requires changes in the patient's current circumstances and relationships when these hinder progress or help to perpetuate maladaptive behaviour. Managing the gamut of potential obstacles to change usually requires flexibility on the part of the therapist and a preparedness to use a variety of interventions that are likely to differ substantially across patients. Sometimes patients will need help in managing their social relationships more effectively, which may require learning new skills and adjusting interactions with others. In other cases, efforts may need to be directed towards changing the social environment either through conjoint sessions with significant others to help them adjust to changes in the patient's behaviour or even by encouraging more radical changes to the social environment by changing social interactions that perpetuate maladaptive behaviours or hinder change.

18.7   Comment

This chapter describes a general way to bring about change in schemas and broad patterns in the way patients think and act. Faced with traits such as submissiveness and thinking styles such as self-invalidation, therapists are sometimes unsure about how to proceed. The stages of change framework provides a structure to guide the process. For example, in one session, Anna described how angry she had been with her partner the previous day because he had a day off work and spent the entire day playing a computer game and made no attempt to help her with household chores and looking after the children. She became increasingly furious but said nothing. In the evening, when she was cleaning up after dinner, he had come to her and asked if she needed help and she said "no." The dialogue proceeded as follows:

THERAPIST: What did he do then?

ANNA: He went back to playing his computer game.

T: What did you do?

A: I carried on cleaning up.

T: Who lost out here?

A: [Stared at the therapist looking puzzled.]

A: I guess I did. He didn't care, he went on playing his stupid game.

T: Hmm!

A: You think he can't win, don't you?

At this point, the therapist has several options about how to proceed. Anna's comment could imply that she thought that the therapist was being critical. However, her tone of voice did not suggest that this was the case and she seemed to be in a thoughtful frame of mind. Another option was to pick up the comment about her partner not being able to win. This was rejected in favour of dealing with the pattern of getting angry about not getting help and then rejecting help when offered because this promised to be the most productive because Anna frequently complained of being exhausted by all the things she had to do. Consequently, the dialogue continued as follows:

T: I was thinking more about what was going on in *your* mind at the time.

A: What do you mean?

T: Well you had been mad all day because he was not helping you but when he did you refused his offer.

A: Well!! I was so mad with him by then … …

T: Yes

A: … … … … I'm passive aggressive aren't I?

Anna has used the term that allows the therapist to use it as well despite its negative connotations. This is the point where beginning therapists wonder about what to do next. The value of the stages of change approach is that it provides a strategy that begins by ensuring recognition and getting a commitment to change.

T: Do you do other things that you consider passive aggressive?

A: [Then recounts several similar instances with other people.]

T: Is this something that causes problems?

A: Yea. No one helps me. When I turn people down they get mad with me and stop offering to help. It means I have to do everything myself.

T: Is this something you want to change?

A: I think I have to.

T: You have to or you want to?

A: Both.

T: OK. What do you think the benefits would be if you weren't so passive aggressive?

A: I'd let people help me. I would not be so mad all the time … I think I'd be less tired all the time … I think I'd get on better with everyone. But do you think it's possible?

T: Well we have managed to deal with similar problems. Why shouldn't we deal with this?

A: Yea, you're right but I don't know how to start.

T: Well perhaps we could start by thinking a bit more about what else you do that you think is passive aggressive so that we both understand the pattern and exactly what you do.

This interaction sets the stage for the next stages of more detailed exploration of the pattern and subsequently to beginning to modulate it by helping Anna to act differently. The framework helps the therapist to organize the process in a systematic way without imposing constraints on what interventions are used or when they are used. The pattern will be dealt with over many months as problems arise or scenarios are presented that provide an opportunity for further work.

Notes

1. Beck et al. (1990), Cottraux and Blackburn (2001), Layden et al. (1993), Young (1994).

2. The framework for conceptualizing change to general patterns of thinking or acting is based on Prochaska and DiClemente's naturalistic description of changes in addictive behaviour (DiClemente, 1994; Prochaska and DiClemente, 1992; Prochaska et al., 1992; Prochaska et al., 1994). Prochaska and DiClemente described change as a six-stage process: pre-contemplation, contemplation, preparation, action, maintenance, and termination. When used to conceptualize change in personality pathology, it is convenient to combine some stages to give a four-stage process (see Livesley, 2003).

3. Beutler and Harwood (2000).

4. Beck et al. (2015), Cottraux and Blackburn (2001), Young et al. (2003), Davidson (2008).

5. This point has been made by many cognitive-behavioural therapists including Layden et al. (1993), Bernstein and Clercx (in press), Rafaeli et al. (2011), Young (1994). This concern led Young to develop schema; see Young et al. (2003), Dimaggio et al. (2015).

6. Cottraux and Blackburn (2001), Young et al. (2003).

7. Young et al. (2003), Bernstein and Clercx (in press).

8. Benjamin (2003).

9. Schoeneman and Curry (1990), Sonne and Janoff (1979), Weiner (1985).

10. Horvath and Greenberg (1994).

Chapter 19

Treating Submissiveness

Discussion of the treatment of specific interpersonal impairments begins with submissiveness because it is often easier to treat than other interpersonal problems. The behaviours and schemas involved are simpler and their exploration does not activate emotional distress to the same degree.

19.1 The Nature of Submissiveness

Maladaptive manifestations of submissiveness include three broad sets of behaviour: subservience, suggestibility, and the need for advice and reassurance. The latter is linked to strong dependency needs that are discussed in the next chapter. The more specific behavioural manifestations of the trait include indiscriminately acceding to others' demands, always deferring to others, placating and appeasing others, consistently seeking to please others, accepting other people's opinions readily, difficulty expressing personal needs, problems voicing one's own opinion, discounting one's own opinions, allowing others to be excessively critical and abusive, being exploited and taken for granted, having difficulty in being assertive, putting others' needs first, putting one's self down, and needing constant advice and reassurance. Some common schemas associated with the trait are listed in Box 19.1. Submissiveness increases vulnerability to abuse and exploitation: all too often these patients go from one abusive relationship to another. This was the case with Anna. In her late teens and early adulthood, she had a series of relationships with emotionally abusive and sometimes physically abusive men. She wryly observed that there was little point in leaving her current marriage because she would only end up with someone similar and sometimes it was best to stick with the devil you knew.

19.1.1 The Origins of Submissiveness

In Chapter 3, it was noted that there is often a discrepancy between patients' overt behaviour and their inner experience. This is frequently the case with submissive individuals with borderline personality disorder (BPD); they present an angry demanding facade that often leads observers to miss their more submissive features and not recognize their inner uncertainty and vulnerability.

Earlier, the origin of submissiveness was explained in evolutionary terms. The small groups in which we evolved were hierarchically organized, creating the need for adaptive mechanisms to manage differences in rank and status. Hence, our remote ancestors developed the facility to avoid the anger of higher-ranking members of the group by showing submissive, placating, and appeasing behaviour. In our more complex contemporary society, social ranking is less obvious but it is there nevertheless in society at

BOX 19.1 Schemas Associated with Submissiveness

Self-deprecation: Believes self to be less important than other people; devalues self, especially in relation to others; assumes others' needs are more important than one's own needs

Anger intolerance: Believes that he/she is unable to cope with the anger or disapproval of others; expects anger or disapproval to lead to rejection; feels guilty and responsible if someone is angry with him/her

Retaliation: Expects others to retaliate to any attempt at being assertive

Conflict avoidance: Intolerance of conflict; places priority on avoiding conflict

Guilt about assertiveness and independence: Feels intense guilt about asserting own interests and wants and about attempts to be an independent or autonomous person

Incompetence: Doubts own ability to cope effectively with people and situations; lacks self-confidence; believes that she/he is helpless and needs continual support and help; feels unable to protect self

Martyrdom: Values making sacrifices for others; always places others' needs first

Approval need: Coping and sense of well-being and self-esteem depend on others' approval

Relationship fragility: Considers relationships to be fragile and unable to withstand expressions of anger and disagreement

large, in the work place, and even in the family. One way or another, we are constantly reminded of status differences between ourselves and others although we do not always see our social encounters in these terms. Status is linked to self-esteem: lower-ranked individuals have lower esteem than higher-ranked individuals at least in the context of their interaction. Hence those with low self-esteem tend to be more subservient and self-effacing.

The link between status and self-esteem helps to explain both the occurrence of submissive behaviour in many patients with BPD and its conflicted nature. Abuse, neglect, and deprivation reduce self-esteem, leading to a tendency to see others as more important, powerful, and knowledgeable than one's self and hence to a tendency to defer to others, submit to their demands, and to be a people-pleaser who is afraid to be assertive. Abusive partners often maintain the pattern by reinforcing the patients' negative self-worth by scorning them for having a mental disorder or being weak and unable to cope. This was the case with Anna: her husband frequently referred to her as a loser, scoffed at attempts to assert herself, and rejected her opinions as being those of someone who was "mental." His behaviour helped to maintain Anna's submissiveness, which often worked to his advantage.

Low self-esteem and submissiveness are exacerbated by dependency needs and attachment problems, leading to a tendency to seek individuals who are seen as stronger in the hope that they will provide the care and attention that these patients desperately desire. However, intense neediness is also coupled with anger arising from the ongoing failure of relationships to meet their needs. The anger in turn is intensified by dysregulated emotions, creating conflict between the need to be subservient due to attachment insecurity and intense anger about past and ongoing neglect. This conflict leads to a surface presentation of angry demandingness that masks underlying neediness and fear, a pattern that is often referred to as hostile dependency.

This conflict characterized Anna. When frustrated, she erupted with intense rage, which created relationship problems and impeded access to the services she needed from the health and social services because she alienated those she turned to for help. Yet, despite the conflicted relationship with her husband, Anna always handed her welfare benefits to him without question even though he spent most of the money on drugs and alcohol, which left her unable to feed her family properly. When asked why she did this, she simply replied "because he asked for it." She accepted without question his statement that he could deal with the money better because she was a "mental case." She also fought constantly with her husband because she was also enraged by his lack of caring but then she became terrified that he would leave. These fears caused her to engage in all kinds of demeaning things to placate him. However, the anger was so intense that it was easy to miss the underlying submissiveness.

Anna's submissiveness was also increased by her beliefs that she deserved to be abused and that meeting other people's demands was the right thing to do. At the same time, the low self-esteem was maintained by constantly acting in a subservient way. This cyclical pattern profoundly affected her life and well-being, causing her to feel abused, used, neglected, and depressed.

19.2 Stage 1: Recognizing Submissiveness and Committing to Change

Change begins by using the two-step process for achieving pattern recognition described previously. First, a current scenario is used to draw attention to the patient's submissive behaviour. If the timing is right, patients readily recognize and accept that they act in this way. However, acceptance is more likely if patients are guided into recognizing the pattern for themselves. Second, other examples of submissive behaviour are identified to help patients to recognize the diverse ways they express this trait. Pattern recognition achieves low-level integration by showing how a wide range of behaviours are connected.

19.2.1 Eliciting a Commitment to Change

Establishing a commitment to change may be as simple as asking "Is this something you would like to change?" or it may require a lengthy discussion of the costs and benefits of change. Some patients may recognize the pattern but not the need to change because they think it appropriate to act in this way and that anything else is unconceivable and even wrong. Anna, for example, readily agreed that she was a "people-pleaser" who could not say no but insisted that this was "the right thing to do." On one occasion, she mentioned feeling exhausted because she "had to babysit again" for a sister who had asked her to babysit because she had received a last-minute invitation. Anna presented the situation as if she had no option but to agree. The therapist noted that the same thing had happened several times recently. Anna agreed but added that she could not do anything about it. The therapist drew attention to the pattern by simply noting that "it seems that you always feel that you have to do whatever people ask." She agreed but quickly added, "What else can I do?"

Since Anna did not appear either to accept that this behaviour created problems or to accept that it was possible to behave differently, the therapist focused only on helping her to recognize other instances of meeting others' requests no matter how inconvenient, such as shopping regularly for her ageing parents – something her sister never helped with – looking after her parents' small garden, and regularly minding a friend's children after school. Although Anna became more aware of the pattern and its costs, she did not want to change because of strong religious convictions that demanded selflessness and helpfulness.

Shortly afterwards, Anna arrived for a routine session distraught. The previous evening, her children had complained that she was never home and her husband expressed concerns about her neglecting the children. These comments caused considerable distress because she was devoted to her children and wanted to give them a very different upbringing from her own. She felt intense conflict due to clashing values – devotion to her family and a faith-based need to help others even at some sacrifice to herself. In session, Anna said that she felt overwhelmed and that everything was out of control. She now accepted that things had to change because she could not do everything even though it felt as if she should be able to. The shame she felt about her children feeling neglected led to a modest commitment to change. As a result, the therapist wondered if it would help if she established some priorities. Anna agreed and said the most important thing was to take care of her children, which meant spending more time at home.

19.3 Stage 2: Exploring Submissiveness

The next step is to increase patients' awareness of the thoughts and assumptions (schemas) that are associated with decisions to act in a submissive way and to recognize how these thoughts help to explain why they feel that there is no alternative but to act in this way.

19.3.1 Tracking Associated Schemas

Since events that trigger submissive behaviour are in most cases obvious, exploration largely involves using scenarios to identify the schemas aroused by the event and track the subsequent flow of thoughts and feelings. Patients usually think that they do not have a choice about how to act for a variety of reasons. We saw how Anna used her religious beliefs to justify her actions. But behind the initial schema lie others that need to be identified such as fear of evoking anger, of guilt, or even of being a bad person. Anna, for example, usually felt guilty and that she was a bad person when someone got angry regardless of the circumstances. Like many patients she seemed to assume that relationships are fragile and cannot withstand disagreement, an attitude that fosters subservient tendencies.

The activation of schemas associated with submissiveness often evokes schemas linked to rejection and abandonment because submissiveness and the attachment system are often activated by the same events. Since attachment figures are usually considered older, more powerful, and wiser than the child, they have higher status. Consequently, contact with an attachment figure is also likely to activate submissiveness. Similarly, events that arouse submissiveness are threatening and hence activate attachment. Under normal developmental conditions, these effects are likely to be modest and unimportant, but with attachment trauma, the effects are more intense, especially when the attachment figure is the abuser and exploits the power difference with the child, leading the child to develop a tendency to show subservient and placating behaviour. This is what happened with Anna. As will be discussed more in the next chapter, attachment trauma and deprivation led to intense dependency needs that caused Anna to try constantly to satisfy the needs of others in the hope that it would cause them to love her and care for her.

Another schema associated with subservience and compulsive caregiving is the sense of being a martyr. The combination of intense unresolved dependency needs and submissiveness often leads to strong needs to care for others as a way to meet personal dependency needs and bolster self-esteem. The inability to say "no," a subservient attitude, and fear of rejection increase this behaviour. Such individuals often feel worthy because they are sacrificing themselves for others. At the same time, they resent having to care for or help others, creating a pattern of hostile-dependency. Anna also showed elements of this behaviour.

19.3.2 Explore the Costs and Benefits of Submissive Behaviour

As with any behaviour, subservience is maintained because it has benefits. Anna understood some of the benefits of her actions – they met her values, made her feel virtuous, and boosted her self-esteem because she felt useful. She also recognized how this behaviour allowed her to avoid negative goals such as avoiding the anger of her family and reducing fears of rejection but it took longer for her to recognize the costs of repeatedly acting in this way – causing her children to feel neglected, the costs to her health, and so on. It was more difficult still to recognize how repeatedly acting in this way made her feel used and exploited as she allowed people to take advantage of her.

19.4 Stage 3: Generating Change

The strategy for treating traits such as submissiveness (see Chapter 4) suggested that the most effective approach is to focus on: (i) reducing the frequency and intensity of submissive behaviour and (ii) promoting more adaptive and less exhausting ways to express this trait. Both methods require the restructuring of associated schemas and the acquisition of new skills and behaviours.

Changes to interpersonal patterns like submissiveness have different implications to the kinds of changes that have been discussed so far. Changes in self-harm and emotional distress are viewed positively by patients and significant others because the patient stops doing things that everyone finds troubling. This is not necessarily the case with behaviours like submissiveness because they lead to changes in interpersonal behaviour that have an impact on other people in the patient's life who may not welcome these changes, especially when it means that the patient stops being so accommodating or is more assertive. Hence it is useful to discuss the likely effects of change on others to confirm the commitment to try new courses of action and help the patient anticipate and deal with how others may react. With Anna, this involved discussing what she wanted to achieve, the things she needed to do to achieve these goals, and how she thought her family and husband would react.

19.4.1 Changing the Frequency and Intensity of Submissive Behaviours

The frequency with which a trait is expressed begins by changing the way situations are interpreted so that the trait is activated less often. The rigid ways in which patients interpret and respond to situations are clearly illustrated by the way Anna saw requests to help in a fixed way and how she assumed that she had no choice about how to respond. Flexibility is built by examining a suitable scenario. With Anna, the scenario discussed earlier of her sister requesting that she babysit again was used to help her to recognize the automatic way she reacted to such requests and to encourage her to see such requests in a broader context. This included encouraging her to examine the merits of such requests rather than responding automatically to them. It turned out that the event was not especially important as her sister only wanted to socialize with a friend she saw regularly. Anna was then encouraged to weigh this against the costs to herself and her family. The latter was not something she ever considered until her children and husband complained. Attention was also given to the frequency of these requests and their impact on Anna. Gradually, she came to recognize that many of her family's expectations were unreasonable, which decreased the sense of obligation she felt to comply.

Increasing flexibility in the interpretation of situations is largely a matter of promoting self-reflection and metacognitive functioning, which seems to get suspended by fear of rejection or of making the other person angry. As a result, patients do not recognize that their own fears and schemas bias them towards seeing things in a particular way or how these schemas lead them to automatically assume that if another person is angry with them it is their fault and that they must have done something. Anna, for example, assumed that when her extended family was upset with her, then it must be her fault. To deal with these problems Anna needed help with being more reflective. She was initially helped to adopt this mode of thinking by encouraging her to react to her family's requests by asking herself three questions: Is this a reasonable request? What are my thoughts and feelings about it? If I do this, what are my children going to think?

Over time, Anna learned to process such requests and to see her submissive behaviour in a broader interpersonal context. She noted the sheer frequency of demands on her from her extended family and that no one else in the family was subjected to the same demands. She began to feel used, which strengthened her resolve to change although it also caused a short-term increase in distress. In the process she became more observant. She began to notice the frequency with which her family put her down: she was subjected to a constant barrage of criticism about her behaviour and appearance and regular complaints about her selfishness and lack of morals. This is where an evolutionary understanding is helpful – Anna was low on the totem pole in her family and her status was maintained by the way her family treated her. Add to this the fact that her husband not only treated her similarly but was also abusive, and it becomes understandable why Anna was so dependent and subservient, and so dysthymic. Of course, she regularly got angry about this treatment and responded with rage, and so she appeared anything but submissive. But, despite the anger she nearly always gave in despite complaining about it.

As different scenarios were examined, Anna came to recognize the complexities of this behaviour. She began to recognize not just the dynamics of these events but also how her continued submissiveness actually encouraged others to treat her as a "doormat," a realization that was a further catalyst to change. To her surprise this worked, which emboldened her to make further changes.

Besides building flexibility in interpreting events, it is also helpful to generate greater flexibility in how submissiveness is expressed. The black-and-white thinking style associated with BPD leads to a tendency to all-or-nothing reactions. Again, this is not something patients readily perceive. Anna, for example, did not seem to realize that she could respond to her family's demands for help with anything other than total agreement. However, as she began recognizing how unreasonable some requests were, she began exploring ways to deal with the situation. Since she was still very fearful of their anger and rejection, it was agreed that the first step would be to defer requests that conflicted with her children's needs and expectations by saying that she would like to help but she could not because of other commitments, but offering to help on another occasion. Even this idea seemed alarming so she practised what to say in-session and in imagination before trying it out.

19.4.2 Modifying Behavioural Expression

With many traits, change is largely accomplished by modifying the way the trait is expressed. This is most apparent with traits such as sensation seeking, which, although not a borderline trait, often occurs in patients with BPD where it can add to crises and interpersonal problems because boredom leads patients into activities and relationships that are stimulating but cause problems. Change usually involves helping the patient to find more adaptive ways to meet the need for excitement. This approach is less directly relevant to changing submissiveness because there are few adaptive ways to show high levels of submissiveness. However, it is sometimes possible to replace some submissive behaviours with more assertive actions and to channel submissive tendency so that the trait is expressed in a more controlled way.

19.4.2.1 Behavioural Experiments Focused on Small Changes

Since it is difficult to change broad patterns such as submissiveness, it is best to make small changes to specific behaviours that evoke less fear that others will react adversely. Any success can be used to build the confidence needed to implement other changes. Not many successes are needed to modulate the pattern.

The component of submissiveness that caused the most problems for Anna was the tendency to agree to any suggestion or request without hesitation and difficulty expressing and satisfying her own needs and wants. Specific examples of these behaviours then became the subject of a behavioural experiment. For example, Anna was regularly invited to meet a friend for coffee. She usually agreed even if inconvenient because she was afraid of losing the friendship. On each occasion, the friend decided where to go and usually chose a particular chain which Anna accepted even though she disliked their coffee. Although this irritated her, she always acquiesced. When discussing a recent invitation of this type, she decided that the next time her friend contacted her she would agree to meet but suggest they meet somewhere else "for a change." She agreed to this behavioural experiment and discussed with the therapist what she could say and tried out several things before finding a form of words that she was comfortable with. This rehearsal is important. It increases the chances of success and provides an opportunity to anticipate the other person's reactions and discuss ways to respond to them. To her surprise, her friend agreed without hesitation.

19.4.2.2 Channelling Submissiveness

Submissiveness can also be restructured by channelling it so that it is expressed in a more controlled and predictable way. When Anna was beginning to change this behaviour, she was asked to provide care for an elderly relative of an acquaintance. This seemed an opportunity to channel her need to care for others and curb her family's demands. Her need to care for others contributed to her submissiveness but it also provided a constructive outlet for her own considerable dependency needs. After discussing the opportunity in therapy, she agreed to work several days a week and the occasional evening. Paid employment boosted her self-esteem and hence reduced feelings that increase submissiveness.

More importantly, it offered an opportunity to structure her caregiving. Now she had what she considered a legitimate reason to decline requests to do things – she was busy looking after her client or she needed to rest enough to have the energy to work.

19.4.3 Building Assertiveness Skills

Changes to the low assertiveness facet of submissiveness can be brought about by teaching assertiveness skills to enable patients to set limits on the demands made of them, express their needs and wants clearly, and make themselves heard in ways that do not evoke unnecessary anger. Lacking these skills, patients are often seen as either extremely timid or demanding and angry, and many oscillate between the two. Part of the difficulty is that assertiveness is often confused with anger so that change begins by helping patients to make this distinction and learn to be assertive before they become angry and upset. Assertiveness may be developed through a specific training programme or by incorporating these interventions in therapy or by using a combination of the two. If specific assertiveness training sessions are provided, it is still useful to incorporate skill building into individual therapy to ensure their application and deal with specific problems and concerns.

19.4.4 Changing Maladaptive Schemas and Self-Reflexive Thinking

Specific behavioural changes need to be reinforced by restructuring the maladaptive schema associated with these behaviours using the restructuring methods described in the previous chapter. Thus when reviewing with Anna her success in dealing with her friend, the outcome was contrasted with her fears that her friend would be angry and reject her. A few demonstrations of the unrealistic nature of these fears are often sufficient to restructure them. At the same time, Anna was encouraged to dispute these ideas when they come to mind. Successful implementation of behavioural experiments can also be generalized to feeling self-esteem and self-efficacy. A benefit of simple behavioural experiments is that they are self-reinforcing; success automatically makes patients feel better about themselves so that all the therapist has to do is to underline their effects.

19.5 Stage 4: Consolidation and Generalization

The previous chapter discussed some general ways to ensure that changes are consolidated and generalized to everyday situations. Besides these strategies, it is also helpful to promote a new narrative to understand submissiveness. Submissive and caregiving tendencies are usually important components of patients' self-narratives and scripts. The script Anna followed involved a deep sense of obligation to meet the needs of others and to be as helpful as possible, which sprung from values and beliefs that Anna held dear. This script was part of the rather fragile identity she had constructed. Exploration of the script also suggested that the sense of obligation stemmed from her belief that her needs were less important than those of others because she was less worthy, a belief that stemmed from her deep shame about being abused and mother not loving her. This narrative along with multiple maladaptive schemas helped to maintain the pattern.

As submissiveness is modulated, it becomes important to consolidate these changes by incorporating them into a narrative that includes such matters as the importance her own and her children's needs, increased self-efficacy and autonomy, greater understanding of the interpersonal aspects of this behaviour, increased recognition of the resilience of meaningful relationships, increased tolerance of others' anger, and decreased fear of rejection and abandonment especially in the context of assertiveness. With Anna, it was also important to help her to re-frame her values so that they were not interpreted so rigidly. This involved incorporating an understanding that her religious beliefs about helping others should not be viewed only in the context of a specific event such as a sister's request that she babysit for her but rather seen within the broader context of the nature of these requests and her commitment to others. Specifically, she began to recognize that her belief did not mean that she did not need to set priorities but rather that she had an obligation to put her children first. We will pick up the theme of narrative construction in Chapter 22; for now we just note its importance and the need to construct new scripts based on new insights into interpersonal patterns.

19.6 Concluding Comments

This chapter is intended to illustrate how the general stages of change framework can be used to treat a maladaptive behavioural pattern. This framework is not intended to be followed in a fixed way nor should it be assumed that all the interventions illustrated will be needed with all cases or that they should be used in the sequence described. It is simply a heuristic device to help the therapist to organize treatment and as a way to remind the therapist of the issues that need to be addressed when seeking to change any behaviour, schema, or way of thinking. It should also be noted that the module will not be required with all patients because many are not as submissive as Anna. However, I suspect that the significance of this trait is sometimes missed because clinicians focus on more overt behavioural features of BPD because these are emphasized by current diagnostic systems and some common therapies. When there is a history of abuse and frequent enmeshments in abusive relationships, it is useful to consider the possibility that these behavioural tendencies lurk in the background.

Chapter 20

Working with the Core Interpersonal Conflict

This chapter discusses the management of the core conflict between need for care, love, attention, and proximity with attachment figures and significant others and fear of rejection both throughout therapy and during this phase of treatment. The conflict arises when psychosocial adversity creates an approach-avoidance conflict in which the natural tendency to seek out attachment figures when threatened also activates fear of approaching these individuals because of the harm that they previously caused. To simplify this discussion, the management of each pole of the conflict will be discussed separately followed by some general comments on treating the overall conflict.

20.1 Neediness and Dependency

The intense dependency associated with borderline personality disorder (BPD) usually arises from deprivation and abuse. However, dependency can also result from overprotective caregiving. Although the two forms of dependency have some common features, they have different treatment implications.

20.1.1 Patterns of Dependency

Overprotectiveness fosters dependency by hindering the development of independence, self-efficacy, and confidence in one's ability to interact effectively with the world, leading to a constant need for guidance and reassurance. This kind of dependency is usually less severe and presents fewer management problems than dependency arising from deprivation, because with overprotective caregiving the child's early needs for care are usually met. Hence the therapeutic task is to foster independence and self-efficacy. Although this pattern can occur with BPD (Allison, a patient who will be discussed in later chapters, showed some of these features), it is less common than dependency arising from deprivation. The latter combines a need for support and reassurance with intense neediness. This presents more management problems because gratification of these needs tends to stimulate them rather than satisfy them, leading to increased demands for care and decreased coping. This outcome is seen in patients with severe BPD who deteriorate as a result of contact with the mental health system. It is as if the care they received, especially if in-patient care is involved, increases these needs, leading to further regression. This eventuality is reduced by adopting a therapeutic stance that provides support while also promoting change and self-efficacy. Nevertheless, some clinicians become overly concerned about patients becoming dependent and regressing in therapy, leading them to fail to provide the support needed to build the alliance. However, a modest degree of short-term dependency on therapy and the therapist need not be a problem, providing it fosters alliance formation and leads to progress. Such dependency can subsequently be managed and resolved as treatment progresses. Dependency is usually only a cause for concern when associated with lack of progress or actual deterioration.

In the early stages of therapy, both kinds of dependency are often expressed as a strong desire for advice and reassurance so that they are largely differentiated by reference to the patient's history. Over time, however, those with dependency arising from deprivation show greater neediness and describe an intense need for care and love in ways that are qualitatively different from these with an overprotective background. Since dependency arising from attachment trauma is the general pattern with BPD, this will be the primary focus of this section with only brief mention of ways to deal with overprotective dependency. The assumption is that the latter pattern will largely be addressed by building self-esteem, self-efficacy, and self-confidence.

20.1.2 Applying the Stages of Change Model

The treatment of dependency can be structured using the *stages of change* approach although it requires modification. First, patients usually think initially that the problem is not their neediness but rather the failure of significant others to meet their needs. Hence, they are more concerned with getting significant others to change or with finding someone who can provide the love and care they seek rather than changing the needs themselves. It usually takes patients considerable time to recognize that this approach does not work and that the only solution is to modify these needs. Until this realization occurs, the focus is more on managing dependency rather than changing it with direct interventions. The general treatment modules seek to do this by establishing a treatment process that minimizes the risk of fostering regression.

Second, changing dependency and neediness is more complex than the other changes that have been discussed. With self-harming behaviour, emotional dysregulation, and submissiveness, change is largely a matter of identifying the problem, eliciting a commitment to change, exploring the behaviour, and taking steps to change it. Intense dependency is a more complex problem and the goal is different. We seek not only to modulate dependency but also to help the patient to accept that some aspects of dependency, especially extreme neediness, cannot be satisfied because it belongs to a different stage of life and that the only solution is to relinquish it. But this understanding only tends to emerge in the final phases of therapy. This may not appear to be so different from the goal with deliberate self-injury; however, ceasing to engage in a relatively specific behaviour is a different proposition from relinquishing a longing that is a core part of the self.

Third, exploration of neediness invariably evokes emotionally laden memories of childhood events associated with neglect, deprivation, and the failure of caregivers to provide love, care, and protection. The means that work on neediness has to be graduated according to the patient's capacity to manage the feelings involved. It also means that the distinction between exploration and change, something that is always a little blurry, is even less clear. However, I will retain the distinction here to organize a description of the change process. It is also a useful structure for therapists to keep in mind when managing the process.

20.1.2.1 Stage 1: Pattern Recognition and Commitment to Change

Since it takes time for dependency needs to be fully recognized and accepted, the initial commitment to change is usually confined to talking about these needs and trying to understand them. With Anna, these needs featured prominently in therapy from the outset because many crises resulted from some kind of failure to meet them. Nevertheless, Anna did not consider these needs to be a problem: she saw the problem as someone's failure to act appropriately and the rage she felt about this failure prevented her from even thinking about her needs. Hence, initially treatment was more concerned with containing the emotions these needs aroused than with understanding them. From time to time, however, especially when exhausted by the impotency of her rage, Anna collapsed into a state of overwhelming despair about her need to be loved and how no one seemed to either care or understand. On these occasions, these needs were acknowledged as something "we need to talk about" but the emphasis continued to be placed on containing the distress. Once she had become more settled, scenarios involving some failure to meet her needs were used to get a commitment to try to understand them.

With other patients, there is a reluctance to recognize neediness because this increases feelings of vulnerability. This leads them to assert their independence and self-reliance by defiantly proclaiming that they are perfectly capable of managing by themselves. This reaction is common in institutional settings where feelings of vulnerability may be interpreted as a sign of weakness that others will prey upon or exploit.

20.1.2.2 Stage 2: Pattern Exploration

Exploration usually involves discussing scenarios that suggest excessive reliance on others or intense neediness to foster awareness of these needs and their impact on relationships and well-being.

20.1.2.2.1 Exploration in the Context of the Therapeutic Relationship

Early in treatment, both forms of dependency often lead patients to seek explicit advice on a wide range of matters with comments such as, "Do you think that I am doing the right thing?" "What should I say to him?" Some highly dependent individuals take this a stage further by insisting that the therapist should provide a solution: "Tell me what to do because you have dealt with these problems before and so you know what's best." In managing such situations, the challenge is to convey an understanding of the intensity of these needs without gratifying them. This requires helping patients to realize that decisions about what to do and how to live their lives can only be legitimately made by the patient themselves although the therapist can help in understanding issues and options. Nevertheless, this kind of input is more likely to be accepted if the therapist acknowledges that this is not what the patient wants and discusses the patient's disappointment. This type of discussion conducted in a supportive and understanding way often helps patients to talk about their needs as opposed to demanding their gratification. At the same time, simple generic interventions such as encouraging modest goals, highlighting changes, and acknowledging assets also help to manage these needs by helping patients build the confidence and self-efficacy needed to counter the regressive pull of intense neediness.

A second way these needs are expressed early in therapy is excessive concern about planned absences or breaks in therapy: "I do not know how I am going to manage when you are away." At this stage, the underlying needs and fears need to be recognized while also enhancing coping. Hence the therapist may acknowledge the patient's concerns about being unable to cope or even survive during the absence but then challenge him/her by noting that the patient has felt this way before and managed in order to affirm the patient's resilience. These concerns can also be discussed again after the absence to reaffirm the patient's ability to manage without the therapist. Such examples provide a starting point for promoting an understanding of how dependency needs are expressed, and, equally importantly, how these behaviours influence interpersonal relationships. For example, patients do not always recognize how these behaviours encourage assertive or controlling individuals to be more dominating or how these behaviours can trigger abuse.

An important practice point linked to positive outcomes is to help patients to understand that the schemas and associated behaviours enacted in therapy are the same as those that create problems in everyday situations. This understanding is promoted by encouraging patients to identify scenarios involving significant others that are similar to those occurring in therapy. The process of working with both within-therapy and extra-therapy events enhances understanding of the impact of these behaviours on everyday relationships. Within-therapy exploration also permits an in-depth examination of these behaviours as they occur.

20.1.2.2.2 Identifying Maintaining Schemas

Overprotective dependency tends to be associated with inadequacy, incompetence, and fear or guilt about showing independence, and shame about being dependent and conversely about wanting to be independent, whereas dependency arising from neglect and abuse is more associated with neediness, feeling flawed or damaged, being unlovable, rage over neglect, shame, and sometimes a sense of entitlement ("I deserve to be looked after"). Usually it takes time to uncover these schemas because they are used automatically and associated with intense affect.

20.1.2.2.3 Accessing and Working with Associated Emotions

Dependency associated with overprotectiveness tends to evoke intense anxiety, fearfulness, and avoidance, which limits exploration and thwarts attempts to act differently. Change is largely achieved by encouraging behavioural experiments to try out new behaviours and using any success to challenge beliefs of incompetence and inadequacy. Dependency associated with neglect and deprivation is also related to intense anger, sadness, loss, and shame. This collage of emotions intensifies demands for care and attention and hinders exploration. The emotions also make it difficult to find suitable ways to satisfy these needs either because they alienate those the patient turns to for help as occurred with Anna or because the patient insists that they are satisfied in particular ways as shown by the way Madison insisted that mother demonstrated caring by being available whenever asked.

The emotions associated with neediness differ in accessibility. Anger and rage are never far from the surface. Underlying them are painful feelings of sadness and loss that can create an intense state of despair and emptiness. Below them lurks shame and associated beliefs of being defective and unlovable. In therapy, it was necessary to work through the different levels of emotion to access sadness and loss, and ultimately shame. A reduction of anger and rage resulting from increased self-regulation of emotion usually permits work on sadness and loss about the neglect or abuse. This work then usually leads to awareness of the shame generated by both the developmental events that lead to neediness and the intensity of these needs.

20.1.2.3 Stage 3: Promoting Change

Restructuring strong dependency needs takes time and interventions switch back and forth between exploration and change as different facets of these behaviours are addressed. In Anna's case, this work was spread over about a year during which exploration of the schemas and emotions associated with dependency gradually made them more accessible to restructuring using the general methods discussed in Chapter 18. These changes modulated the behaviours sufficiently to allow a more systematic focus on these problems in therapy.

20.1.1.3.1 Recognizing Strengths and Promoting Self-Efficacy

Dependency behaviours are maintained and even accentuated by beliefs of incompetence and inadequacy. Hence change is achieved both by challenging these beliefs directly and by using any change such as decreased self-harm and improved emotional self-regulation to foster counterbalancing schemas of self-efficacy and positive expectations about change. With Anna, throughout therapy any change was used to challenge her doubts about being able to manage without help and to reinforce the fact that she had made changes she had not thought possible. Her belief in her capacity to change was also enhanced by noting repeatedly that she seemed to spend a lot of time between sessions thinking about her problems and commenting on the depth of her understanding and how this was helping her to get a handle on her difficulties and to identify the things she needed to do to change. This focus on reinforcing self-reflection was very useful in helping Anna to relinquish some aspects of her intense neediness especially for love and attention, as will be discussed later.

20.1.1.3.2 Reducing Demandingness

Some of the intensity of dependency needs arises because these needs are consistently frustrated. This occurs for many reasons including the patient's conflicts about these needs. They are also frustrated by the way patients seek help. We came across this idea briefly when discussing crises when it was suggested that patients learn to request help rather than demand it. This point usually needs to be made frequently because the anger generated by intense neediness continually frustrates effective help-seeking. In effect, patients need to learn the old adage that you attract more bees with honey than with vinegar. Although they recognize the significance of this idea, it takes considerable time, multiple repetitions, and the exploration of multiple scenarios before it becomes part of their behavioural repertoire.

20.1.1.3.3 Sublimating Dependency Needs

Altruistic, caregiving behaviour is a powerful antidote to regression and a useful way to contain neediness. As therapy progresses beyond the regulation and modulation phase, opportunities arise to manage dependency by encouraging patients to meet these needs by caring for others rather than by being cared for. This issue was briefly discussed in the previous chapter on managing submissiveness. The benefit of this sublimating of dependency needs is occasionally seen on in-patient units following a crisis admission. As the crisis settles, some patients begin to help other patients, especially those less able to fend for themselves, and these activities seem to help them to reintegrate.

At various times, I have referred to the role of work in the recovery process. When discussing the early sessions, reference was made to the value-building structure into the patient's day. With increased stability, this can be taken further by encouraging patients to find employment even if only voluntary work. Working creates structure and builds self-worth. It encourages a more outward-looking perspective to compensate for an intense inner focus. It also provides opportunities to channel dependency needs into more useful outlets by encouraging patients to seek work caring for others, or if the patient has major interpersonal difficulties, it may be better to work with animals such as volunteering at an animal shelter. What matters is that they find a way to sublimate their dependency needs and develop an interest outside themselves. Modulating dependency in this way often makes it more amenable to other interventions.

20.1.1.3.4 Relinquishing Neediness

Ultimately, patients need help in accepting that neediness cannot be satisfied and needs have to be given up. However, they have to reach this understanding for themselves because it is unlikely to be accepted very readily if it comes from the therapist and any mistiming of the suggestion often evokes intense anger that is difficult for the patient to process and to accusations that the therapist simply does not understand. Realization of the necessity of relinquishing neediness occurred late in Anna's treatment. Throughout therapy, she talked about her longing to find someone to look after her and love her. Behind most interpersonal encounters lay an intense, excruciatingly painful longing to be loved that originated in childhood deprivation. As therapy progressed, Anna talked increasingly of her longing for mother to show love and affection. Unfortunately, mother always seemed indifferent to Anna's distress and hypercritical of her behaviour. From time to time, Anna felt hopeful that mother was beginning to be supportive and that the gulf between them was being bridged, but each time her hopes were dashed and she crashed into despair.

Occasional interviews with Anna's mother suggested that she felt little affection for Anna probably because she triggered painful memories from mother's childhood. Indeed, Anna's periodic attempts to engage mother caused her to withdraw even more. This situation continued through the first two years of treatment. As crises settled and emotional control increased, Anna talked more openly of her longing and her anger at mother's behaviour. However, the anger was always tinged with hope that mother would change. Anna also came to recognize the intensity of her needs and likened them to those of a little girl, noting that she still felt small around mother. She began to find other outlets for her needs by helping others in a controlled and planned way. By this time, mother had moved to another city and Anna saw her less frequently. Then suddenly problems with her husband came to a head and mother suggested that Anna go to stay with her while she decided what to do. Anna was ecstatic. Here at last was the opportunity to be reconciled with mother and to have relationship she longed for. She left almost immediately.

Unfortunately, things did not work out. Anna terminated the visit and she returned to her husband. In a subsequent therapy session, she discussed what happened and it was clear that she had given it much thought. Although mother had invited her to stay, Anna felt unwelcome and mother was cold and hypercritical. She showed little empathy for Anna's situation and seemed unable to offer support. Anna had talked things over with her father who was more supportive. He discussed the situation with Anna's mother but he was unable to get her to soften her stance. The relationship between Anna and her mother deteriorated until Anna left. After describing events in detail, the following dialogue occurred:

ANNA: I was so angry – why invite me and then treat me like that. But then I thought what's the point. What's the point, she won't change. So, I have given up on her. She is never going to love me. I am not even angry about it anymore

THERAPIST: You're not? [checking whether this is simple avoidance because in the past Anna's rage was intense].

ANNA: No!

THERAPIST: What happened to it?

ANNA: I realized she couldn't do it. I used to get mad, really mad, because I thought that she did not love me and that she was holding back. I thought she was deliberately treating me in that way. Then it suddenly hit me – she can't. Now, I feel sad for her. [Note how anger is giving way to sadness – see earlier discussion on the layering of emotions.] I realized that I don't need her. I used to think I did. Now it doesn't matter anymore. It did but it doesn't now [she shrugged her shoulders dismissively].

THERAPIST: The time has passed. [Note, Anna's previous comment suggests that she is beginning to realize that mother cannot provide what she has longed for and that she does not need her love and attention. This allows the therapist to take this realization just a little further by beginning to put this need in the past as a step towards helping Anna to accept that it ultimately needs to be relinquished.]

ANNA: Yes. I don't need her anymore. We'll talk. I'll keep in touch in the same way but I won't be looking to her for help.

Anna's realization that mother cannot meet her needs and, more importantly, that she does not need her resulted from extensive preparatory work that created a context that allowed Anna to see mother differently – that she was not withholding as Anna had previously thought but rather that she also had problems that prevented her from loving Anna. She began to see things from mother's perspective and to recognize that mother was also struggling with issues that were outside her control. This allowed her to be more empathic and also more objective. Earlier efforts to promote self-reflection allowed Anna to think about and process what happened in a way that allowed her to control the pain and distress generated by her longing for mother's love. It is also clear just how far Anna has come in building trust not only in therapy and the therapist but also in her own abilities and judgement. The content of the session suggests that Anna had given extensive thought to what had happened in the time since leaving mother's home and seeing the therapist again. In the session, the therapist was largely being used as a sounding board as Anna recounted the conclusions of extensive self-reflection. All the therapist had to do was to reflect key points and add the occasional comment to deepen Anna's understanding.

20.1.1.3.5 Working through the Sadness

Of course, Anna's new realizations did not end here. Considerable time was spent dealing with the consequences of this incident. But the focus changed. Whereas Anna's feelings about her mother were previously dominated by anger and rage, they were now largely feelings of sadness and loss. In a subsequent session, when Anna wept inconsolably about mother's inability to love her, she said that it felt as if there was a little girl inside her who longed for her mother to love her and who desperately sought to please everyone in order to get them to love her. She recalled how hard she had worked as a young child to do things that would cause mother to love her. On one occasion, she had carefully tidied mother's bedroom in the hope that it would make mother happy but mother criticized and mocked her efforts. She remembered how she had carefully memorized the way mother arranged objects on her dressing table so that she could put them in exactly the same place in future. But nothing ever seemed to work. Mother could never be pleased or placated.

The surprising feature of this phase of treatment was that despite being extremely distressed within sessions, Anna otherwise functioned well and her general adjustment continued to improve. Gradually, she came to accept that she would never have the mother she had longed for, and to her surprise, she found this liberating. Rather than focusing on the past and what she did not have, she began to think more about what she had and what she wanted. It should be noted that at this point in treatment, sessions were once a month but Anna spent a considerable amount of time between sessions thinking about what had been discussed and reflecting in depth on her childhood experiences, her current feelings about mother, and her current situation.

The next session also revealed the depth of the work Anna was doing between sessions. She started by noting that she had been thinking more about mother's inability to love her and that in addition to the fact that Anna reminded her of events from mother's own childhood that impeded her capacity to show love, she also decided that mother felt threatened by her because "my dad loved me." She added that she had always been father's favourite. Such a comment could be interpreted in various fanciful ways but the simplest explanation seems to be that mother was needy herself and needed to be the centre of attention. Consequently, she was unable to tolerate the fact that Anna, a child she did not love and rejected, was loved by her husband. On various occasions, she forced her husband to choose between her and Anna, the last time being when Anna had stayed with her and her father had attempted to get mother to treat Anna differently.

Between sessions, memories of childhood had flooded back. Anna recalled how mother had expected her to care for a younger sister even though she was not much older and that she had to do the grocery shopping from a young age. She also recalled they were never supposed to bother mother so if one of them got hurt mother got very angry with them for causing problems. She recalled having an acute pain in the night and being terrified of waking mother and mother taking her to the hospital and on the way threatening her that she had better be really ill. On another occasion, mother had hit her so hard she broke her arm. Mother blamed Anna saying that it was her fault because she should not have made her so mad. Even an uncle who came to help blamed Anna for what she had done to mother. Anna said that now she realized that no matter what happened, mother made herself into the victim, and everyone else in the family bought into the idea.

As she recalled these events, Anna became increasingly sad and sobbed inconsolably that she was only a child. However, it never felt as if she was a child. Mother had never let her be a child. She never helped her, let her do what she wanted, and generally neglected her. She recalled that an older neighbour who seemed to understand what was happening used to meet her as she walked home from school alone and take her to her own home and cuddle her. As she sobbed, Anna linked these events to her life. She noted that the men she chose were like her mother and that she treated them in the same way. She constantly sought to please them as she did her mother in the hope they would love her but they never did and like mother they constantly pushed her away. The only exception was Marty. She felt loved by him but he was like her father, and eventually he left. As she looked back, she noted that they were all like children. She did everything for them as she had done to her family but they rarely reciprocated. It all felt so sad.

Then Anna took a slightly new direction. She said that as she thought about never feeling like a child, she realized that she had not been nurtured and had not learned to nurture herself. She added:

> I do everything for everyone because I want to be loved and I want everyone to nurture me but they don't. The only way to heal myself is to nurture myself. And, that's what I'm doing. I'm peeling away the layers to understand what really happened and now I realize it was not my fault. I didn't create it. I loved my mum, I idolized her. I wanted her to love me. I was so in love with her, I wanted to please her. I do that with everyone.

And so Anna began to link her need for love with her people-pleasing submissiveness discussed in the previous chapter. She continued, "I thought I was a monster who did not deserve to be loved. But then I thought how bad can a seven-year-old child be?" Anna went on to say that she realized that she had to learn to nurture and love herself. She added that her children were teaching her because they were nurturing her and she was able to let them. To which the therapist commented, "And you are nurturing them." Anna said, "Yes, they feel loved." Anna was recognizing that her children provided what she had been searching for – someone to love and be loved by. She was also recognizing that this was sufficient.

The description of this session does not do justice to the emotions involved. This was an intense emotional session in which Anna experienced the intensity of her sadness and the painful realization of what she had missed. However, she quickly regrouped when the session ended.

20.1.1.3.6 Working through the Shame

In the sessions in which Anna described anger and sadness linked to her longing for mother to love her, she touched on underlying schemas of being bad and unlovable – a monster who did not deserve to be loved. As work on the sadness continued, she talked more about these schemas and the associated feeling of shame became more accessible.

Shame plays an important part in maintaining neediness and the anger it evokes. As Anna continued to work through her longing for mother to love her and the anger and the sadness it created, she began to experience intense shame because mother did not love her. At the same time, she began to link the shame to core schemas of being bad and unlovable. She also began to recognize the extent to which she had blamed herself for mother's behaviour and how this shame dominated her relationships. The shame also seemed to keep alive Anna's hopes that mother would eventually love her. Part of her felt that if only she could change and stop being a bad girl, mother would eventually love her. It also protected her from the painful realization that mother was actually incapable of doing so.

Shame, unlike anxiety and most other negative emotions, is not managed primarily using emotion-regulation strategies but more by bringing it into the open where it can be discussed, experienced, tolerated, and processed in the here-and-now of therapy. When brought into the open in this way, shame tends to fade. The therapist's acceptance and empathy play a major role in this process. Essentially, the patient learns from the therapist how to show self-compassion and to realize that there is nothing to be ashamed about. As Anna eventually put it, "Why should I be so ashamed? I did nothing wrong. I was a child.

I was not supposed to care for her. She was supposed to care for me." It seems that experiencing shame in the context of a relationship that conveys empathy and compassion allows the shame to be processed and understood rather than split off and avoided.

20.1.2.4   Stage 4: Generalization and Consolidation

At this phase of treatment, there is little distinction between the exploration, change, and generalization stages of change. Most of the work that Anna did to change her dependency behaviour and begin resolving feelings about mother also involved changing her everyday interactions with others. She also began the long, and sometimes painful, process of constructing a new narrative, a necessary achievement if the changes that she was making were to become incorporated into her life.

Anna's original narrative about herself and mother was one of rage at mother's failure to be loving that led to angry demands that mother, and everyone else in her life, change and that others provide what mother failed to do. This made her preoccupied with the past and prevented her from seeing and seeking other ways of meeting her needs and other ways of living a satisfying life. Slowly, a different narrative took shape that incorporated acceptance of the past as something that could not be changed but which does not need to dominate her life. She began to talk about what she could do to make her life rewarding, which allowed her to see opportunities that she had not recognized before. We will return to the issue of narrative construction in the next chapter. However, this work illustrates the point made several times previously that change involves more than learning new skills or restructuring maladaptive schemas and modes of thought. It also involves creating new narratives and scripts that allow people to see themselves and their social lives differently and establish new ways of living.

20.2 Rejection-Sensitivity

The other pole of the core conflict is rejection-sensitivity, a complex amalgam of schemas associated with the interpersonal traits of attachment insecurity, submissiveness, and fear of disapproval/need for approval. Each trait is organized around a specific social fear – loss of, or abandonment by, attachment figures; threat arising from others who are considered more dominant or important; and fear of social disapproval or exclusion. The schemas linked to attachment insecurity that contribute to rejection-sensitivity primarily involve fears and expectations of rejection, abandonment, and loss of significant others and beliefs that abandonment is intolerable and likely to be catastrophic. Submissiveness contributes schemas linked to fear evoking anger. Finally, the trait need for approval/fear of disapproval contributes such schemas as a need to be accepted, fear of rejection and disapproval, and fear of exclusion. The result is a multifaceted combination of schemas that exerts a powerful influence on interpersonal relationships.

20.2.1 Overview of the Change Process

Like work on modulating and changing neediness, changes to rejection-sensitivity are spread throughout therapy and the nature of this work changes as therapy progresses. However, the goal of change differs. With neediness, the ultimate goal is to relinquish the more primitive aspects of dependency needs, whereas with rejection-sensitivity, the goal is to reduce these fears. This is achieved both by building competing schemas and by restructuring the schema itself and the events that arouse it.

Early in therapy, rejection-sensitivity arises primarily in the context of crises triggered by fear of abandonment. During this phase, the focus was largely on identifying fear of rejection and discussing the feelings it evokes in the context of the patient's relationships with specific individuals. The concern always at this stage is to contain distress but as therapy progresses the patient is increasingly encouraged to challenge and dispute these beliefs.

The schema is also activated in the context of the therapeutic relationship and this requires more active attention because it may threaten the alliance and therapy. Anna, for example, raised concerns about the therapist abandoning her in the first few sessions both directly and indirectly by noting that people always left and that this had happened with a previous counsellor. This was discussed as fully as Anna's mental state permitted. Her concerns were also validated by noting that they were understandable given her previous experiences. However, fear of rejection is largely managed by establishing a corrective treatment process. Changes to rejection-sensitivity largely involve the use of interpersonal methods for changing schemas discussed in Chapter 18. Throughout therapy, the continuous corrective experience provided by a treatment process organized around generic interventions effectively challenges and disconfirms fears of rejection. At the same time, patients are encouraged to use standard cognitive methods for reviewing and challenging evidence supporting and negating the interpretation of some events that evoke rejection fears.

As therapy progresses, the depth at which rejection, dependency needs, and the need for love and care are expressed progressively increases and begins to incorporate memories of neglect, abuse, attachment trauma, and earlier feelings of rejection along with increasing awareness of the different emotions linked to these experiences. This progress seems to be related to two therapeutic developments. First, work on the more intense experiences and feelings associated with rejection-sensitivity and neediness requires improved emotion regulation. In fact, the rate at which emotion dysregulation improves seems to determine the overall rate of therapeutic progress. It is not just that emotion-regulation skills are needed to stop the painful feelings associated with rejection and neediness from spinning out of control but also the struggle to deal with unstable emotions is exhausting, leaving little energy or appetite for dealing with painful interpersonal issues. Second, exploration and change of rejection-sensitivity and neediness require considerable trust in the therapist and therapy, which takes time to build. I briefly mentioned the importance of trust when discussing strategies for changing intense dependency as illustrated by the treatment of Anna. However, we need to consider this issue in a little more detail because it is fundamental to change in core interpersonal and self pathology.

20.2.2 Trust: A Prerequisite for Change

Given the importance of trust, we need to consider what we actually mean by trust and the factors that generate it. Trust is built primarily through therapist–patient interaction rather than through interventions that seek to restructure the schemas involved. It is built through multiple relationship experiences that consistently challenge the patient's feelings of distrust and model a different way of relating. This starts with the therapist providing a consistent relationship experience and treatment process. This demonstrates the therapist's commitment to the patient and treatment and offers tangible evidence of the therapist's responsiveness and availability that help to counter fears that the therapist will be like previous attachment figures who were neither available nor responsive. Promotion of trust continues with the therapist showing a genuine interest in understanding the patient and his/her experiences and in validating these experiences. Trust is deepened when the patient experiences a sense of being understood by the therapist, especially feeling understood in the context of the treatment relationship. This requires the therapist to communicate understanding and acceptance of the way the patient relates to the therapist and the complexities of this relationship. Trust is also enhanced by the therapist being open to ideas with regard to both understanding the patient's problems and concerns and in exploring these concerns and how they can be changed. Finally, throughout therapy events occur in which patients behave, either wittingly or unwittingly, in ways that test the therapist's commitment to the therapy and patient. At these times, maladaptive schemas and associated interpersonal patterns get reenacted in treatment, and when the therapist behaves differently from the patient's expectations, these beliefs are disconfirmed and associated behaviours are weakened. In the process, trust increases.

However, the kind of trust that is needed to make fundamental changes in interpersonal and self pathology is more than simply being able to rely on the therapist's responsiveness, availability, empathic understanding, and commitment. The additional component is more a sense that the therapist can be relied upon to behave in a genuine way without any hint of subterfuge and, equally importantly, relied upon to act with the patient's best interests in mind. This is linked to what has been called existential trust or distrust[1] – acceptance of the fact that the therapist's communications and actions are genuine and authentic. This kind of trust takes time to develop. When patients have been exposed to the kind of attachment trauma that Anna experienced, it is simply not adaptive to relinquish the schemas, beliefs, and relationship patterns that it inculcated too easily. They developed to protect the person from these experiences and minimize their consequences. Even though maladaptive, it probably seems prudent to the patient to change them slowly and only when it is abundantly clear that it is safe to do so.

20.2.3 Rejection-Sensitivity in the Later Stages of Treatment

By the time therapy reaches the current phase, rejection-sensitivity is usually less intense. It was modulated by the treatment process and by consistently encouraging patients to dispute these beliefs using simple cognitive methods. It also loses some of its intensity when the patient's emotional life becomes more settled because intense emotions seem to drive rejection fears. They also cause others to act in ways that threaten rejection and hence confirm the schema. This is what happened with Madison.

20.2.3.1 The Effect of Increased Emotion Regulation

Increased emotion regulation led to a substantial decrease in Madison's abandonment anxiety. Consequently, relatively little therapeutic work was done on interpersonal problems other than helping her to dispute her fears of rejection and abandonment as they occurred with her parents and more importantly with her boyfriend. This work was sufficient and her fears lost much of their intensity. This is probably because the rejection-sensitivity was largely driven by Madison's emotional state whereas with Anna it was largely the result of attachment trauma so that improved emotional control had less impact. What seemed to matter more was change in the intensity of her need to be loved and cared for, an issue I will return to later.

Improved emotion regulation does not just free the energy needed to effect other changes; it also changes the way other people respond to the patient. With Madison, many of the experiences of rejection she experienced from boyfriends occurred because they could not cope with the intensity of her feelings or her moodiness. As these settled, she experienced fewer rejections and more positive reactions from her boyfriends, which reduced the panic she felt about possible rejection.

20.2.3.2 Strengthening Counterbalancing Schemas and Processes

Rejection-sensitivity can also be modulated by promoting schemas and personality processes that help to counterbalance or reduce fear of rejection. Since such fears increase low self-esteem and low self-worth, any development that increases feelings of self-worth reduces the probability that rejection fears will be aroused. As Madison's ability to self-manage her emotions increased, her previous self-confidence was re-established, which enabled her to see that she had assets, which helped to put her fear of rejection into perspective.

Fear of rejection was also closely linked to feeling unloved and unlovable. Changes in these schemas also help to modulate rejection-sensitivity. Madison originally interpreted her parents' difficulty being supportive during crises as an indication that they did not care about her. Rumination over these events and about boyfriends ending relationships led to the more generalized belief that she was unlovable. As the emotionality settled and other people's behaviour changed as a result, she came to see that the difficulty her parents and boyfriends had with her was not that they did not love her but rather that they could not deal with her moods and rage. This allowed her to recognize that she was not unlovable but rather unmanageable when in a crisis. As a result, the schema began to lose its absolute quality and gradually faded in significance.

Although these changes led to a substantial decrease in rejection anxiety, the fear continued to lurk in the background and came to the fore whenever a minor problem in her relationship with her boyfriend occurred because of her tendency to catastrophize. However, the problem was readily managed by encouraging her to dispute with herself. Hence therapy quickly moved to the integration and synthesis phase, which was also comparatively brief and was largely concerned with consolidating her emerging self-narrative and with helping her to re-establish her life.

20.2.3.3 The Impact of Changes in Dependency and Neediness

Strong dependency needs make the fear of rejection more alarming. Hence any decrease in dependency needs automatically leads to a decrease in rejection-sensitivity. This is largely what happened with Anna. As the intense need to be loved by mother and by the men she was involved with faded and was replaced with more adaptive ways to express these needs, her preoccupation with being rejected and rumination over previous abandonments faded as well. These events fell into perspective when she realized that the men she longed to be cared for had problems of their own that prevented them from having truly intimate relationships. These relationships became increasingly less important and she ruminated less about them as she began to move on by thinking about how she could build a life for herself and her children. Little needed to be done by way of therapeutic intervention other than to support the process and reinforce the changes she was making.

20.3 Core Conflict

Now that the two poles of the conflict between neediness and rejection-sensitivity have been discussed, we need to consider whether anything else is needed to address the conflict itself. It most cases not a lot. As the different poles of the conflict are understood and restructured, the conflict comes to have less influence on the patient's relationships. Usually all that is needed is to clarify the nature of conflict and help the patient to understand the conflict in the context of his/her life and current circumstances. In most cases, the significance of the conflict was probably noted during assessment and the patient's attention was also probably drawn to this pattern relatively early in treatment in a very general way by noting that there seems to be a pattern to the patient's relationships involving quickly getting involved with someone and then becoming disappointed and backing off.

The conflict often gets expressed early in therapy in a muted form. In most early sessions, Anna was overwhelmed but she was also very wary. Occasionally, a session occurred in which she was a little less distressed and able to open up a little more about her concerns especially about her relationship with her husband. These sessions revealed the flashes of insight that blossomed later in therapy. Such sessions were inevitably followed by a more difficult session in which Anna was upset and angry and reluctant to talk about what was happening. Simple interventions noting the difference between the two sessions and enquiring about whether Anna had also noted the change were often dismissed or explained as reflecting her exhaustion from struggling with her feelings and what was going on in her life. It was only much later that she was able to talk about how sharing things made her feel vulnerable and caused her worry about whether the therapist would give up on her like her previous therapist did.

Most of the work on the conflict focused on one pole or the other. It was as if Anna did not connect the two poles but rather saw them as separate problems. This changed in the interpersonal phase. As she began exploring her needs in relationship with mother and recalled more about childhood events that left her feeling unloved and rejected, she also began to connect these needs to her various partners and how she had felt rejected by them. At this time, the therapist provided information about the conflict and its components and how the need for love and care was related to rejection-sensitivity.

Continued exploration of the conflict as described in previous sections was also used to consolidate Anna's understanding of the way the conflict had dominated her adult relationships and how she sought to satisfy needs that mother had not met in her relationships with men. This work went well beyond merely identifying and labelling the conflict to beginning to help Anna to construct a new understanding of the theme that had organized much of her life, an understanding that also helped her to see that other options were available and that she did not need to follow the same script for the rest of her life. In working on the core conflict, efforts to help Anna to change maladaptive interpersonal patterns merged with work on constructing a more adaptive self-structure. This is the theme of the next three chapters.

20.4 Concluding Comments

No matter how much we emphasize that therapy is a collaborative process and that the patient is responsible for change, it is difficult to escape the idea that therapy basically involves the therapist intervening in some way that ultimately brings about change. The idea is understandable. This is what therapists do. The idea is also consistent with the notion that change is the result of events that are external to the person. However, it is not all that therapists do nor is it the only change process that occurs in therapy. Personality is not just the result of the impact of environmental events on heritable influences. Developmental change also arises from processes that are intrinsic to personality. A rich array of processes including self-reflective thinking and metacognitive processes are used to organize and re-organize environmental inputs and heritable factors into the complex structures and systems that constitute personality.

These intrinsic processes are disrupted in BPD. Intense unstable emotions probably interfere with their functioning by reducing the informational value of emotions and by overwhelming organizing mechanisms. They are also likely to be impeded by the rigidity that characterizes cognitive functioning in the patients and by their profound distrust of social communications. As these problems are addressed in therapy, these intrinsic orga-nizational processes begin to function again, generating changes in personality as schemas and interpersonal patterns are restructured and reorganized. This seemed to be what happened in therapy with Anna. It was noted earlier that the therapist did not need to do much more than support and reinforce the work Anna was doing between sessions to restructure her dependency needs and change how she related to others.

Note

1. The term "existential distrust" is used by Fonagy and Luyten (in press) to describe a core impairment in personality disorder involving a fundamental distrust of interpersonal communications acquired in the context of dysfunctional attachment relationships.

Introduction

The final phase of therapy seeks to construct a more adaptive self and a life worth living. Systematic work on these issues probably only occurs with relatively few patients. Most therapies that proceed beyond the crisis management phase terminate after emotion regulation improves and after some initial work on interpersonal problems. However, evidence suggests that even after apparently successful treatment many patients still have difficulties. Hence this phase is important if treatment is to achieve something more than symptomatic improvement and if patients are to be helped to live more satisfying lives.

Therapeutic work on constructing an adaptive self differs from the work of earlier phases of treatment that were largely concerned with exploring, strengthening, and restructuring already existing behaviours and schemas. Now the task is not to analyse but rather to synthesize – to construct a new self structure and narrative. This means that integration is now not only an approach to treatment but also a treatment goal – to promote integrated and coherent personality functioning.

The task of enhancing the self may seem vague and difficult, and therapists may be unsure how to proceed. This is often because the treatment literature does not offer an explicit model of the self to guide therapeutic work. However, a practical approach is to use the three-component structure outlined in Chapters 2 and 3: (i) the self as experiencing subject or knower, (ii) self as known to the person, which consists of knowledge about the self, and (iii) the self as agent and centre of self-regulation: an idea that recognizes the importance of self-directedness. At this point, the reader may wish to review earlier material before continuing with the text because this structure is the basis for the treatment strategies discussed. The model suggests that comprehensive treatment should seek to strengthen the self as knower, promote differentiation and integration of self-knowledge (self as known), and promote self-directedness (self as agent).

However, work on these issues does not begin with the final phase of therapy. Multiple changes generated throughout treatment form the foundation that contributes to the process by increasing self-knowledge, self-understanding, and self-reflection, and by modifying maladaptive ways of thinking that hinder self-development. Now the task is to build on these achievements by helping patients to (i) consolidate the effects of earlier work on the three components of the self, (ii) construct a more integrated self, (iii) formulate a more coherent self-narrative, and (iv) develop a life worth living by building a personal niche that provides opportunities for a contented and rewarding life. These are the themes of the next three chapters.

Building a More Coherent Self

This chapter has three sections. The first reviews how routine therapeutic work also facilitates self-development. The second discusses how to reconcile and integrate different self-representations and self states. The final section examines the importance of self-directedness in promoting integration.

21.1 Setting the Stage: The Contribution of Earlier Therapeutic Work

The three-component structure of the self – the self as knower, known, and agent – used to organize this phase of treatment also provides a useful way to think about how routine interventions impact the self.

21.1.1 Strengthening the Self as Knower

Strengthening the self as knower is crucial in constructing a more coherent self and a life worth living. Unless patients trust their basic feelings and wants, there is no basis for elaborating a sense of who they are and what they want from life. Earlier, it was noted that our sense of self is based on our subjective experience of (i) personal unity and coherence, (ii) personal continuity across time, (iii) clarity and certainty about self-knowledge, and (iv) authenticity and conviction about basic emotions and wants. Experiences of unity and continuity anchor us to our world and provide the sense of stability and permanence needed for self-development. We also need to feel a sense of certainty and authenticity about our experiences, especially our emotions, if we are to interact effectively with the world. When we do not trust our basic experiences, we are deprived of the information needed to make decisions, leaving us uncertain about how to act and creating an existential distrust of the information we receive from others. Since all aspects of the self as knower are impaired in borderline personality disorder (BPD), construction of a more adaptive self begins by strengthening these features.

Patients' certainty about the authenticity of basic experiences is increased by validation and its effects may be increased by drawing patients' attention to how they are becoming more certain about their experiences and more confident in their judgements. Simple comments such as, "You seem to be more sure about your feelings," or "You seem to doubt yourself less" reinforce confidence and strengthen the self as knower. Authenticity is also enhanced by promoting self-efficacy because people feel more authentic when they believe that they are the authors of their own behaviour, that they can control their own destiny, and that their actions arise from their own internal states such as wants and feelings rather than from external factors such as the actions of others.[1] People also feel more authentic when they believe that they have a choice about how to behave and that their actions are consistent with their basic nature. Therapists can use these ideas to build self-efficacy and hence feelings of authenticity by helping patients to recognize that they have options, encouraging them to exercise this choice, and to see that they, not other people, are responsible for how they feel and what they do.

Earlier work also modulated behaviours that cause patients to doubt their basic feelings. Especially important are reducing emotional lability and maladaptive modes of thought such as self-invalidation, catastrophizing, and externalizing. Unstable emotions cause patients to doubt the genuineness of their feelings because they are so variable and intense and because these fluctuations undermine their sense of unity and stability. Hence greater stability increases confidence in personal experiences and qualities. We saw this with Madison. When her emotions became more stable, she was able to construct a new narrative that helped her to manage her emotions more effectively and incorporate them into a global self-narrative. Changing such modes of thought as self-invalidation and externalization also facilitates self-development by removing doubts about the genuineness of personal experiences.

21.1.2 Enhancing the Self as Known

Patients with BPD have poorly defined interpersonal boundaries, limited self-knowledge, and a poorly integrated self. Much of the general work of therapy addresses these problems. Boundary development is promoted by the therapist's focus on consistency and patients acquire much of their understanding of how to maintain boundaries by observing how the therapist goes about this task. Most interventions automatically enhance self-knowledge about wishes, needs, schemas, and behavioural patterns – the raw material for constructing an adaptive self. This knowledge is subsequently transformed and elaborated by self-reflective processes to create new forms of self-understanding. Particularly important is earlier work that promotes reflective thinking because this forms the foundation for self-development.

Integration is promoted throughout therapy by interventions that draw things together in various ways. First, the basic strategy of linking events–thoughts–feelings–actions integrates by organizing experience into meaningful temporal sequences. Second, integration is fostered by helping patients to recognize patterns to their behaviour and to see meaningful connections among behaviours that were apparently unrelated. This begins by connecting different forms of self-harm and continues by drawing together diverse behaviours into broad interpersonal patterns such as submissiveness, neediness, and rejection sensitivity. These developments are enhanced by meaningful explanations of the relationships among events and behaviours. A simple example is helping patients to connect deliberate self-harm to emotional distress, which in turn is connected to interpersonal events that evoke feelings of rejection. Such statements are like meaning bridges:[2] they connect two or more things such as events, feelings, actions, cognitions, or personality features. These kinds of constructions are especially helpful in promoting an integrated self. A third way earlier work promoted integration is by constructing narratives about specific problems such as self-harm, unstable emotions, interpersonal problems, and trauma. These narratives not only help to modulate the behaviours in question but also lay the groundwork for constructing a more adaptive self-narrative.

21.1.3 Increasing Self as Agent

The development of self-directedness is a slow incremental process especially with regard to the ability to set and work towards long-term goals. Like other aspects of self-development, strengthening of the agentic self begins early in treatment with initial steps to establish and attain short-term treatment goals. Any success increases self-efficacy – a prerequisite for self-directedness. Success can also be used to encourage patients to take ownership of changes that occur and to help them to recognize that they have the resources and ability to change their lives. As a result of these interventions, patients should enter this phase of treatment with a stronger sense of self-efficacy and agency that can then be used to encourage an interest in setting future goals and directions.

21.1.4 Summary

This brief review of the contributions of routine therapeutic work to self-development is intended to alert the therapist to opportunities to enhance the self throughout therapy and also to draw attention to the fact that although the self is complex, the interventions needed to build a more adaptive self are relatively straightforward. If we can establish basic conditions such as trust in the genuineness of one's basic mental state and remove impediments to self-development such as persistent self-invalidation, lack of self-efficacy, and emotional avoidance, the basic mechanisms used to construct the self can then begin to function again. These mechanisms can then be enhanced with simple interventions that help to integrate self-knowledge and construct adaptive narratives.

Although much of the work promoting integration to this point in treatment has been relatively low-level integration achieved by connecting and linking events and experiences and by drawing things together by identifying behavioural patterns, patients often note the benefits of this work. For example, one patient noted that she was feeling better and more together. She added that she had been feeling better for some time but feeling "together" was new and it made her feel more settled. Such comments are important. Since they hint at the emergence of greater coherence in personality functioning, they need to be highlighted whenever they occur even if only by reflecting on them or asking what the patient thinks has helped him or her to feel more "together." Besides these low-level integrations, more systematic attempts were occasionally made to promote higher-level integration by constructing narratives. The next sections and the next two chapters discuss how to further this work by reconciling and integrating different representations of the self and promoting self-directedness (the rest of this chapter) and by combining specific narratives into a global understanding of the self (Chapter 22) and establishing a life worth living (Chapter 23).

21.2 Reconciling and Integrating Different Views of the Self

Adaptive self systems are integrated. The different items of self-knowledge (primarily self-schemas) that constitute the self as known are connected to form a matrix: the richer the connections within this matrix, the greater the sense of integration and coherence. Patients with BPD have a poorly integrated self structure: the connections among items of self-knowledge are impoverished. Also in many cases, self-knowledge is organized into distinct clusters with few connections between clusters. The different clusters give rise to distinct self-states, each characterized by a specific constellation of thoughts, feelings, actions, and interpersonal behaviour. An important task for this phase of treatment is to integrate and reconcile these different self-states.

21.2.1 Self-States

Multiple, poorly integrated self-states are an important feature of severe BPD.[3] Although self-states vary widely across patients, states such as out of control, paralysed, shut down, blank, filled with rage, terrified, frightened, a mess, jealous, and incompetent are common. For example, earlier descriptions (see Chapters 3 and 5) of the self-states of a man in his early forties referred to two distinct self-states, one of a loving family man who cared deeply for his wife and three young children, and the other characterized by an intense state of despair, self-loathing, and emptiness. These states were not only characterized by different emotions and schemas, but also represented different experiences of the self in relationship to his world and different patterns of social interaction.

In the family-man state, he was caring, attentive, and worked hard to support his family. When in this state, his wife and family loved him dearly for his caring and kindness. However, when in the self-loathing state, he felt an intolerable sense of inner emptiness, which caused him to feel morose, to want little to do with his family, and to lash out in rage. In this state, which could last for days or even weeks, he had little recall of his more normal state and hence felt that the despair would last forever. Occasionally, he moved into a third, equally dysfunctional, acting-out state in which he was sociable and engaged in various sensation-seeking activities that caused him to neglect his family. The patient had no idea about what caused a change from one state to another.

The existence of self-states indicates the failure to develop appropriate connections among the different elements of self-knowledge so that some aspects of the self are relatively separate or split off from other parts.

At this point, we need to review briefly earlier discussions of the differences between adaptive and maladaptive self systems because we all have different images of ourselves and see ourselves differently in our different roles in life. Indeed, it was noted in Chapter 2 that an important feature of adaptive self systems is the ability to use the self matrix to construct momentary working selves – representations of the self designed to help us manage the specific situations in which we find ourselves. Hence we need to be clear about the differences between momentary working selves, an adaptive aspect of self-functioning, and self-states, a feature of a maladaptive self system.

The two differ in several ways. First, working selves are adaptive because they are context-sensitive: that is, they are constructed to help us to manage specific situations. Hence, the working self changes when the situation changes. In contrast, self-states are unrelated to context and often continue when the situation changes. Second, momentary working selves are relatively temporary whereas self-states are relatively enduring. Third, momentary working selves are experienced as aspects of the self and felt to be part of an overall sense of self whereas self-states are experienced as distinct and unrelated.

21.2.2 Changing and Integrating Self-States

Changes to self-states are brought about in two ways. First, the specific schemas, emotions, and behaviours that constitute a self-state can be restructured using the *stages of change* framework described previously as part of the routine work of the exploration and change phase of treatment. Restructuring the different components of a self-state is likely to change both the activation and intensity of the state. Second, the overall state can be changed by (i) constructing a general understanding or narrative that explains the connections between the different components of the state, what triggers the state, how the state impacts relationships, and the factors that help to maintain the state; and (ii) integrating different self-states by building connections among them.

21.2.3 Identifying Self-States

The occurrence of distinct self-states is usually first noted when assessing patients although these states are only fully recognized and confirmed as therapy progresses. During the assessment, Anna said that sometimes she felt as if she were different people. When asked what she meant, she said that she seemed to behave in extreme ways and that she suddenly changed from one extreme to another for no apparent reason. For example, on some occasions, she was overwhelmed and could not do anything and at other times she was filled with uncontrollable rage.

During the early part of therapy, these states were encountered in the context of emotional crises. In one session, Anna said that she had spent most of the previous three days in bed. When asked what had happened, she said that she suddenly felt overwhelmed and unable to cope so she went to bed and had wept most of the time. However, she was so distressed in the session that there was little opportunity for further exploration. A similar event occurring shortly afterwards evoked less distress within the session, which allowed greater exploration. Anna said that she had felt overwhelmed and spent several days in bed because she had been "running around like a chicken without a head" until she became exhausted. She also felt so unloved and uncared for that she could not cope any longer. She went to bed filled with despair and curled up like a ball because she felt so alone and so terrified of being abandoned. She also felt suicidal because it was as if she had always felt this way and always would. Anna referred to this as her unloved, needy state. On other occasions, she was filled with uncontrollable rage and lashed out at everyone. In this angry state, she resented the demands made of her and did not care about anyone or anything. She also felt bored with her life, which caused her to become more angry and demanding. It also became apparent early in therapy that Anna had a third state that differed from the other two in which she experienced a powerful need to care for others, especially her children, and devoted her time to them to the exclusion of everything else.

When working with patients to describe and explore self-states, it is important to do so in a way that brings things together and avoids further fragmentation of the self. This can occur when self-states are treated by the therapist as if they represented distinct and unrelated personalities rather than different aspects of the self. For example, therapists occasionally encourage patients to give a first name to these states, which increases the distinctiveness of these states and hence further fragmentation of the self when the goal is to connect the different states and integrate self structure.

21.2.4 Exploring Self-States

As therapy progresses, a decrease in emotionality enables more detailed exploration of self-states because the feelings generated are less disruptive. Exploration usually involves examining a specific scenario to (i) identify triggering events, (ii) track the flow of schemas and emotions, (iii) identify typical actions and behaviours, and (iv) identify the consequences in terms of the impact of the state on self and others.

21.2.4.1 Anna's "Unloved" Self-State

Detailed exploration of Anna's self-states began with the unloved, needy state during the latter part of the regulation and modulation phase when she presented a typical scenario of being unable to function for a few days. This revealed that the state was typically triggered by events that caused her to feel neglected, abandoned, or rejected. Since she was hypersensitive and saw rejection and criticism in events that others would dismiss as insignificant, the state was easily evoked. Feeling sad also seemed to play a part in activating the state because it increased her sensitivity.

As the state progressed, the rejection schema in turn evoked the schema of feeling unloved and the dependency needs discussed in the previous chapter and eventually the acute distress these schemas evoked gave way to exhaustion and quiet despair. It was at the point that Anna usually felt that there was nothing else to do but withdraw to her bed. When discussing schemas (Chapter 18), the idea of non-verbal schema was introduced and illustrated with a schema that Anna referred to as her "little Harley" state. This schema came to dominate the state giving rise to a prolonged period of intense, silent misery.

Anna's behaviour also changed as the state progressed. In the early phases of therapy when her relationship with her husband was better, Anna responded to feelings of rejection by being clingy and demanding reassurance. At that time, her husband tried to reassure her and to help her with household chores but this never seemed to be sufficient. Eventually he gave up, leaving Anna even more distraught. On other occasions, when she stayed in bed, he or other family members would visit her and ask if they could do anything. Anna always rejected such offers saying that she was alright. This behaviour was another expression of the core conflict between neediness and rejection, discussed in the previous chapter. It also shows how this conflict which originated in the past is continually reinforced and maintained in the present.

21.2.4.2 Benefits of Self-State Exploration

Fleshing out an understanding of self-states in this way takes time so we need to consider the benefits of this process. Most patients are only aware of the intensity of their feelings when in a given state and relatively unaware of why they feel this way. When Anna was confined to her bed, she seemed to exist in an amorphous state of loneliness and despair and she had little understanding of how she came to be this way. Exploration gives structure to this experience. This is useful because it provides a perspective on the experience that gradually allows patients to accept their self-states and view them more objectively. It also helped Anna to see that there was a sequence to what happened – when she felt rejected she felt an intense sense of desperation and fear that gradually led her to feel overwhelmed that led to her moving into a withdrawn isolated state that was almost timeless. As she thought about a recent scenario, Anna realized what happened to end the state – her daughter came to see if she was alright and to ask for her help. The state suddenly came to an end because she suddenly felt that she was neglecting her children, an example of how altruism counters regression.

This understanding also allowed Anna to begin taking charge of her self-states. Previously she saw herself as a victim and thought that there was nothing she could do about these states. Once she recognized what triggered this state, she began to use emotion-regulating skills whenever she felt the first sting of rejection and cognitive strategies to challenge and re-evaluate her perception of events. She also came to understand how she perpetuated the state by refusing offers of help and rejecting expressions of concern. Previously, she had not recognized that she did anything to either cause or perpetuate these states. Understanding how her behaviour influenced others and how their actions maintained these states reduced both self-blame and her tendency to blame others for her problems. This also encouraged her to think about what else she could do to change this behaviour. To her surprise, Anna began to recognize that people, including her husband, offered to help more than she realized. Also, the realization that sometimes this self-state ended because her children needed her help was a surprise and led to increased concern about her children and renewed efforts to ensure that their lives were different from her own.

An understanding of structure of self-states is also needed to begin integrating these states and building a richer network of connections within self-knowledge. To discuss how this can be achieved, I need to describe briefly the other self-states that Anna experienced.

21.2.4.3 Anna's Other Self-States

Early in therapy, Anna's angry state was also apparent. In this state, she was filled with intense rage and seemed compelled to attack the other person. As with the "unlovable" state, this state did not only consist of uncontrollable feelings, but also involved resentment about not having her needs met and about the demands made of her. She was also scornful and dismissive of others and cared little about how her moods and actions affected them. The rage was also tinged with boredom and frustration; she was bored with her life and frustrated at being unable to do much about it. The state was also triggered by any perceived slight, rejection, criticism, and threat of abandonment that then became the focus of her attention and was used to attack or denigrate the person she considered responsible. Again, Anna's hypersensitivity to such events meant that the state was easily triggered and often the trigger seemed to lie more in how she interpreted situations as opposed to the actual event itself.

An interesting feature of this state is the way it affected information processing. As the state progressed, Anna's attention narrowed until it became totally focused on Anna's interpretation of the triggering event and the other person's behaviour. Sometimes the trigger was not something the other person did but rather Anna's assumption that the person had done something and even that he or she was likely to do something. With the narrowing of attention, Anna did not stop to question her interpretation. Instead, she became oblivious to other information and to the context of the interaction. As a result, nothing the other person said or did had any impact. It was merely used to fuel her rage. This narrowing of attention and relentless anger occurred repeatedly with her husband. It also occurred in therapy usually when the therapist would not do something Anna wanted such as prescribing inappropriate medication. The only course of action was for the therapist to disengage from the interaction but remain highly attentive to what Anna was saying. This combination of non-engagement and attentiveness usually helped the rage to settle. However, in everyday circumstances it is difficult for people to disengage in this way; people get defensive or seek to explain their actions which usually leads to the confrontation escalating.

Anna also experienced a third self-state in which she was preoccupied with caring for her children which went beyond normal parental protectiveness to involve a preoccupation with ensuring their lives were very different from her own and with taking every step to protect them. When in this state, Anna was almost totally absorbed with her children's welfare, leaving little time or energy for anything else, which usually led to her feeling exhausted.

21.2.5 Integrating Self-States

Much of the work on exploring and modifying the schemas associated with self-states occurs earlier in therapy. At this juncture, the goal is to integrate self-states and promote a more cohesive self structure. Since the nature of self-states and their importance vary substantially across patients, it is difficult to define a set of interventions for general use. However, three general ways to establish connections among self-states are to (i) identify common elements, that is, features such as schemas and behavioural patterns that are shared by several states; (ii) establish transitions by identifying what causes a shift from one state to another; and (iii) construct higher-order bridges in the form of meaning structures that explain the relationships among states or account for the development of these states.

21.2.5.1 Common Elements

The simplest form of integration is to identify features such as schemas and behavioural patterns that are shared by two or more states. This is useful because patients usually feel that their self-states are unrelated, which exacerbates their sense of fragmentation. This impression begins to break down when common features are recognized. For example with Anna, discussion of a recent experience of her unloved state included a discussion of the angry state whereupon the therapist commented in both these states Anna felt unloved and that no one cared for her. Anna, in a sense, agreed by commenting, "Well they don't." The therapist added, "In both states you feel no one cares, no one loves you. So they are not quite as different as they feel." Anna responded, "You're right. I had not thought of that." This led the therapist to ask whether there were other ways in which they were similar and to Anna noting that they both ended up in the same way – feeling overwhelmed and exhausted. She also noted that, "In both (states) I do things that make it worse for myself. Why would I do that?" The therapist noted that, "That's a good question. Do you have any ideas?" Anna pondered that and decided that she got scared and pushed people away and fought with them until she wore herself out.

Anna also noted that both states were triggered by an event that made her feel rejected, which caused her to wonder why she sometimes reacted with anger and sometimes by getting upset and overwhelmed. Eventually, she decided that the outcome depended on how she felt at the time. When she was feeling normal or even irritated, she reacted by getting into a state of rage, but when she was sad or felt alone, she became increasingly needy. It also became clear that all three states ultimately led to the same outcome, feeling overwhelmed and unable to cope.

The strategy used to explore and integrate self-states is in itself integrative because it automatically draws the different states together. It is useful to compare the discussion with Anna to the cautionary comments made earlier against using an exploratory process that increased the distinctiveness of self-states giving the example of applying a name such as Little Anna or Jane to these states that emphasizes their distinctiveness.

21.2.5.2 Transitions among States

Integration is also promoted by identifying what causes a shift from one state to another. This is seen with the way Anna's needy state often ended by her children indicating that they needed her help, which caused a switch from silent despair to the hyper-attentive state. The connection not only drew the two states together but also allowed Anna to begin to manage the unloved state. For a while, whenever she thought she was moving into this state, she controlled it by making herself busy doing things for her children. She also began to recognize that sometimes the rage state shifted rapidly to the needy state when her husband, tired of her anger and how nothing he did seemed to make a difference, withdrew, which activated her fear of rejection. At that point, she panicked about whether she had gone too far and driven him away.

21.2.5.3 Higher-Order Bridges

Probably the most effective form of integration is the construction of a higher-order meaning system that encompasses all states and explains their occurrence. Two general forms of over-arching construct are (i) an explanation of self-states in terms of the core conflict of neediness versus rejection-sensitivity and (ii) a developmental explanation in terms of childhood experiences. Both were used in treating Anna.

The core conflict was used initially to explain some aspects of Anna's self-states, especially her needy state. Although work on her self-states largely occurred while also working on dependency as discussed in the last chapter, I have discussed them separately in the interests of clarity. Anna spontaneously noted that her current feelings of neediness were almost identical to how she felt when she was little. As a child, she longed for mother to love her and strove desperately to gain her affection by doing whatever possible to please her. She behaved in the same way with almost everyone in her life, especially men. Anna also recognized that her state of rage occurred when she felt that her needs were not being met and that no one cared about her. This construction allowed her to begin to see parallels between her relationships and how she felt about herself, which helped to draw things together at a time when she needed to feel more integrated and less fragmented. Equally importantly, this construction initiated further work on trying to understand these states and how they affected her relationships.

More complete integration of the self-states resulted from the exploration of childhood experiences and deprivation described in the previous chapter. This allowed Anna to elaborate her understanding of the needy state in terms of the feelings she had as a child and her intense longing for mother to love her. Longing to be loved dominated the needy state and her relationships with men. This understanding gave Anna greater access to her memories of childhood experiences of physical and emotional abuse and also made them more believable. Anna noted that she had always known mother was abusive but had not really believed it because her father and other relatives denied the abuse and regularly told her how much mother loved her, something father continued to do. Gradually, she came to accept that the abuse really happened and came to terms with how angry mother was. Anna recalled how mother became enraged even over the relatively minor things that Anna and her siblings did. She also remembered more examples of the enormous effort she had made to make mother love her but no matter what she did mother was never satisfied or pleased.

As she recalled these events, Anna suddenly paused and with a look of shock said, "Hell! I'm just like her."

The realization struck home and she repeated, "I am just like her, that's what I do with Matt (husband). When I get into that state there is no pleasing me." This insight allowed Anna to understand how the needy and rage states originated in childhood and how similar they were to the way mother behaved. Subsequent work, between and within sessions, led her to conclude that her needy state had not really changed since childhood, an understanding that consolidated the realization that these needs belonged in the past. She also understood more about how her rage state was similar to that of mother and how, when she was in this state, she treated people in exactly the same way as mother did. This integrated these states within a general framework. Further work also allowed Anna to understand that the intense, and at times compulsive, need to care for others represented both an attempt to get people to love her and a way to meet her own needs. At this point, work on interpersonal issues and self pathology are inextricably intertwined.

21.3 Promoting Agency and Self-Directedness

Although integration has been discussed so far in terms of building cognitive links within self-knowledge, this is not the only source of integration. Long-term goals and goal-directed action also contribute to coherence by organizing and directing action across time. For most people, the long-term goals they set and the directions they would like their life to take are an important part of who they are and the self-narratives they construct. Goals make life meaningful and work on attaining these long-term goals promotes a sense of unity by harnessing a variety of abilities and personality characteristics in the interests of goal attainment.

The impairment in self-directedness associated with BPD is sometimes largely functional: it is difficult to sustain the effort needed to achieve goals when extensive energy is devoted to trying to control distress as was the case with Madison. However, in many cases it is also part of core self pathology: uncertainty about wants and feelings make it difficult to establish lasting goals. Since, self-directedness is part of an adaptive personality system, an important task of the later phase of treatment is to help patients to establish goals as part of the process of constructing a life worth living. Unfortunately, it is difficult to stimulate goal setting through direct therapeutic action. Rather, once impediments to self-directedness are addressed during treatment, an interest in goals tends to increase automatically.

As maladaptive patterns change, patients often become frustrated because despite feeling better, their lives are often not very different. Having lived largely in the present, they have difficultly changing their perspective and imagining a different kind of future. A major task in the middle and later stages of treatment is to help patients to imagine future possibilities and marshal the resources needed to achieve them. Goals also become important because previously patients were often more concerned with avoiding situations and outcomes that they feared rather than achieving positive goals. This fear crippled motivation and initiative. As these fears resolve, the need to establish positive goals and develop a sense of purpose comes into focus. Although patients need to establish long-term goals for themselves, therapists can facilitate the process by encouraging patients to think about the future, helping them to identify simple and practical goals that can create a sense of direction, and encouraging them to pursue interests. These issues will be considered in more detail in the next two chapters.

21.4 Concluding Comments

This phase of therapy is challenging for therapists because of the lack of established procedures and intervention protocols and because progress often depends on the occurrence of specific events in the patient's life that provide opportunities to promote self-development. This is clearly illustrated by the development of self-directedness. Since long-term goals can only be generated by patients themselves, the process of establishing goals largely depends on the occurrence of events that force them to re-evaluate their lives and to recognize the value of having a sense of direction and purpose. Therapists need to be alert to events, no matter how minor, that provide opportunities to facilitate change. For example, one patient who despite feeling better for some time could not motivate herself to change her life until she was repeatedly wakened by noisy neighbours, which forced her to realize that she needed a place of her own so that she could have peace and quiet. Since the phrase that she used of "wanting a place of her own" seemed to the therapist to suggest that she had a partly formed dream of having her own home, the therapist simply reflected it. The patient explained that she had been thinking that she needed to "get on" with her life and that to do this she needed somewhere better to live. This led to a discussion of what she meant by "getting on with her life" and what she needed to do to get a place of her own. She thought the first step was to get a job. The noisy neighbours seemed to have crystallized a sense of discontent that was hovering in the background for some time (see Chapter 12) into a desire for her own apartment. The patient arrived for the next session tired and grumpy. Her neighbours kept her awake several times in the previous week, which consolidated her desire to get a job and move. In the week, she had seen an employment counsellor who had helped to organize her résumé and made useful suggestions about seeking employment.

The incident illustrates the organizing and integrating effects of long-term goals. The patient's desire to move resulted in her changing relatively quickly from passivity to actively seeking to reorganize her life. However, the point that I want to stress is that many of the changes that need to occur during this phase of treatment are dependent on events outside therapy and that it is important for therapists to have a clear understanding of what needs to be done to help patients to construct a life worth living. We will never know what would have happened had the therapist not reflected the patient's desire for a "place of her own" – something similar would probably occurred later – but it set in motion a series of changes, each relatively minor, that moved the patient's life in a new direction.

Notes

1. DeCharms (1968), Ryan et al. (1995), Sheldon et al. (1997), Wild (1965).
2. Stiles (2011).
3. Horowitz (1998), Livesley (2003), Ryle (1997).

Chapter 22

Promoting an Adaptive Self-Narrative and Flexible Working Selves

Throughout this volume, I have noted the importance of stories in making sense of our experiences, regulating our mental states, mobilizing our resources, and organizing our transactions with the world. Throughout therapy, patients are helped to construct new narratives about diverse aspects of their lives, experiences, relationships, and personality. Now, the task is to combine these narratives into a more global conception. This is not something that can be achieved in a formal way – it is not a matter of simply getting patients to write a new narrative. Rather, it needs to emerge as part of the process of therapy so that it is fully integrated with other aspects of personality functioning. Since there is little research to guide therapists on how best to help patients construct a self, we need to be clear about the functions of self-narratives and have a broad understanding of what they should include.

22.1 Function and Structure of Self-Narratives

Our self-narrative organizes what would otherwise be a jumble of experiences into an overarching map of our lives, our world, and our place in it, which explains who we are and how we came to be this way. Narratives give meaning to self-knowledge and make it available as a resource for organizing action and regulating experience.[1] They provide a high level of integration by (i) describing the relationships among life experiences, personality features, and behaviour; (ii) showing how events and experiences are related across time; (iii) providing thematic coherence and continuity by highlighting important themes that span the epochs of our lives; (iv) connecting events to personal qualities – traits, beliefs, and values – in a way that weaves an understanding of the interplay between our personality and life experiences; and (v) providing a form of explanatory coherence[2] by including a developmental perspective on the experiences that shaped our lives and personality and, perhaps, how our personality has shaped our experiences and interactions with the world. This description of the contribution self-narratives make to integration illustrates the kinds of narrative understanding we need to promote in therapy.

But self-narratives are not just stories about a person's life. They also incorporate scripts – elaborate schemas that embody knowledge about events and situations, making it accessible to manage the problems of everyday living. A simple example is a restaurant script that consists of knowledge about restaurants and what should be expected of them that helps us to act appropriately when visiting a restaurant. We encountered the idea of such mini-narratives or scripts when discussing crises when it was suggested that patients develop more effective ways to seek help and by helping them to develop a script about how to present in emergency departments. Self-narratives also have a regulatory function. As noted when discussing emotion processing, narratives help to regulate emotions by providing a nuanced understanding of emotional events that allow the person to see events from different perspectives and respond to them more flexibly.

To fulfil these diverse functions, self-narratives need to be multifaceted.[3] They encode a wide range of experiences into more specific scripts that guide our behaviour in the various roles and environmental contexts we occupy. Hence they are integral features of the self as agent. Once formed, the agentic self also contributes to integration because efforts to attain goals require us to coordinate our talents, abilities, interests, personal qualities, values, and resources.

With the establishment of long-term goals, self-narratives incorporate a vision for the future. Most people's sense of who they are includes ideas about the person they would like to be and how they would like to see their lives unfold. This adds to their sense of personal unity by extending the self into the future. Few patients have managed to articulate a vision for their future, a limitation that adds to their constricted lifestyle and passivity. This is most apparent in patients with chronic suicidal ideation: because they assume that one day they will kill themselves, they do not need a vision of a future self. Their tendency to live in the present and difficulty integrating events across time adds to the problem. This is probably the most insidious aspect of chronic suicidal ideation. As one patient noted, "I have a problem and I don't know what to do about it. I always thought I would kill myself and so I did not think about the future. I just lived day to day. Now I know I will not kill myself. So now I have a future but I don't know what to do with it." This comment also nicely illustrates the limitations of focusing solely on promoting new skills and restructuring maladaptive cognitions: this patient also needs a narrative of a future self – a realistic story of how she can live the rest of her life. In constructing this story, she begins to take charge of her future. Instead of being a pawn of fate, she becomes an agent, controlling her own destiny.

22.2 Fostering a Coherent Self-Narrative

The following section illustrates some general ideas that may be useful in working to construct a more coherent script with examples for the treatments of Anna, Madison, and Allison, a patient we are meeting for the first time.

22.2.1 Introducing the Problem

At some point in the later part of therapy, we need to broach the idea of developing a new sense of self and getting a life. The idea of getting a life usually strikes a chord with most patients. Indeed, as emotion regulation improves, patients usually become more outward-looking and often comment on the need for a more satisfying life. However, the idea of constructing a self-narrative is often more difficult to explain. It is probably best simply to alert patients to the task by noting that they seem to be developing a better understanding of themselves and discussing the benefits that derived from giving meaning to experience and reconciling inconsistencies in how they think about themselves, their situation, and relationships.

22.2.2 Reminiscing about Therapy

Much of the work on constructing a global self-narrative is achieved while reviewing therapy and reminiscing about the changes made and their impact, a process that deepens the therapeutic relationship. When discussing the alliance, it was noted that when people recall shared experiences they feel a deepening sense of connection and intimacy. Hopefully, these experiences in therapy will further reduce patients' fears of intimacy and mutuality and encourage generalization to everyday relationships. Reminiscing also deepens the trust needed to develop a new self-view and way of living. It also offers opportunities to promote integration by connecting events across time and highlighting changes that contribute to a new sense of self.

22.2.3 Combining and Extending Narratives

Reviewing progress and reminiscing about therapy provides opportunities to build connections among more specific narratives constructed earlier in therapy to create a more global understanding. Reminiscing in everyday life activates the storytelling mode and creates an openness to ideas and possibilities. The activation of the storytelling mode in therapy makes it easier to recall older narratives and weave them together.

Many aspects of a coherent self-narrative are constructed in the mind of the therapist but end up in the mind of the patient. The process begins when the therapist establishes more integrated personality functioning as a treatment goal and takes form initially with the case formulation, which represents the therapist's initial understanding of the patient's life and disorder. As observed when discussing Madison's treatment, formulation and reformulation can have a substantial settling effect presumably because they draw things together and make them meaningful.

The initial formulation also forms the starting point for constructing a global self-narrative. The next step is to elaborate components of the formulation into specific narratives. This begins by constructing a new narrative about how crises unfold and alternative scripts for seeking help in crises and continues by constructing a narrative about emotions and emotional life. Narrative construction accelerated when dealing with interpersonal problems with the formation of scripts to guide interpersonal interaction and new ways of thinking about the interpersonal world. Now we are concerned with combining these achievements into a more coherent and richer self-narrative that embodies an understanding of the changes achieved in therapy in order to consolidate these changes and ensure that they continue when treatment ends.

22.2.3.1 Clinical Example: Madison

This work was relatively straightforward with Madison presumably because she had less severe personality pathology. Once emotion regulation improved, therapy progressed quickly. Several narratives were constructed during therapy and reviewing the changes that had occurred provided an opportunity to establish links among them. This was not the work of a single session. Rather it was spread over some months interspersed with discussion of the major changes she was making in her life, issues around a new relationship that was very different and more stable than previous ones, and experiences resuming her studies.

The first narrative constructed was a new script about how to approach her parents for help in a crisis. This was quickly followed by a reformulation of crises that allowed Madison to understand how events were often triggered by feelings of rejection and escalated because she ruminated angrily about the unfairness of it all and fears of being unlovable. When reminiscing about these events in therapy, the narrative about crises was linked with the narrative about help-seeking in crises. Madison came to see how rumination about being unloved generated intense uncontrollable rage that led her to seek help from parents in an enraged state. She ruefully commented that "I must have been very difficult" and "it must have been very difficult for mum all along." This narrative was subsequently linked to new narratives constructed during the interpersonal phase that included the understanding that it was not that mother did not love her but rather that mother had also been struggling with her own problems during long periods of Madison's childhood and often felt overwhelmed. Madison noted how similar they were.

As these narratives were reviewed, Madison commented that she and her mother were getting along now and that she thought that her dad was proud of how well she was doing at university. Also, for the first time ever, her parents liked her new boyfriend. Clearly, Madison was constructing a new self-narrative that integrated the past, often by restructuring it. At the same time, her life was moving on and therapy was drawing to an end.

22.2.4 Provide Summaries

In addition to narrative construction, it is often helpful for therapists to facilitate the process with summary statements that draw things together by offering a broad perspective on a set of problems or events. Sometimes these summaries are used to discuss new treatment goals, but at this stage of therapy, they provide a new perspective on critical issues. Summaries are especially useful when patients are struggling to make sense of a complex issue or when they feel stuck. This is illustrated by the following vignette based on the treatment of Allison, who is being introduced to illustrate the process because major summary statements were not used with either Anna or Madison.

22.2.4.1 Clinical Example: Allison

Allison was the youngest child of parents who were a little older than average. Although she had a brother, he was much older and left home while Allison was quite young. As a result, she was raised like an only child with overprotective parents. Mother in particular was preoccupied with Allison's well-being. She was an anxious, fearful person who rarely went out and lived a constricted lifestyle dominated by an anxious concern for Allison and a desire to avoid a world she considered threatening, attitudes that she instilled in Allison from an early age. Rather than teaching Allison how to deal with problems and anxieties, mother taught her to be cautious and avoid risk. Allison learned these lessons well, leading to mildly enmeshed mother–daughter relationship that was intensified by the fact that father was remote and often absent.

Allison was a gifted child and had the opportunity in her pre-teens to attend a boarding school for gifted students in another country. She was delighted with this opportunity even though it meant being away from home. The idea of being away home did not cause Allison any significant difficulties. Rather, she looked forward to the opportunity to develop her talent. Nor does she not recall being upset or even homesick when she started at the school. However, school was stressful primarily because she was not sure what to do or how to deal with the situations she encountered. The demands to excel and competition from her peers were overwhelming. There was little of the support that she was used to. During the first year, she developed various somatic complaints. In the second year, her mood became more unstable and volatile. She also started cutting herself. Things deteriorated until she was forced to leave the school and return home. The effects were devastating. Symptomatically, she deteriorated, resulting in repeated hospital admissions. Gradually, her condition stabilized but did not improve substantially. Nevertheless, she finished high school, doing well enough to proceed to university. She eventually completed a degree, although it took much longer than usual, and pursued graduate studies, which were also extended due to frequent crises, hospital admissions, and periods of intense distress that made studying impossible. The therapy that she received as a teenager and young adult seemed to assume that her problems were related to separation anxiety and desire to return to mother.

Let us flash forward to Allison in her mid-30s. She is in the final phases of therapy that has lasted about four years. She had left home a few years earlier and had completed her studies and has been working for several years in a demanding professional position. Her mood is stable but she often feels anxious and distressed, which she manages without any disruption to her work. She has not engaged in deliberate self-injury for several years although she thinks about it occasionally. Nevertheless, she continues to live a restricted life. Despite being successful at work, she is haunted by a pervasive sense of incompetence and she worries endlessly about becoming ill again. She has few friends and no interests or activities that she enjoys. She continues to feel intense guilt about her independence and worries extensively about mother's well-being.

During this phase of therapy, Allison had been reviewing her relationship with mother and her earlier treatment. She was ashamed about being unable to cope with being away from mother and her failure at boarding school and having to return home overwhelmed by disappointment. These events were discussed over many sessions because her previous therapists' (she saw more than one during her teenage years) interpretations of what happened at the school still troubled Allison. The assumption that her difficulties were due to separation anxiety was reasonable and in many ways a standard way to understand such events. However, the formulation had the unintended consequence of reinforcing beliefs of vulnerability, incompetence, and failure instilled by mother, which resulted in a self-narrative about incompetency and inability to manage life's challenges, a narrative that continued to frame her life by making her fearful of engaging in the world despite her successes at work. These discussions, and other events occurring in therapy, suggested an alternative perspective on what happened at the boarding school, and since Allison seemed to be stuck, this seemed an opportune time to discuss it.

The therapist first commented that since the previous session, he had been mulling over their recent sessions and wondered whether what happened in her early teens could be looked at in another way and what Allison thought of this idea. The therapist then suggested that rather than Allison having separation anxiety – something she could not recall experiencing – her difficulties seemed to suggest that she had not learned how to cope with problems on her own or how to deal with the world nor was she equipped to handle the problems that everyone faced as part of everyday life. Moreover, mother taught her to avoid the world rather how to be in the world. This was then elaborated by talking about how mother had not helped her to establish friendships or taught her how to deal with friends and peers but rather discouraged friendships and had never encouraged Allison to invite friends home. In fact, mother discouraged any form of independence. It was not that Allison could not cope without mother as much as mother could not cope without Allison because mother herself had difficulties living in the world. This summary took until the end of the session.

When the therapist was offering this re-framing summary, Allison said little but was very attentive.

Allison arrived for the next session looking pensive. She said that she had thought about what the therapist had said ever since. She had been surprised by the therapist saying that he had been thinking about her problems. She had not expected this. She always thought of herself as a non-entity, so it was a shock that someone actually thought about her. She went on to add that the summary surprised her because it was "a very compassionate way of looking at what happened." Allison explained that the idea that she was anxiously attached to mother and desperate to return to her made her feel that she was to blame for what happened and that she was a weak person who was unable to manage on her own. The explanation she had been offered as a teenager also made her feel criticized. Now she realized that the shortcoming was also her mother's, something she had always thought but never really accepted. This lifted a weight off her shoulders – "I'm not totally to blame for what happened."

Allison also commented that the summary felt "more real" to her. She explained that at the age of 14 years she had felt forced to accept the earlier explanation of her problems even though it did not "feel right." She assumed that the doctors and nurses must have been right and hence she struggled to believe their formulation even though she felt uncomfortable with it. This now raises the prospect that Allison is now acting in the same way – accepting the therapist's re-framing of her experiences because she felt she had to agree with therapist. Allison did not think that this was the case. The summary felt right. Moreover, she recalled disputing the previous formulation with several therapists but did not feel that they listened.

This point is interesting when viewed in the context of earlier ideas about the self as knower and the importance of trusting the authenticity of one's intuitions about basic mental states. As a teenager, Allison's intuition was that her therapists' explanation of her problems was not quite accurate but nevertheless she felt obligated to reject her intuition in favour of the explanation offered. This probably added to doubts about her own judgement and to a lack of self-confidence.

22.2.4.2   Working with Summaries

Although summaries can have a major impact by re-framing the patient's understanding of events, other benefits result from working through the summary in therapy so that the ideas become incorporated into the patient's self-narrative. With Allison, this work extended over many sessions, until it progressively became incorporated into new self-narrative and formed the basis for Allison "getting a life." Note here that therapy sessions were now only occurring about once a month. The frequency of sessions across therapy will be discussed in the final chapter.

The summary helped Allison to recall how inept she felt when she first went to boarding school. Originally, she attributed this to simply being incompetent but now she recognized that she had simply not learned basic life skills, which made her feel inadequate compared to her peers. This did not end the ruminations about being incompetent but it helped to modulate them. Now, she could see just how she was unprepared to handle the independence suddenly thrust on her. For example, she recalled that shortly after joining the school, she developed a minor medical problem that required her to see a physician. This meant that she had to take public transit alone across an unfamiliar city. She did not know what to do. She had never used public transport before and had no idea how to go about it. Nor had she ever been to see a doctor on her own. The prospect was overwhelming for a shy young teenager who had lived a sheltered life. She did not go. As a result, the problem got worse until it began to interfere with her school work. In retrospect, Allison thought that this was the beginning of her problems.

She recalled other similar events. This reactivated the intense shame that she felt at the time about what she saw as personal shortcomings, limitations, and vulnerabilities. In short, she saw herself as flawed. This provided an opportunity to work through shame again at a more intense level. The process also allowed some restructuring of how Allison interpreted the situations that evoked shame and the narratives that maintained it. Increasingly, she focused less on what she considered personal shortcomings and more on recognizing and feeling some compassion for the 12-year-old girl that she was who felt overwhelmed because she was thrust into situations without the necessary resources. This was a helpful development because previously most of the things Allison did were accompanied by constant self-criticism and self-denigration with little sense of self-compassion.

As she reworked her understanding of the teenage years, Allison initially felt a surge of anger towards mother, which added to her guilt over struggles to be independent. Gradually, she began to process the anger by recognizing that what had happened at the boarding school was more complex than mother failing to teach her life skills. Her own personality and reactions added to the problem. Whereas others would have sought help and viewed such matters as using public transport as simple problems that were readily solved, she reacted with shame so that rather than asking for help, she hid her difficulties. She also came to recognize that she and mother had similar problems with anxiety. The compassion that she was learning to feel about herself began to extend to mother. Although this led to a more integrated understanding of her life and her relationship with mother, it also caused a temporary increase in what might be called separation guilt – guilt about living an independent life, an issue that will be discussed in the next section.

At this point, it is instructive to compare the narratives that Allison constructed about her anxiety and emotional distress with that constructed by Madison (Chapter 17). Although both women had similar problems, they formed very different narratives. Madison accepted that she had these problems, saw them as something to be overcome, and as a result learned not only how to control her feelings but also how to use them. Her narrative helped her to control her anxiety and rebuild her life. In contrast, Allison's narrative of incompetence and vulnerability added to her difficulty in managing her emotions and led to a constricted lifestyle. This prompts the question of why their narratives were so different. The answer seems to lie in differences in developmental experiences and their other personality traits. Although both had highly anxious mothers, their mothers dealt with their anxiety very differently. Madison's mother, who seemed to have less severe problems, was proud of the fact that she had learned to manage her anxiety and that it did not control her life. She held herself up as a role model for Madison to emulate. In contrast, Allison's mother was crippled by anxiety and led a cloistered life and encouraged Allison to do the same.

In addition, although Madison and Allison had similar borderline traits, their other personality characteristics differed and these differences influenced how they responded to their emotional problems and treatment. Madison was relatively outgoing and self-assured.

This allowed her to feel confident that she could manage her anxiety and overcome her problems once she understood them. As a result, she was able to rebuild her social networks quickly once her emotional distress settled, which helped to consolidate her gains. In contrast, Allison was more introverted and even socially avoidant, which undermined her self-confidence and added to her sense of vulnerability and caution.

This vignette also provides an opportunity to review several issues discussed earlier. First, the summary illustrates the diverse and idiosyncratic pathways along which borderline pathology develops and hence the need for caution in applying general models to individual patients – although separation anxiety may contribute to some cases of borderline personality disorder (BPD), it did not appear to play a major role in Allison's case. Second, it illustrates the point that skill building is not sufficient; patients also need adaptive narratives. Third, it illustrates the importance of considering the overall personality. It is not sufficient to focus exclusively on diagnostic criteria and related traits; other traits have a substantial impact on outcome. In Allison's case, it was important to take into account the impact of shyness and social avoidance. Finally, it demonstrates how BPD results from a complex interaction between heritable personality traits and life events.

In conclusion, the use of summaries to help patients construct a more adaptive self-narrative involves several steps. First, the therapist needs to recognize that a reformulation is likely to be helpful at that time. Second, the reasons for the new formulation need to be fully explained. Third, the patient's feedback needs to be sought and discussed in depth and the formulation should be modified as needed to accommodate the patient's input. Fourth, the summary needs to be worked through to help the patient to incorporate the formulation into his or her emerging self-narrative. This may require the patient to engage in new behaviours to consolidate these changes.

22.2.5 Encouraging Action That Consolidates Self-Development

Behavioural experiments are also useful in fostering self-development. Again, these interventions are illustrated by the case of Allison. As Allison elaborated her self-narrative, she was encouraged to think about what kind of life she would like and to construct a narrative that included a "future self." It quickly became apparent, however, that two schemas were obstructing her ambitions and causing her to doubt whether she should actually pursue some of her desired goals: guilt about being independent and a pervasive sense of incompetence.

Elaboration of the summary statement led Allison to revisit the conflict that had dominated her life – that of living an independent life. She had always recognized the conflict and how mother had sought to limit her independence but did not seem to be fully aware of its impact. This illustrates the point made when discussing self-knowledge in Chapter 11 – that we often know things without being totally aware of their emotional significance. Now, Allison began to realize the full impact of the conflict and the many ways mother stymied her efforts to have a life of her own. Yet, she still felt intense guilt about doing anything that caused mother to feel anxious – and since mother saw disaster lurking everywhere, she felt anxious about virtually everything Allison did. Ironically, the development of greater compassion for mother's problems added to the guilt she felt about having an independent life. This guilt also was increased temporarily because Allison felt sad that her mother unlike herself had not received treatment but this was short-lived because she quickly recognized that mother had similar opportunities but did not take them.

As these issues were explored, Allison came to recognize that mother's anxieties were endless and inconsistent with Allison having any kind of independent life for herself. Basically, mother felt anxious unless she knew where Allison was every moment of the day and she worried constantly about her safety even when doing routine tasks. Nevertheless, it remained difficult for Allison to do anything that would cause mother anxiety; as a result, her life remained constricted. At this stage of therapy, progress often depends on chance events that may be quite minor. Hence therapists need to be alert for any event that provides an opportunity to promote change. In Allison's case, one such event was a colleague at work commenting that she had joined a choir. This reawakened Allison's earlier interest in music and with the therapist's support she decided to join the choir despite mother's fear that this meant she would be out alone at night. This action helped to reinforce the idea of having a life and doing things despite mother's disapproval.

A similar opportunity occurred shortly afterwards when again a colleague at work talked about a recent hiking trip and responded to Allison's interest by inviting her to join her on her next hike. Allison was reluctant, and when she mentioned the idea to mother, she had reacted with alarm regaling Allison with stories of people who had been injured while hiking, others who had got lost, and even some who had been attacked by bears. This added to Allison's realization that mother's fears were endless and that even if she lived a totally sheltered life, mother would still worry. While discussing this in therapy, she decided to go hiking with her colleague, which subsequently became a regular occurrence and even progressed to overnight trips. Gradually, she came to terms with the fact that mother would worry no matter what she did. In the process, her guilt faded, a development assisted by her growing understanding of how mother used her anxiety to instil guilt and to control the people in her life.

These developments helped to consolidate Allison's new self-narrative and the idea of getting a life for herself. Further progress occurred when the hiking trips came to an end because the colleague moved. This created an enormous dilemma – Allison really enjoyed hiking and it had become part of her life but mother was alarmed at the prospect of her hiking alone. She decided to continue but not tell mother. After a few trips, she told mother, who reacted in the predictable way but there was little she could do. Subsequently, Allison started making overnight trips alone. The impact on her sense of self was considerable. Now she began to see herself as an independent woman able to survive in the backwoods alone, a far cry from the timid teenager afraid of getting on a bus in a strange city.

Allison's relationship with mother also changed. Guilt and anxiety gave way to a more caring attitude that also recognized that there were limits to what she could do to help mother. Whereas in the past she saw herself as responsible for mother's anxiety, she now recognized there was little she could do about it. She began to see mother as an ageing parent whom she could help without sacrificing her own life.

22.2.6 Incorporating Changes into Self-Narratives

As patients begin developing new interests and behaviours, it is useful to ensure that these are put into words because this makes them more real and ensures that their significance is recognized so that they are incorporated into the patient's self-narrative. This is one reason patients sometimes do not want to talk about traumas and painful events – if these events are not put into words, it is easier to continue pretending to oneself that the events did not happen and to deny their significance.

Core schemas such as Allison's incompetence schema resist change so that it often takes considerable time to restructure and incorporate the restructured schema into a new self-narrative. It is as if patients selectively ignore progress that conflicts with well-established beliefs. Often it takes something unusual or intense to shake things up and open the patient to accepting the significance of the changes that have occurred. Thus, Allison continued to see herself as incompetent despite having improved substantially, completing her studies and obtaining full-time employment, holding down a stressful professional position for several years, being able to make complex presentations to large groups of colleagues despite having been afraid of public speaking, and receiving glowing evaluations of her work. Her view of herself as incompetent continued to be rigidly held along with the belief that she should avoid being assertive because she was unlikely to be successful and others would ridicule her efforts. Attempts to restructure the schema by challenging its categorical nature had softened it a little but it took a specific event to catalyse a change.

Allison noted that a few days earlier, the administrator she reported to had circulated some administrative changes that substantially affected her, which were also at odds with the organization's policies. Allison was furious. But whereas in the past she would have fumed and done nothing, on this occasion she sent an email to her manager, pointing out the problems with the proposal. Immediately, she felt alarmed about what she had done and began catastrophizing about the consequences. Later that day, she received a reply. She was surprised by the conciliatory tone of the email and by the fact the supervisor thanked her for drawing her attention to the problems with the changes she had proposed and which were now withdrawn. The supervisor also congratulated Allison for being so thoughtful and knowledgeable and expressed appreciation for her work generally. Allison was stunned. Faced with a written email, it was difficult to hold on to her categorical belief about being incompetent, which left her feeling confused and anxious but also delighted at the recognition. The event and its implication were discussed over several sessions and previous work on challenging the schema was reviewed.

Although this event permanently diminished the stranglehold the incompetency schema held over her life and sense of self, Allison was not quite ready to relinquish it. However, the categorical nature of the schema was replaced by a recognition and, more importantly, acceptance of the idea that she had areas of competence – a major shift – while retaining the belief that she was interpersonally incompetent. As these issues continued to be worked on in sessions that were now about every four to six weeks, Allison came to one session noting that things were going well. She was feeling much less anxious and more in control of her life. These changes were worked through in several subsequent sessions and she began to work over the material between sessions more than she had in the past to the point that she began one session noting that she was feeling much less anxious because she had decided that she "had the resources to cope with most of the things that were likely to happen" to her.

22.2.7 Incorporating the Idea of Having Personality Disorder

A final aspect of narrative construction that we need to consider is whether and how to incorporate the idea of having personality disorder. This is a complex issue. On the one hand, patients need to accept that they have had these problems and hence incorporate their understanding of them into their narratives. On the other hand, it is not helpful to incorporate ideas that are negative or which place unnecessary constraints on how they behave and how they see themselves. The problem is that both personality disorder and BPD have negative connotations. Indeed, the very term "personality disorder" is often misunderstood and tends to evoke harmful ideas about being damaged or flawed. As one patient commented, "they say I have personality disorder but I don't like that. It suggests that I am a bad person but I think I'm a nice person." We need to avoid our patients thinking about themselves in this way, which is a further reason to ensure that adequate information about the disorder is provided throughout treatment.

These problems are one reason why I do not use the term BPD. As noted in the Preface, I have used the term in this book because it is familiar and because I have no doubts about the pathology involved. It is the label that is the problem. It is not very meaningful. The term "borderline" lost its original meaning of being at the borders of neurosis and psychosis long ago. Also, as I argued earlier, the DSM criteria offer an incomplete description of the psychopathology involved. Hence I tend to tell patients that the primary problem is emotional dysregulation and that unstable emotions affect both how they think about themselves and how they interact with others. How patients are helped to incorporate these ideas into their self-narrative depends on the treatment outcome.

In patients with good outcomes who have few residual problems, it seems appropriate that they understand that they had a discrete episode from which they have recovered. Such cases are probably comparatively few. More common are patients who although recovered have relatively high levels of anxiousness and emotional lability that may lead them to be more anxious and emotional than the average person. This is the narrative that Madison constructed. She accepted that she worried more than the average person and was more emotional but she saw this as a liability that she could manage and that she could also use to motivate her studies and sporting activities. This seemed a constructive way to see things.

Patients with more severe disorder whose recovery is less complete need help in constructing a different narrative that recognizes any ongoing problems but does so in a way that does not prevent them from having a satisfying life. One patient who was comfortable with the idea of having BPD commented at the end of therapy that,

> I am still borderline. I am still vulnerable in social situations but I can manage it. I will always have problems with relationships but I'll be fine if I do not live with anyone again and do not spend a lot of time with people. I am fine with that. I am not really a people person. People bore me. I have lots of interests and things I like to do on my own and now I feel it's OK to be like that.

This also seems a reasonable narrative. And, she was right. Some years later, she was doing fine and living a life she considered contented pursuing interests she had not been able develop previously.

22.3 Generating Flexible Working Selves

Integrated modular treatment assumes that the self consists of a relatively stable body of self-referential knowledge that is organized through the formation of links between different items (self-schemas and experiences) and through the construction of global self-narrative. This structure is used to construct and reconstruct momentary working self, designed to help us manage the situations we encounter (see Chapter 2). The body of self-knowledge that constitutes the self as known contains extensive information that can be used to guide effective interaction with the world. Momentary working selves are the vehicle for applying this information resource to given situations. Throughout treatment, self-knowledge is progressively increased and integrated. Now we need to consider how to encourage patients to use this knowledge to construct adaptive working selves. Patients tend to use their limited and poorly integrated self-knowledge in rigid ways and have difficulty matching their working selves to specific situations. Instead, they tend to see themselves in the same way across situations. Allison, for example, saw herself as incompetent, inadequate, and vulnerable, regardless of the situation.

Although there is literature on how to enrich self-narratives, at the time of writing, I was not aware of any literature dealing with the treatment implications of the idea of the working self. Consequently, this section is limited to a few ideas that I have found helpful. However, the most useful thing that therapists can do is to be mindful of the importance of promoting flexibility in constructing working selves so that opportunities to promote flexibility are recognized. This is important because the idea of constructing a working self is often counter-intuitive to therapists who are familiar with traditional ideas of the self as fixed. It should be noted here that the idea of working self should not be confused with the idea of self-states discussed in the last chapter. Working selves unlike self-states are transient constructions that are designed to help us to function effectively in a given situation.

The first step in promoting flexibility is to explain the idea of the working self by pointing out how people see themselves differently in the different roles they occupy. This is usually best done when discussing a scenario that provided an opportunity to discuss how the patient saw him- or herself at the time. For example, the idea was explained to Allison when she described how incompetent she had felt when she was asked to explain a project to some colleagues at work. She said she was anxious because she was not very good at public speaking and she was afraid that her colleagues would see her incompetence and that she would be humiliated. The therapist recalled that she had talked about feeling this way about herself in the previous session when talking about a social event with some friends and acquaintances. Allison said she always felt that way. The therapist commented:

> It seems that you see yourself in the same way in most situations and this is the way you have seen yourself for most of your life. It hasn't changed. We've talked a lot recently about how your life has changed and the changes you've made but these changes haven't changed how you think about yourself. It is as if your ideas about yourself are frozen ... as if you have not kept up with your own progress.

Subsequently, more information was provided about the value of being more flexible in how we think about ourselves in different situations and how the image we construct of ourselves helps us to deal with situations more effectively. At the same time, the idea was linked to previous discussions of the value of flexibility in interpreting and reacting to events.

Once the idea of working self is understood, the next step is to discuss how the patient sees him- or herself in different situations and relationships with the purpose of encouraging greater awareness of how the self is seen across situations. In the course of discussing a few examples, recurrent maladaptive or stereotyped content is highlighted and thereby challenged. Similarly, any differences in self-attributions across situations that seem helpful and adaptive are reflected and explored. The goal of this process is to promote narratives that are relevant to the situation and the interpersonal context.

22.4 Concluding Comments

Although most current therapies for BPD pay little attention to narrative construction, it is a useful way to consolidate and generalize change and promote more integrated functioning because narrative and self are closely interconnected.[4] The act of telling a story about who and what we are, and our experiences of ourselves and others, contributes to our sense of self and structures our identity by linking our experiences of ourselves across time. Storytelling is a facility that comes naturally to people and hence it can be used in this final phase of therapy as a natural way to promote a sense of personal coherence and integration.

Notes

1. Dimaggio et al. (2015), Osatuke et al. (2004), Stiles (2011).

2. Habermas and Bluck (2000) describe four factors contributing to the global cohesiveness of adolescent narrative identity that are useful to bear in mind when helping patients to construct an adaptive self-narrative – temporal, biographical, causal, and thematic – which influenced my discussion of the value and function of self-narratives. See also McAdams and Janis (2004) for a further discussion of these issues.

3. Dimaggio et al. (2015).

4. Bruner (2004), Angus and McLeod (2004).

Chapter 23

Getting a Life, Constructing a Personal Niche

Most patients with borderline personality disorder (BPD) live constricted lives that offer few opportunities to engage in activities and relationships that are satisfying or offer opportunities for personal growth and fulfilment. The struggle with painful emotions causes patients to shut down and their behavioural horizons to shrink (see Chapter 15), and even when distress subsides, this constricted way of living often continues. For treatment to be successful, patients need to build a life worth living. This requires both a coherent sense of self and an environment that supports the changes they have made and provides opportunities for further growth. This chapter considers the second requirement – how to help patients create a personal world that supports a more adaptive and rewarding life.

23.1 The Idea of a Personal Niche

Although the environment is an important part of a person's life, it is often neglected in therapy because it is implicitly assumed to be independent of the person. But this is not the case. Healthy individuals do not react passively to the environment. Instead, they actively shape their world over time to create a personal niche that is congenial to them.[1] They seek out situations and individuals to establish a niche that organizes their lives; offers outlets for needs, abilities, talents, and aspirations; supports their interests; and provides opportunities for personal satisfaction and a contented way of living. Successful niches enable people to act in accordance with their basic nature, thereby promoting feelings of authenticity, cohesion, and integration.

The idea of a personal niche also draws attention to the intimate relationship between the self and the environment. We saw earlier the importance of the social environment in constructing the self and how self-knowledge and self-understanding are acquired through interaction with others. However, as discussed in the previous chapter, the self is not a static structure: once formed, the self is actively involved in coordinating the internal conditions of the person with the external environment and in managing the relationship between the individual and his or her world. Healthy individuals gradually create a personal space that supports adaptive activity and provides opportunities for self-expression. This requires that niches promote feelings of safety and security and provide the structure, resources, and flexibility to allow people to express themselves in unique ways. Niche construction is an ongoing process. We continually reshape our niche to meet the ever-changing circumstances of our lives.

Adaptive niches also connect people to the world they occupy. Those with adaptive and satisfying lifestyles feel a sense of connection to their world that creates feelings of stability and belongingness as opposed to feelings of alienation and disconnection. Niches also provide a supportive social network that helps to connect individuals to the community and add to feelings of security and stability.

These ideas suggest that treatment should help patients construct a niche that allows them to express their inherent qualities and to spend time in situations and relationships in which they can express themselves and feel genuine and avoid situations that activate vulnerabilities and conflicts. Many patients, however, do the opposite. Rather than finding satisfying forms of self-expression, they continually struggle to mould themselves to the perceived expectations of others and engage in relationships and activities that accentuate their problems. Niche construction is linked to positive outcomes; long-term studies of patients without treatment suggest that those who did well managed to find an adaptive niche that created security and a sense of identity.[2]

23.2 Niche Construction

Helping patients to shape their environment and create a satisfying personal niche is not complicated. First, it involves the therapist recognizing the importance of a personal niche in supporting adaptive behaviour. However, some therapies neglect the importance of niche building probably because they are primarily concerned with changing "inner" mental structures or overt behaviour rather than helping patients to modify their social environment. In some ways, psychotherapy has placed more emphasis on helping patients to adapt to their environments than on helping them to construct a more congenial world.

Second, niche construction depends on helping patients to recognize the need to get a life. This is something most patients intuitively understand although they may have difficulty articulating it. Some also feel that they do not have the right to a better life because they are so undeserving. It is almost as if they need permission to live differently – a feature that is common in those who have been abused. Their guilt and shame make them feel undeserving of anything better.

Third, niche building also involves helping patients to recognize that an alternative way of living is possible. For many patients, a constricted lifestyle and rigid thinking combine to obscure their ability to see that alternatives are available and a more satisfying life is an option. The idea of building their social world may be especially difficult to understand for patients who feel that the world is threatening and fearful and that they are powerless. With these patients, it is often helpful to review how the niche that they have occupied has often encouraged maladaptive rather than adaptive action or exposed them to people who helped to perpetuate their problems. For example, work on niche construction effectively began early in therapy with one patient with a fringe lifestyle and many drug-using acquaintances when she made the chance remark about how difficult it is to change when surrounded by people who consistently use drugs. This led to a discussion of how these relationships contributed to her difficulties and eventually to considering the benefits of spending more time with non-drug-using friends. Although this seems obvious, it was not something she had considered. Feelings of demoralization and alienation caused her to feel dependent on these relationships and prevented her from seeing that a different lifestyle was possible and more importantly that she had some choice about the amount of time she spent with friends.

Fourth, creating a niche involves creativity on the part of the therapist in recognizing opportunities to encourage courses of action conducive to niche formation. The following sections discuss some of the strategies therapists can use to help with the process. Although many of these strategies are used throughout therapy, they are implemented more consistently during this phase of treatment.

23.2.1 Encourage Activity

A simple way to facilitate niche construction is to encourage greater activity. The more active patients are, the more likely they are to encounter opportunities to engage in rewarding activities. In the early phases of therapy, activity was encouraged to provide some structure to the patient's day. Later as emotion regulation increased, it was encouraged to counter the effects of the constricted ways of living that often accompany intense emotional distress and emotional avoidance. Now, it is encouraged to help patients to become more engaged with their world and more open to new inputs, and to increase the probability of events occurring that provide opportunities for self-development and self-expression.

23.2.2 Develop Interests

The importance of interests in promoting change was noted when discussing the contribution of positive emotions (see Chapter 17). Interests were considered a form of positive emotion that tends to emerge with improved emotion regulation that can be used to promote other positive emotions. Interests are also important in developing new behaviours and building a new social life. Earlier it was noted that Madison's reawakened interest in sport facilitated her recovery through the development of new activities and relationships. In the previous chapter, a similar process occurred with Allison who returned to her interest in music and later developed an interest in hiking, which contributed to a new self-narrative and a more congenial lifestyle.

The nature of these interests is unimportant; it is the pursuit of an interest that matters. The positive feelings involved lead to greater openness to new experiences while pursuit of the interest increases activity, creating further opportunities for growth. This is illustrated by another patient who commented towards the end of treatment that she came across a documentary on rocks and fossils when changing television channels, which reminded her of a childhood fascination with rocks. She decided to watch the documentary rather than the intended program. In therapy, she described the documentary with great enthusiasm, which was unusual because previously nothing had really interested her. She recalled childhood visits to a local museum with a large mineral and fossil collection. She wondered if the collection still existed. With the therapist's encouragement, she contacted the museum and was delighted to find that the museum needed volunteers. Note here that one positive emotion – interest – led to another, delight. Volunteering quickly led to an invitation to accompany a museum geologist on field expeditions and hence to regular contact with other volunteers. Her social life increased and she began to establish a small social network and she felt less isolated. The example illustrates the value of chance events in fostering positive emotions and how this can set in motion a chain of events that accumulate in helping to build a new niche.

23.2.3 Develop a Social Network

The social world of many patients shrinks during the height of their difficulties, partly due to decreased interest and social avoidance and partly because friends get burned out by the patient's distress. Recovery involves helping patients to re-establish their social life, which may require considerable effort to overcome the patient's fear of further rejection and re-establish confidence in their ability to relate to others. Anna, for example, as she began to improve, started to interact with other parents when she took her child to school. After chatting to another parent for some weeks, the woman suggested that they go for coffee. Anna declined because she thought the woman would find her boring. Although this action was another aspect of Anna's avoidant pattern, it also reflected a deep-seated fear of being uninteresting. Since at this stage of treatment, stability had been attained and Anna was more reflective, it was possible to challenge this avoidance and encourage Anna to make contact with the woman again and return the invitation. She did this and the shared coffee became a regular event. With a series of such small steps, Anna began to socialize again and began to establish a social network that helped to create a sense of belonging that added to her growing sense of stability. For the first time in years, Anna began to feel connected to the world.

23.2.4 Build Links with One's World

As therapy was drawing to an end, Allison suddenly decided that she needed to be more involved in her community. This seemed a healthy development. I have noted several times the intimate connection between the self and the environment. We all have a need to put down roots and feel connected to, and be part of, our world; it creates a sense of belongingness that adds to our sense of personal unity and permanence. The nature of these roots does not seem to matter. For most people, these roots are social – feeling part of the community and neighbourhood. But they can take other forms. The same sense of belongingness may be provided by taking care of one's world as in looking after the immediate environment or creating a personal space such as a garden. Allison thought initially that she would volunteer with the local food bank but then decided she would join a local environmentalist group that was active on some local environmental projects. This seemed a good solution because it combined her new need to be part of her community with her interest in the outdoors. At the same time, these activities brought her into contact with other people and added to her social network. Anna also decided she wanted to contribute to her community as therapy was drawing to an end and she too decided to volunteer at a food bank several mornings each week.

23.2.5 Manage the Social Environment

Although people modify their environments in many ways, there are limits to which this is possible and the social world of most people includes relationships that are unavoidable. This was the case with Anna who was unable to leave her marriage for many legitimate reasons. In these situations, it is still helpful to encourage patients to become more active in managing the relationship to reduce adversity. This helps them to feel less trapped and more in charge of their lives. In Anna's case, several strategies were used to reduce the frequency of angry confrontations and violent arguments. Anna learned to communicate to her husband in a less critical and demanding way. She also began to set limits when he made unreasonable demands rather than acquiesce to the point that she became overwhelmed with rage. To her surprise, he seemed to accept this and the stress within the marriage decreased. This allowed her to make a greater effort to see things more from his perspective. Although the relationship aspect of her personal niche could not be radically changed, these changes allowed Anna to remodel it so as to make things easier.

23.3 Case Examples

Rather than discuss in detail ways to help patients to construct a niche, it may be more useful to consider how niche construction occurred in the treatment of Madison, Anna, and Allison. The following case material illustrates the many factors that accumulated over time to help these patients create a more supportive social world. With Madison, the therapist needed to do little other than support positive developments and nurture the process. Things were different with Anna because she had more severe problems and a more complex social situation.

23.3.1 Madison

With Madison, the process of constructing a niche was relatively spontaneous. The decrease in emotionality led quickly to renewed interests and later to Madison returning to her studies. These developments led naturally to new relations and new opportunities. All the therapist had to do was to nurture the process by taking an active interest in each development and guiding the process a little. As emotion lability settled, Madison's interest in sports returned. The therapist encouraged this by taking an active interest in her initial plans to resume playing as a way to promote positive emotions. As her interest grew, opportunities arose to use this activity to facilitate important aspects of self-development and niche construction. Regular participation in the sport brought Madison into contact with new people with different lifestyles from her previous acquaintances and with men who were more stable and more interested in stable relationships. Her social network increased and became peopled with individuals with fewer problems.

Continued participation in the sport led to an opportunity to teach it to youngsters with disabilities, which increased her self-esteem and made her feel more connected with her community. Shortly afterwards, she extended her community work by other volunteering work. She initially did this because she thought that regular volunteer work would help her to prepare to return to her studies after several years' absence – an idea the therapist supported. These developments, which occurred relatively quickly over a few months, substantially changed Madison's outlook and sense of well-being. Her life changed from being driven by intense emotions and an intense inner focus on distress to being more outward-looking and less reactive. Success in the sport and in the social context enhanced her self-esteem and re-established her self-confidence.

23.3.2 Anna

With Anna, niche construction was handled differently. Shortly after the end of the prolonged regulation and modulation phase during initial work on interpersonal issues, the therapist raised the issue of the importance of Anna getting a life. There were several reasons for this intervention. To this point, Anna's life had been dominated by her disorder.

The previous five years had consisted of one hospital admission after another and little else in her life apart from looking after her children and helping her family. There was little in her life that gave pleasure or satisfaction and she never seemed to have any fun. Also her life was dominated by a preoccupation with the past. Hence, the decrease in distress provided an opportunity to help her think about the future. It was not expected that the comment would have any immediate effect – it was more an attempt to plant a seed in the hope that someday it may begin to germinate.

Anna initially reacted with shock but, despite being surprised by the idea, she reacted positively. After a pause while she processed the idea, she said, "You are absolutely right. That's what I need. I don't have a life and I have never had one." She then talked about what getting a life would mean for her. The problem was she did not have the financial resources to separate from her husband. Nevertheless, she noted that things were changing. She now had a part-time job that was enjoyable and satisfying. Besides the satisfaction of caring for others – something that she valued strongly as noted when discussing submissiveness and dependency (Chapter 19) – the work also gave her a measure of financial independence. Note also that enjoyment and satisfaction Anna got from her work were new emotions for her. Like all positive emotions, they increased a sense of communion with others and a sense of connection to the world – reactions that were discussed in detail to highlight how these experiences were new and how they made Anna feel differently about herself.

These discussions, spread over many months, helped to consolidate the idea that Anna was building a new life for herself – a personal niche that was more rewarding. The positive features of these developments were mitigated to some degree by continued relationship problems that seemed too severe to resolve through conjoint sessions. Nevertheless, stress in the relationship decreased as Anna began to feel better about herself and changed the way she interacted with her husband. These changes led the therapist to tentatively raise the idea of Anna building a life for herself outside the relationship. Anna thought this as a good idea and noted that in fact this was occurring. Together Anna and the therapist reviewed the positive features of the relationship. These included the fact that her children were attached to her husband and that he was attentive to them, which provided them some stability. Anna also noted that he provided some security and a roof over her head and that he made few demands of her. She did not think that she could expect much else because her husband clearly indicated that he had no intention of changing.

The idea of a life outside the relationship while also continuing the relationship seemed appealing and indeed the only viable option. Her job was satisfying and resulted in her beginning to make friends. These people were different from her previous acquaintances, something Anna liked because they had not known her when she was really distressed and hence there was no baggage to these relationships. Some of these women also had young families and had suggested that they all get together with their children some weekend to do things they all enjoyed. In the course of one of these outings, Anna learned that some of her new friends were active members of a local church and they invited her to join. This reactivated her religious beliefs. Her family had been very religious when she was growing up and she attended church regularly. This ended in early adulthood when her problems became more severe.

Joining the church community consolidated Anna's new niche and her connection with the community. She met new people and established a social network that was supportive.

She no longer felt so isolated and alone. At the same time, the renewal of her religious faith and values contributed to her growing sense of identity. Shortly after these developments, some earlier initiatives to obtain employment-related training for the kind of community care work she liked came to fruition. She was thrilled with this prospect and was anxious to accept the opportunity.

While these developments were occurring, Anna also began to think more about her relationship with her husband. As a result, the relationship began to change. In one session, she stated that she realized how she pushed him away although she really wanted to be with him. This was a new development. When she started therapy, she commented that her husband treated her better than any of her other partners but then things seemed to go awry and he experienced a variety of serious personal difficulties. Now Anna was beginning to recognize that problems in the relationship contributed to her husband's problems. She said that she had come to realize that "I can't expect him to treat me well unless I treat him well, and I don't." She explained how she was like her mother and that she treated her husband the way her mother treated everyone. She criticized him about everything and if he did something to help her she criticized him for not doing it properly just like her mother criticized her. She added that she thought that she did this because she was afraid of being hurt and as a result she "walled up" so that no one could get close to her. However, it caused him to withdraw. She also realized that she wanted her husband to love her unconditionally just like she wanted mother to love her. Anna explained that she had come to these conclusions about two weeks earlier and as a result she had been treating her husband differently and that she had even told him she loved him and wanted to be with him. This led to a substantial change in their relationship and currently both were feeling much happier.

In subsequent sessions, Anna reported that the changes in her relationship with her husband had continued and that they were getting along much better. These changes led to a modest revision in Anna's plans to develop a life for herself and to construct a personal niche. She decided to continue developing relationships and a social life and to continue with her plans to get training to work as a care assistant but she also wanted to continue working on her relationship with her husband who was delighted with the changes that were occurring and supported her efforts to get additional training.

23.3.3 Allison

Many aspects of niche building with Allison were included in the discussion of narrative construction in the previous chapter. This is how it is with most cases – narrative construction and niche building occur simultaneously. An important part of narrative development involves encouraging patients to act in ways that are consistent with their new narrative and to engage in behavioural experiments that lead to changes to their environment that contribute to a new niche, and vice versa. With Allison, narrative and niche construction occurred almost entirely in the final phase of therapy. The regulation and modulation phase was prolonged in part by the narrative she had constructed of being incompetent, vulnerable, and needing to live a cautious and sheltered life. During this time, her life consisted almost entirely of attending classes and studying at home alone apart from regular visits to see her parents.

This constricted pattern did not change when she got a job and it continued even when therapy adopted a more interpersonal focus. Changes only began to occur when Allison joined a choir and started hiking. Both events represented a substantial break with the past. Hiking in particular transformed her life and became a major source of satisfaction and pleasure. When hiking she felt a sense of connection to the environment and to nature that she had not felt before. It was also a world in which she felt competent. This competence began to spread to other areas – she felt less anxious and less stressed at work, she became more confident socializing, and she started volunteer work. She decided that this was the life she wanted; she did not need many friends and an active social life was not appealing. This was a very different sort of niche from that of either Anna or Madison but it was one that Allison was comfortable with.

23.4 Concluding Comments

The work of therapy in creating a new personal niche is straightforward, requiring little in the way of complex interventions. In some ways this simplicity is misleading because success depends on the therapist having a clear understanding of what niche building involves. In a sense, the therapist's strategy and mindset changes a little during this phase of treatment. Previously, the work of therapy was couched in terms of the collaborative exploration of the patient's problems and pathology (see Chapter 7). Now, this is supplemented by a process that we could call guided development in which the therapist highlights behaviours and events that could contribute to self-development and niche construction. This is clearly illustrated by Madison – greater emotional stability allowed the normal processes of self-development and the drive to succeed to reinstate themselves. All the therapist had to do was to hold a watching brief over progress and give things a nudge in the right direction from time to time by highlighting developments that seemed important. With Anna, the therapist needed to be more active in promoting niche formation due to the complexities of her situation and the greater severity of her psychopathology. Similarly with Allison, extensive work was needed to enable niche construction by restructuring narratives and schemas that impeded the process. The second thing these patients' therapists did was to take an active and ongoing interest in any new development in order to validate their efforts and maintain motivation.

Notes

1. Willi (1999).
2. Paris (2003).

Chapter 24

Termination and Overview
The Treatment Process across Time

The main treatment methods and strategies required for an integrated and trans-theoretical approach to treating borderline personality disorder (BPD) have now been discussed as they apply to the different domains of personality pathology. Now all that remains is to discuss one final issue – termination – and to revisit some key issues such as the duration of therapy, pathways of care, and the flow of therapy across time, based on an understanding of the overall structure and process of integrated modular treatment (IMT).

24.1 Termination

As with most aspects of IMT, the decision about when and how to end therapy should be collaborative. Usually, the probable duration of therapy is discussed in general terms when establishing the treatment contract so that from the outset of therapy there is a general understanding about when and how treatment will end. If this discussion does not occur prior to treatment because the patient is too decompensated as was the case with Anna, it should occur as soon as possible to reduce any anxiety the patient may have about the therapist terminating treatment – a common fear. For example, Anna mentioned her concern about the therapist abandoning her early in treatment because this had occurred in previous therapies. Consequently, during an early session when Anna was in a less-decompensated state, the therapist explained the treatment would probably take several years and that this should be reviewed jointly as therapy progressed.

With most patients, the duration of therapy is discussed again whenever new treatment goals are established as therapy progresses. A more detailed discussion of termination usually occurs when frequency of therapy is discussed when treatment progresses beyond the regulation and modulation phase because the frequency of sessions can often be reduced at this time, an issue that will be discussed later. This approach to termination means termination is approached gradually and the patient is prepared for therapy ending well in advance. At each step in the process, the patient's concerns are addressed and it is emphasized that the decision to end therapy will only be reached after a joint discussion. This allows patients who are anxious about treatment ending to feel more in control of the process and to set a pace that they are comfortable with. During the final phases of therapy, specific issues are addressed to make the transition smoother and ensure that changes are maintained when therapy ends. This includes a continuation of the review of therapy that began earlier along with further work on developing strategies to ensure changes are maintained after termination.

24.1.1 Review Therapy

The process of reminiscing about therapy and the changes made that were discussed in Chapter 22 as a way to construct a new self-narrative is also an important part of termination. Reviewing progress helps to consolidate change and provides a further opportunity to work through key issues. With personality disorder, repetition of key points is often necessary to ensure changes are implemented. It is also important to ensure that patients appreciate the extent of the changes they have made and take credit for their progress. Since change is often gradual, it is easy to lose sight of how things have changed. Patients who have kept a journal throughout treatment can be encouraged to look back at early entries and the therapist can refer to clinical notes to remind the patient of what things were like in the first few sessions.

24.1.2 Maintenance of Change

The review of how the patient has changed should not only cover changes in symptoms and specific problems but also cover changes in modes of thought and ways of looking at problems such as increased self-understanding, ability to analyse and solve problems, self-reflection, and self-validation because these are critical to the maintenance of change. As therapy moves into conclusion, these skills should be explicitly reviewed and the patient helped to recognize the way that they may be applied in future. Particular attention should also be paid to habitual self-deception mechanisms so that the patient is alerted to the way these contribute to problems. Coping mechanisms that are critical for the individual can be highlighted and problems in their application should be discussed. This provides an opportunity to anticipate problems that the patient is likely to encounter in future so that strategies can be developed for the patient to use should these problems arise.

24.1.3 Managing Anticipated Problems

The fear of negative emotions that most people with BPD develop usually subsides as emotion regulation improves. However, these fears often return as termination approaches, causing renewed sensitivity to everyday stressors and assumptions that effective treatment means that negative feelings should never occur. Such patients need to be helped to accept that emotional fluctuations are normal and life inevitably has its ups and downs and that even strong emotional reactions do not herald a return of the disorder. It is especially important to address catastrophic expectations about the possibility of a serious relapse and to help patients differentiate between the anxieties and stresses of normal life and the kinds of emotional distress that they experienced at the height of their problems. Simply bringing these fears into the open is often sufficient to defuse them.

This occurred with Madison who immediately jumped to the conclusion that she was relapsing whenever she felt anxious. A further discussion of how everyone experiences stress and that she is likely to react to stress a little more intensely than others helped her to put her concerns in perspective. It also provided an opportunity to review how she had acquired a variety of ways to manage her emotions – skills that she did not have when she started therapy. It also provided an opportunity to review how she tended to think in catastrophic ways and how she had learned to challenge this way of thinking. This changed the focus to what she needed to do whenever she began to feel anxious. As a result, she constructed a simple checklist to remind her to step back and look at how she was reacting, to question whether she was interpreting the situation correctly, and to challenge maladaptive thoughts – something she found very effective.

24.1.4 Change as an Ongoing Process

As treatment draws to a conclusion, it is useful to promote the idea that change is an ongoing process that does not stop when therapy ends. It is also helpful to inform patients that improvement usually continues following treatment because some changes take time to consolidate and also because skills acquired in treatment are strengthened by continued practice. One of the benefits of reducing the frequency of sessions in the later part of therapy is that it provides an opportunity for patients to discover that they can manage effectively without frequent sessions and that they have the resources to work out things for themselves.

It is also helpful to work with patients to identify issues that they can continue working on. Such a discussion with Anna led her to decide that she needed to work more on controlling her anger. A discussion of how she might do this led to her deciding that she would develop ways to remind herself to reflect on what was happening rather than simply reacting. She also decided that she needed to spend more time on continuing to develop a life for herself. To ensure that this occurred, the therapist suggested that she might think about allocating some time each week for activities that she found enjoyable and to continuing to reflect on her life and the progress she had made. Another way to promote continued development is to work with the patient to set specific long-term goals and discuss the steps that need to be taken to achieve them.

24.1.5 Attribution of Change

The maintenance of change is influenced by how patients explain the reasons for the changes they have made. Research on behavioural change shows that when people attribute changes to internal factors such as their own efforts, the changes are more likely to be maintained than when they are attributed to external factors such as a response to external pressure.[1] Extending these findings to therapy suggests that changes are more likely to persist when patients attribute their success to increases in personal effectiveness and learning new skills, and when they take credit for their progress. However, patients are sometimes reluctant to "own" responsibility for their success, tending instead to attribute success to the therapist's efforts. Nevertheless, it is also important that patients also acknowledge the therapist's contribution because this prevents the negative consequences that can arise when patients believe that they had to do everything for themselves.[2] Recognition that progress resulted from a collaborative patient–therapist effort also helps to reinforce the value of a collaborative approach to relationships, which also helps to maintain progress.

24.2 Duration of Treatment and Treatment Pathways

This section explores different ways to deliver IMT. Since the primary focus of the volume has been to describe an integrated and comprehensive approach to treating BPD, IMT has been presented as a form of long-term therapy, lasting from two to five or more years, in order to show how an extensive array of interventions taken from different therapeutic models can be combined over time to treat all aspects of borderline pathology. However, it is important to recognize that IMT does not need to be used in this way; the principles underlying the approach are applicable to therapies of all durations and to delivery through individual and group therapy. Moreover, the phase of change structure makes it easy to adapt IMT to different treatment contexts and different durations. Also the general therapeutic modules form the basis for establishing an effective treatment milieu on units that provide inpatient treatment as part of either heath care or forensic services.

24.2.1 Treatment Duration and Phases of Change

The phase of change structure of IMT suggests four basic treatment options:

1. Brief therapy with treatment covering the safety and containment phases with a primary focus on symptomatic improvement. Treatment would largely involve crisis management with emphasis placed on returning the patients to their previous level of functioning with the use of generic interventions, primarily containment. However, some simple cognitive-behavioural interventions could also be incorporated to teach self-management of deliberate self-harm and emotional distress. With patients who do not want longer-term therapy, a viable option is to provide intermittent crisis management provided by the same clinical team and ideally the same therapist. This would provide continuity and allow patients to learn basic emotion-regulating skills over time. This is not an ideal option, but in some settings and with some patients, it may be all that is possible.
2. Short-term therapy would also include modules used in the regulation and control phase, especially patient education, awareness, and self-regulation. Ideally, it would also be helpful to include a focus on enhancing emotional processing but this may not be possible with many patients in short-term treatment.
3. Longer-term therapy would also incorporate the exploration and change phase and hence address interpersonal impairments and the core interpersonal conflict.
4. Long-term therapy would cover all phases and hence all domains. However, as noted when discussing the last two phases of treatment, these phases overlap substantially because the pathology involved leads to both interpersonal and self problems, so the distinction between longer-term and long-term treatment is largely a matter of the extent to which these problems are addressed.

Although it is difficult to put fixed time periods for these different treatment options because response differs widely across patients, approximate durations are about five to ten sessions for crisis intervention, twenty to thirty sessions for short-term therapy, and fifty-plus sessions for longer-term therapy and an additional twenty to thirty sessions for long-term therapy. With longer-term and long-term therapy, sessions would not necessarily but probably be weekly. If a group modality is used to deliver IMT, these estimates provide a reasonable guideline for the length of the different groups.

24.2.2 Pathways of Care

Although in most clinical setting BPD is usually treated in relatively fixed ways with weekly sessions being the norm, there are good reasons to be more flexible in delivering care. Patients with BPD differ enormously in problems and pathology and in their life circumstances, which need to be accommodated for effective treatment. Multiple treatment pathways are feasible but we have little empirical information on the best ways to provide treatment. Under these circumstances, it seems best to avoid rigid protocols and to tailor treatment delivery to the needs of individual patients. The phase structure of IMT provides useful ways to think about the different pathways that individual treatment may take and how therapy should be delivered at each phase of change.

24.2.2.1   Typical Treatment Pathway

Typically when therapy begins with the patient in an acute crisis state, regular weekly appointments are established. However, I like to see patients who have frequent crises and make regular use of emergency services twice weekly initially in an attempt to contain the crises and reduce the need for brief inpatient admissions because these tend to be very disruptive and make it more difficult to engage the patient in therapy. This is then reduced to weekly sessions once crises are contained and the patient becomes more stable. The pattern of weekly appointments is continued to the end of the control and regulation phase or beginning of the exploration and change phase. With most treatments, the achievement of greater emotional self-regulation is a good time to review treatment in terms of the progress made and what else if anything needs to be done. If the decision is made to continue therapy, new goals are established and the frequency of sessions is reviewed.

The common pattern of weekly sessions is largely based on clinical tradition, and it seems unlikely that such an arrangement is necessary for all patients throughout therapy. Often, greater stability makes it possible to reduce the frequency of sessions especially for patients who are making good progress. The interpersonal problems and self pathology that are addressed at this point in therapy respond relatively slowly and patients need time to reflect between sessions and apply the understanding gained in each session to everyday relationships. Although clinical lore holds that in-depth psychotherapeutic work requires intense therapy in terms of frequency of sessions, there is no evidence that this is the case and I am increasingly convinced that weekly appointments are unnecessary and may actually seem to hinder implementation of change. It is noteworthy that Anna's intense work on resolving her dependency needs and constructing a more effective self-narrative and personal niche occurred when sessions were once a month – just under twenty sessions spread over two years. The low frequency of sessions did not appear to hinder this work and may actually have contributed to its effectiveness. Similarly, Allison's work on constructing an adaptive niche and a new sense of self (see Chapters 22 and 23) took just over twenty sessions spread over about thirty months. With this arrangement it is possible to offer the benefits of long-term therapy in a more cost-effective way. Thus Madison's treatment lasted over three years but only involved eighty-nine sessions.

24.2.2.2   Alternative Treatment Pathways

The first three phases of change (safety, containment, and regulation and control) form a common treatment pathway for all patients with BPD (and for all forms of personality disorder involving emotional dysregulation) so that the attainment of effective emotion-regulation skills is a nodal point in therapy, calling for a collaborative review of subsequent treatment options. Some patients opt to terminate therapy at this point because emotional stability was their primary goal in which case a termination date is set and therapy begins to focus of work of termination as discussed earlier. This may also be a point to either terminate treatment with those patients with severe personality disorder who are considered unlikely to benefit from continued therapy or change the focus of therapy.

24.2.2.2.1 Support and Rehabilitation

For some patients with severe disorder, this may be a time to consider a more supportive or rehabilitative approach that acknowledges the severity of the underlying impairments and focuses on helping the patient to manage ensuing problems. This requires a frank but supportive discussion of treatment options with a focus on helping patients recognize and accept their vulnerabilities and manage their lives accordingly without these vulnerabilities leading to a seriously constricted and unsatisfying way of living.

For example, one patient with a long history of emotional instability and highly conflicted relationships who had achieved greater emotional stability and ceased to show any form of suicidality decided that her interpersonal difficulties were unlikely to change because she had been this way for so long. She also decided that she had neither the energy nor the desire to work on changing. She thought that she would be fine if she did not live with anyone again because she was so vulnerable in close relationships. After exploring these problems in several sessions, a new contract was discussed with less frequent appointments and a focus on helping her to maintain the progress she had made and to build a more congenial lifestyle that provided social support without any close relationships. Over time, she managed to do this in a variety of ways that led to a sense of contentment that she had not experienced previously.

This kind of mixture of supportive and rehabilitative therapy does not need to be intensive. Usually sessions can be monthly or even less frequent. Treatment focuses on using the skills and strategies acquired earlier to deal with everyday events. Gradually, the frequency of sessions is reduced and therapy terminated. However, a few patients with severe pathology seem to function better from continued contact with the therapist and many can be maintained by an appointment every three or four months or even once a year. The knowledge that there will be regular meetings seems to help patients to cope better because there is always an opportunity to "save" things to discuss in the next session, which seems to prevent problems from becoming overwhelming. There is also the option to add in occasional extra sessions should more serious problems occur. Interestingly, even with such occasional contact, patients seem to continue to improve over time.

24.2.2.2.2 Work on Interpersonal and Self Pathology

For other patients, the attainment of emotion stability is the jumping-off point for further therapy that addresses core interpersonal and self problems. Relatively few treatments seem to progress this far. This is unfortunate because the evidence shows that even after successful treatment of emotional dysregulation substantial problems remain, and many patients have severely compromised social adjustment. At the very least, these patients should be helped to establish a way of living that is more rewarding. One reason why this does not happen is that it is often assumed that these problems require intensive therapy. However, this may not be the case. As I have tried to show with the cases of Anna and Allison, substantial changes can be achieved with less-intensive but carefully structured therapy, provided the groundwork is laid in the early phases of treatment.

Although the early phases of therapy are primarily concerned with improving the self-management of suicidality and emotional dysregulation, it is important not to be too preoccupied with skill building and cognitive restructuring that the importance of building self-reflection is overlooked. Particularly important is early work of building the ability to understand the mental processes of self and others and constructing meaning systems. These are important developments that not only influence the capacity for self-regulation but also form the basis for changing core interpersonal and self pathology. Improved emotional regulation permits these processes to function more effectively and therapy to begin addressing core problems. This was clearly illustrated by therapy with Madison who was able to rebuild her life relatively quickly once emotional control was achieved. Nevertheless, effective treatment of self and interpersonal problems requires motivation and the capacity for self-reflection that are not present in all patients.

24.2.2.3 Stepped Care and Phased Treatment

An alternative way to deliver therapy for BPD that warrants attention especially by mental health and forensic treatment programmes is stepped care. With stepped care, more intensive treatment is only provided to those who do not benefit from simpler first-line treatments.[3] Application to BPD would involve intermittent or phased treatment with all patients requiring treatment receiving brief therapy based on the common treatment pathway described earlier. Subsequently, those patients requiring additional therapy would be channelled into either the supportive/rehabilitation pathway or longer-term therapy.

This seems to be viable model given limited resources. My only reservation is a concern about the possible effect of intermittent or stepped treatment on the treatment relationship. Although the relationship is important in therapy for most mental disorders, it is especially important with BPD because the disorder primarily involves relationship problems. Hence an important component of therapy is the use of the relationship to effect change. An empirical question is whether this is possible with an intermittent or phased model.

24.3 Concluding Thoughts on the Treatment Process

In concluding our discussion of integrated treatment, it may be helpful to reconsider briefly two important aspects of the treatment process – the nature of the alliance and the kinds of change we seek to achieve with IMT.

24.3.1 The Alliance through Time

IMT is structured around generic change mechanisms with a special emphasis on the treatment relationship. Over time, the alliance changes and deepens but this progression is not consistent and there is usually considerable fluctuation within and across sessions especially in the early phases. However, by the end of the control and regulation phase, the alliance is usually more consistently positive with a deepening sense of trust. Sometimes this changes as interpersonal problems linked to abuse and trauma come to the fore because they evoke shame and hence a resurgence of fears of rejection. As these feelings are accessed and worked through, the alliance improves again and trust usually increases further. The emergence of trust is an important therapeutic development (see Chapter 20). Trust now becomes something deeper than being able to rely on the support and availability of the therapist. It involves confidence in the therapist, especially in the therapist acting with the patient's best interests in mind. The experience of this form of trust is itself therapeutic. It represents a major attitudinal shift that enables the patient to resolve substantive interpersonal problems. This was seen in the treatment of Anna. It was Anna's confidence and trust in the therapist that allowed her to face and work through the distress, anger, and shame she felt about the failure of mother and the men in her life to provide the love and nurturance that she so badly sought, and ultimately to give up her intense neediness.

These developments shed additional light on the role of the treatment relationship in the change process. They establish the therapeutic conditions needed for change, provide a continuous therapeutic experience that challenges many of the core schemas and relationship patterns of BPD, provide a corrective model of how adaptive relationships work, and provide the security and trust needed for greater openness and flexibility in how patients experience themselves and their relationships, which enables them to make fundamental changes.

24.3.2 Change Reconsidered

One of the reasons why therapy is so complex and takes longer than we would like is that the changes we seek to bring about are complex and varied. Some treatment approaches understandably focus on changing the more overt manifestations of BPD such as self-harming behaviour, dysregulated emotions, and maladaptive cognitions and maladaptive cognitive processes such as maladaptive modes of thought and impaired metacognitive functioning. However, besides these kinds of change, patients also need help in organizing and structuring their experience. Emotions, relationships, and the self tend to be experienced as chaotic and disorganized. This is why emotion regulation is so critical to the change process. It is difficult to help patients to structure their experiences when their emotions are disorganized. Structuring experience also requires an additional form of change – the construction of meanings systems ranging from simple explanations of maladaptive behaviour to broad narratives that seek to explain a wide range of phenomena. As we have seen, increasing emphasis is placed on the construction of narratives as treatment proceeds.

Narrative construction is part of yet another form of change that is central to treating personality disorder – the promotion of more coherent personality functioning. The model of BPD underlying treatment stresses the importance of conceptualizing disorder in terms of disorganized personality functioning and not merely as a set of symptoms or problems. Hence the latter half of therapy in particular is concerned with promoting different levels of integration, culminating in the construction of a more adaptive self-narrative and personal niche. This involves a final kind of change – environmental change, something that is emphasized more by IMT than by most therapies.

The conception of personality as a complex system considers the environment to be an important feature of the system and not as something totally distinct from the person. Adaptive individuals are assumed to seek out and create environments that support adaptive behaviour and furnish opportunities to express and satisfy their basic personality characteristics. This leads to the assumption that changes in personality are more likely to last if accompanied by changes in life circumstances and, conversely, that it is difficult for change to last if the environment that contributed to the formation of maladaptive behaviour remains the same. To consolidate change, patients need to be encouraged to restructure their environments and to seek situations that are conducive to the changes being made or to learn how to relate to the environment in ways that avoid confirming old schemas or undermining new ones.

24.4 Concluding Comments

Looking back across this volume, I am a little concerned that in attempting to describe the treatment of BPD in a straightforward and easily understood way, I may have made it look too easy. It isn't. Treating BPD is difficult and challenging, and it can be stressful and frustrating. Nothing is ever as straightforward as texts like this can seem to suggest. However, it is always interesting, and no matter how long you have been doing it, there are always new things to learn, new mistakes to make, and new problems to challenge one's knowledge and understanding. More vexing, there are always patients who defeat one's therapeutic skills. No matter who we are, where we work, or how experienced we are, we all continue to have our early dropouts and treatment failures. Although we have learned much in recent decades about how to treat BPD, and how not to treat it, we know much less than we think we know. Our knowledge remains limited, and much of what we take for knowledge is little more than clinical lore unsubstantiated by evidence.

However, my disquiet stems from a basic paradox in treating BPD and indeed any form of personality disorder; although personality disorder is enormously complex and hence we need equally complex conceptual models to understand it, treatment itself and the interventions needed are relatively straightforward. The challenge is to use our treatment methods with the consistency and frequency needed. If there is a single rule in treating BPD, it is "keep it simple and keep it consistent." Managing this paradox when treating patients is itself a challenge. We need a sophisticated understanding of the patients we treat but we need to be able to represent this understanding in a straightforward and jargon-free way not only to ensure our patients understand their problems but also to ensure that we have arrived at the clarity of understanding needed to intervene effectively. I have attempted to deal with this problem by presenting frameworks for understanding both BPD and therapy that capture the complexity of both in ways that are consistent with the evidence while also seeking to avoid complex terminology and unsubstantiated theoretical speculation. However, since our knowledge remains limited, these frameworks are at best temporary constructions designed to be easily modified to accommodate new findings.

It seems fitting that in conclusion I return to the issue raised in the first chapter and barely mentioned since – the spirit or tone of therapy. Although this aspect of therapy is difficult to describe without resorting to platitudes, it is the aspect of therapy that I consider most critical to success. If we get the tone of therapy right, everything else tends to fall into place.

Notes

1. Older studies on behavioural change in healthy individuals showed that changes were more likely to persist if these changes were attributed to internal factors and the individual's own efforts rather than external factors (Heatherton and Nicholls, 1994; Schoeneman and Curry, 1990; Sonne and Janoff, 1979).

2. Horvath and Greenberg (1994b).

3. For reviews on stepped care in psychotherapy, see Bower and Gilbody (2006) and Newman (2000).

References

Ackerman, S.J., Hilsenroth, M.J., Baity, M.R., & Blagys, M.D. (2000). Interaction of therapeutic process and alliance during psychological assessment. *Journal of Personality Assessment*, **75**, 82–109.

Adler, J.M., Chin, E.D., Kolisetty, A.P., & Ottomans, T.F. (2012). The distinguishing characteristics of narrative identity in adults with the features of borderline personality disorder: An empirical investigation. *Journal of Personality Disorders*, **26**, 498–512.

Akhtar, S. (1992). *Hidden structures: Severe personality disorders and their treatment*. Northvale, NJ: Aronson.

Allen, J.G. (2013). *Mentalizing in the development and treatment of attachment trauma*. London. Karnac

Allen, J.G., Newsom, G.E., Gabbard, G.O., & Coyne, L. (1984). Scales to assess the therapeutic alliance from a psychoanalytic perspective. *Bulletin of the Menninger Clinic*, **48**, 383–400.

Allport, G.W. (1961). *Pattern and growth in personality*. New York: Holt, Rinehart & Winston.

American Psychiatric Association. (2001). Practice guideline for the treatment of patients with borderline personality disorder. *American Journal of Psychiatry*, **158** (suppl), 1–52.

Amrhein, P., Miller, W.R., Yahne, C.E., Krupsky, A., & Hochstein, D. (2004). Strength of client commitment language improves with training in motivational interviewing. *Alcoholism: Clinical and Experimental Research*, **28**, 74A.

Amrhein, P., Miller, W.R., Yahne, C.E., Palmer, M., & Fulcher, L. (2003). Client commitment language during motivational interviewing predicts drug use outcomes. *Journal of Consulting and Clinical Psychology*, **71**, 862–878.

Angus, L.E., & McLeod, J. (Eds.), (2004a). *The handbook of narrative and psychotherapy: Practice, theory and research*. Thousand Oaks, CA: Sage.

Angus, L., & McLeod, J. (2004b). Toward an integrative framework for understanding the role of narrative in psychotherapy process. In L.E. Angus & J. McLeod (Eds.), *The handbook of narrative and psychotherapy: Practice, theory and research* (pp. 367–374). Thousand Oaks, CA: Sage.

Appelbaum, A.H. (2006). Supportive psychoanalytic psychotherapy for borderline patients: An empirical approach. *American Journal of Psychoanalysis*, **66**, 317–332.

Appelbaum, S.A. (1973). Psychological mindedness: Word, concept and essence. *Journal of Psychoanalysis*, **54**, 35–46.

Arnevik, E., Wilberg, T., Urnes, O., Johansen, M., Monsen, J., & Karterud, S. (2009). Psychotherapy for personality disorders: Short term day hospital psychotherapy versus outpatient individual therapy: A randomized controlled study. *European Psychiatry*, **24**, 71–78.

Arntz, A., Appels, C., & Sieswerda, S. (2000). Hypervigilance in borderline disorder: A test with the emotional Stroop paradigm. *Journal of Personality Disorders*, **14**, 366–373.

Ayduk, O., Mendoza–Denton, R., Mischel, W., Downey, G., Peake, P.K., & Rodriguez, M. (2000). Regulating the interpersonal self: Strategic self-regulation for coping with rejection sensitivity. *Journal of Personality and Social Psychology*, **79**, 776–792.

Ayduk, O., Mischel, W., & Downey, G. (2002). Attentional mechanisms linking rejection to hostile reactivity: The role of "hot" versus "cool" focus. *Psychological Science*, **13**, 443–448.

Ayduk, O., Zayas, V., Downey, G., Cole, A.B., Shoda, Y., & Mischel, W. (2008). Rejection sensitivity and executive control: Joint predictors of borderline personality features. *Journal of Research in Personality*, **42**, 151–168.

Baer, R.A., Smith, G.T., Hopkins, J., Krietemeyer, J., & Toney, L. (2006). Using self-report assessment methods to explore facets of mindfulness. *Assessment*, **13**, 27–45.

Bamelis, L.L.M., Evers, S.M.A.A., Spinhoven, P., & Arntz, A. (2014). The results of a multicenter randomized controlled trial on the clinical effectiveness of schema therapy for personality disorders. *American Journal of Psychiatry*, **171**, 305–322.

Bandura, A. (1977). Self-efficacy: Toward a unifying theory of behavioral change. *Psychological Review*, **84**, 139–157.

Barlow, D.H., Farchione, T.J., Fairholme, C.P., Ellard, K.K., Boieseau, C.L., Allan, L.B., et al. (2011). *Unified protocol for transdiagnostic treatment of emotional disorders*. Oxford, UK: Oxford University Press.

Barnicot, K., & Priebe, S. (2013). Post-traumatic stress disorder and the outcome of dialectical behaviour therapy for borderline personality disorder. *Personality and Mental Health*, **7**, 181–190.

Barnow, S., Stopsack, M., Grabe, H.J., Meinke, C., Spitzer, C., Kronmüller, K., & Sieswerda, S. (2009). Interpersonal evaluation bias in borderline personality disorder. *Behaviour Research and Therapy*, **47**, 359–365.

Bartak, A., Soeteman, D.I., Verheul, R., & Busschbach, J.J.V. (2007). Strengthening the status of psychotherapy for personality disorders: An integrated perspective on effects and costs. *Canadian Journal of Psychiatry*, **52**, 803–810.

Batchelor, A. (1995). Client's perception of the therapeutic alliance: A qualitative analysis. *Journal of Counseling Psychology*, **42**, 323–337.

Bateman, A.W., & Fonagy, P. (1999). The effectiveness of partial hospitalization in the treatment of borderline personality disorder – a randomized controlled trial. *American Journal of Psychiatry*, **156**, 1563–1569.

Bateman, A.W., & Fonagy, P. (2000). Effectiveness of psychotherapeutic treatment of personality disorder. *British Journal of Psychiatry*, **177**, 138–143.

Bateman, A.W., & Fonagy, P. (2001). The treatment of borderline personality disorder with psychoanalytically oriented partial hospitalization: An 18-month follow-up. *American Journal of Psychiatry*, **158**, 36–42.

Bateman, A.W., & Fonagy, P. (2004). *Psychotherapy for borderline personality disorder: Mentalization-based treatment*. Oxford, UK: Oxford University Press.

Bateman, A.W., & Fonagy, P. (2006). *Mentalization-based treatment for borderline personality disorder*. Oxford, UK: Oxford University Press.

Bateman, A.W., & Fonagy, P. (2008). 8-year follow-up of patients treated for borderline personality disorder: Mentalization-based treatment versus treatment as usual. *American Journal of Psychiatry*, **165**, 631–638.

Bateman, A.W., & Fonagy, P. (2009). Randomly controlled trial of outpatient mentalizing-based therapy versus structured clinical management for borderline personality disorder. *American Journal of Psychiatry*, **166**, 1355–1364.

Bateman, A.W., & Fonagy, P. (2013). Impact of clinical severity on outcomes of mentalisation-based treatment for borderline personality disorder. *British Journal of Psychiatry*, **203**, 221–227.

Bateman, A.W., & Fonagy, P. (2015). The role of mentalization in treatments for personality disorder. In W.J. Livesley, G. Dimaggio, & J.F. Clarkin (Eds.), *Integrated treatment for personality disorder* (pp. 148–172). New York: Guilford Press.

Baumeister, R.F. (1989). Social intelligence and the construction of meaning in life. In R.S. Wyer, Jr., T.K. Srull, et al. (Eds.), *Social intelligence and cognitive assessments of personality. Advances in social cognition* (Vol. 2, pp. 71–80). Hillsdale, NJ: Lawrence Erlbaum Associates, Inc.

Baumeister, R.F. (1991). *Meanings of life*. New York: Guilford Press.

Baumeister, R.F. (1994). The crystallization of discontent in the process of major life change. In T.F. Heatherton, J.L. Weinberger, et al. (Eds.), *Can personality change?* (pp. 281–297). Washington, DC: American Psychological Association.

Baumeister, R.F. (1998). The self. In D.T. Gilbert, S.T. Fiske, & G. Lindzey, *Handbook of social psychology* (4th ed., pp. 680–740). New York: McGraw-Hill.

Baumeister, R.F., & Heatherton, T.F. (1996). Self-regulation failure: An overview. *Psychological Inquiry*, **7**, 1–15.

Beck, A.T., Freeman, A., & Associates. (1990). *Cognitive therapy of personality disorders.* New York: Guilford.

Beck, A.T., Freeman, A., Davis, D.D. (2015). *Cognitive therapy of personality disorders* (3rd ed.). New York: Guilford Press.

Beck, A.T., Freeman, A., Davis, D.D., & Associates. (2004). *Cognitive therapy of personality disorders* (2nd ed.). New York: Guilford Press.

Benjamin, L.S. (2003). *Interpersonal reconstructive therapy: An integrative, personality-based treatment for complex cases.* New York: Guilford Press.

Bennett, D., Parry, G., & Ryle, A. (2006) Resolving threats to the therapeutic alliance in cognitive analytic therapy of BPD disorder: A task analysis. *Psychology and Psychotherapy: Theory, Research and Practice,* **79**, 395–418.

Bernstein, D.P., & Clercx, M. (in press). Schema Therapy. In W.J. Livesley & R.L. Larstone (Eds.), *Handbook of personality disorders* (2nd ed.). New York: Guilford.

Beutler, L.E., & Harwood, T.M. (2000). *Prescriptive psychotherapy.* Oxford: Oxford University Press.

Binks, C.A., Fenton, M., McCarthy, L., Lee, T., Adams, C.E., & Duggan, C. (2006). Pharmacological interventions for people with borderline personality disorder. *Cochrane Database of Systematic Reviews,* **1**, CD005653.

Black, D.W., Blum, N., Pfohl, B., & St. John, D. (2004). The STEPPS group treatment program for outpatient clients with borderline personality disorder. *Journal of Contemporary Psychotherapy,* **34**, 193–209.

Blum, N., Pfohl, B., St. John, D., Monahan, P., & Black, D.W. (2002). STEPPS: A cognitive-behavioral systems-based group treatment for outpatient clients with borderline personality disorder – a preliminary report. *Comprehensive Psychiatry,* **43**, 301–310.

Blum, N., St. John, D., Pfohl, B., Stuart, S., McCormick, B., Allen, J., Arndt, S., & Black, D.W. (2008) Systems Training for Emotional Predictability and Problem Solving (STEPPS) for outpatient clients with borderline personality disorder: A randomized controlled trial and 1-year follow-up. *American Journal of Psychiatry,* **165**, 468–478.

Blum, N.S., Bartels, N.E., St. John, D., & Pfohl, B. (2012). *Systems training for emotional predictability and problem solving (Second Edition): Group treatment program for borderline personality disorder.* Coralville, IA: Level One Publishing (Blums Books).

Borden, E.S. (1994). Theory and research in the therapeutic working alliance: New directions. In A. Horvath & L.S. Greenberg (Eds.), *The working alliance* (pp. 13–37). New York: John Wiley & Sons, Inc.

Bordin, E.S. (1979). The generalizability of the psychoanalytic concept of the working alliance. *Psychotherapy: Theory, Research and Practice,* **16**, 252–260.

Bower, P., & Gilbody, S. (2006). Stepped care in psychological therapies: Access, effectiveness and efficiency. *British Journal of Psychiatry,* **186**, 11–17.

Bradley, R., & Westen, D. (2005). The psychodynamics of borderline personality disorder: A view from developmental psychopathology. *Development and Psychopathlogy,* **17**, 927–957.

Bruner, J. (2004). The narrative creation of the self. In L.E. Angus & J. McLeod (Eds.), *The handbook of narrative and psychotherapy* (pp. 3–14). Thousand Oaks, CA: Sage Publications.

Budge, S.L., Moore, J.T., Del Re, A.C., Wampold, B.E., Baardseth, T.P., & Nienhaus, J.B. (2014). The effectiveness of evidence-based treatments for personality disorders when comparing treatment-as-usual and bona fide treatments. *Clinical Psychology Review,* **34**(5), 451–452.

Buie, D.H., & Adler, G. (1982). The definitive treatment of the borderline personality. *International Journal of Psychoanalytic Psychotherapy,* **9**, 51–87.

Carlson, E.A., Egeland, B., & Sroufe, L.A. (2009). A prospective investigation of the development of borderline symptoms. *Development and Psychopathology,* **21**, 1311–1334.

Carver, C.S. (2012). Self-awareness. In M.R. Leary & J.P. Tangney (Eds.), *Handbook of self and identity* (2nd ed., pp. 50–68). New York: Guilford.

Carver, C.S., & Scheier, M.F. (1981). *Attention and self-regulation: A cognitive theory approach to human behavior.* New York: Spring-Verlag.

Carver, C.S., & Scheier, M.F. (1998). *On the self-regulation of behavior.* Cambridge, UK: Cambridge University Press.

Castonguay, L.G., & Beutler, L.E. (2006a). Common and unique principles of therapeutic change: What do we know and what do we need to know? In L.G. Castonguay & L.E. Beutler (Eds.), *Principles of therapeutic change that work* (pp. 353–369). New York: Oxford University Press.

Castonguay, L.G., & Beutler, L.E. (Eds.), (2006b). *Principles of therapeutic change that work.* New York: Oxford University Press.

Chanen, A.M., Jackson, H.J., McCutcheon, L.K., Jovev, M., Dudgeon, P., Yuen, H.P., et al. (2008). Early intervention for adolescents with borderline personality disorder using cognitive analytic therapy: Randomised controlled trial. *British Journal of Psychiatry,* **193,** 477–484.

Cicchetti, D., Cummings, E.M., Greenberg, M.T., and Marvin, R.S. (1990). An organizational perspective on attachment beyond infancy: Implications for theory, measurement, and research. In E.M. Greenberg, D. Cicchetti, and M.T. Cummins (Eds.), *Attachment in the preschool years* (pp. 3–50). Chicago: University of Chicago Press.

Clark, L.A. (1993). *Manual for the Schedule for Non-adaptive and Adaptive Personality (SNAP).* Minneapolis: University of Minnesota Press.

Clarke, S., Thomas, T., & James, K. (2013). Cognitive analytic therapy for personality disorder: Randomized controlled trial. *British Journal of Psychiatry,* **202,** 129–134.

Clarkin, J.F., Levy, K.N., Lenzenweger, M.F., & Kernberg, O.F. (2007). Evaluating three treatments for borderline personality disorder: A multiwave study. *The American Journal of Psychiatry,* **164**(6), 922–928.

Clarkin, J.F., Yeomans, F.E., De Panfilis, C., & Levy, K.N. (2015). Strategies for constructing a more adaptive self-system. In W.J. Livesley, G. Dimaggio, & J.F. Clarkin (Eds.), *Integrated treatment for personality disorder* (pp. 397–418). New York: Guilford Press.

Clarkin, J.F., Yeomans, F.E., & Kernberg, O. (1999). *Psychotherapy for borderline personality disorder.* New York: Wiley.

Costa, P.T., & McCrae, R.R. (1990). Personality disorders and the five-factor model of personality. *Journal of Personality Disorders,* **4,** 362–371.

Costa, P.T., & McCrae, R.R. (1992). *Revised NEO Personality Inventory (NEO-PI-R) and the NEO Five-Factor Inventory (NEO-FFI) professional manual.* Odessa, FL: Psychological Assessment Resources.

Costa, P.T., & Widiger, T.A. (Eds.), (2002). *Personality disorders and the five factor model of personality* (2nd ed.). Washington, DC: American Psychological Association.

Cottraux, J., & Blackburn, I.M. (2001). Cognitive therapy. In W.J. Livesley (Ed.), *Handbook of personality disorders* (pp. 377–399). New York: Guilford Press.

Cottraux, J., Note, I.D., Boutitie, F., Milliery, M., Genouihlac, V., Yao, S.N., et al. (2009). Cognitive versus Rogerian supportive therapy in borderline personality disorder. *Psychotherapy and Psychosomatics,* **78,** 307–316.

Crawford, M.J., Koldobsky, N., Mulder, R., & Cottaux, P. (2011). Classifying personality disorder according to severity. *Journal of Personality Disorders,* **25,** 321–330.

Crawford, T.N., Cohen, P.R., Chen, H., Anglin, D.M., & Ehrensaft, M. (2009). Early maternal separation and the trajectory of borderline personality disorder symptoms. *Development and Psychopathology,* **21,** 1013–1030.

Critchfield, K.L., & Benjamin, L.S. (2006). Integration of therapeutic factors in treating personality disorders. In L.G. Castonguay & L.E. Beutler (Eds.), *Principles of therapeutic change that work* (pp. 253–271). New York: Oxford University Press.

Damasio, A. (1994). *Descartes' error: Emotion, reson, and the human brain.* New York: Putman.

Davidson, K. (2008). *Cognitive therapy for personality disorders* (2nd ed.). London: Routledge.

Davidson, K., Norrie, J., Tyrer, P., Gumley, A., Tata, P., Murray, H., et al. (2006). The effectiveness of cognitive behavior therapy for borderline personality disorder: Results from the BOSCOT trial. *Journal of Personality Disorders,* **20,** 450–465.

De Bonis, M., De Boeck, P., Lida-Pulik, H., Hourtane, M., & Feline, A. (1998). Self-concept and mood: A comparative study between depressed patients with and without borderline personality disorder. *Journal of Affective Disorders*, **48**, 191–197.

DeCharms, R. (1968). *Personal causation: The internal affective determinants of behavior*. New York: Academic Press.

DiClemente, C.C. (1994). If behaviours change, can personality be far behind? In T.F. Heatherton, & J.L. Weinberger (Eds.), *Can personality change?* (pp. 175–198). Washington, DC: American Psychological Association.

Dimaggio, G., Popolo, R., Carcione, A., & Salvatore, G. (2015). Improving meatacognition by acessing autobiographical memories. In W.J. Livesley, G. Dimaggio, & J.F. Clarkin (Eds.), *Integrated treatment for personality disorder* (pp. 173–193). New York: Guilford Press.

Dimaggio, G., Semerari, A., Carcione, A., Nicolò, G., & Procacci, M. (2007). *Psychotherapy of personality disorders: Metacognition, states of mind, and interpersonal cycles*. London: Routledge.

Dimaggio, G., Semerari, A., Popolo, R., & Lysaker, P.H. (2012). Autobiographical memory and menatilizing impairment in personality disorders and schizophrenia: Clinical and research implications. *Frontiers in Psychology*, **3**, 1–4.

Distel, M.A., Trull, T.J., Derom, C.A., Thiery, E.W., Grimmer, M.A., Martin, N.G., & Willemsen, G. (2008). Heritability of borderline personality disorder features is similar across three countries. *Psychological Medicne*, **38**, 1219–1229.

Doering, S., Hörz, S., Rentrop, M., Fischer-Kern, M., Schuster, P., Benecke, C., et al. (2010). Transference-focused psychotherapy v. treatment by community psychotherapists for borderline personality disorder: Randomized controlled trial. *British Journal of Psychiatry*, **196**, 389–395.

Domes, G., Czieschnek, D., Weidler, F., Berger, C., Fast, K., & Herpertz, S.C. (2008). Recognition of facial affect in borderline personality disorder. *Journal of Personality Disorders*, **22**, 135–147.

Domes, G., Schulze, L., & Herpertz, S.C. (2009). Emotion recognition in borderline personality disorder: A review of the literature. *Journal of Personality Disorders*, **23**, 6–19.

Downey, G., & Feldman, S.I. (1996). Implications of rejection sensitivity for intimate relationships. *Journal of Personality and Social Psychology*, **6**, 1327–1343.

Downey, G., Mougios, V., Ayduk, O., London, B.E., & Shoda, Y. (2004). Rejection Sensitivity and the defensive motivational system. Insights from the startle response to rejection cues. *Psychological Science*, **15**, 668–673.

Duggan, C., Huband, N., Smailagic, N., Ferriter, M., & Adams, C. (2008). The use of pharmacological treatments for people with personality disorder: A systematic review of randomized controlled trials. *Personality and Mental Health*, **2**, 119–170.

Dulit, R.A., Fyer, M.R., Leon, A.C., & Frances, A.J. (1994). Clinical correlates of self-mutilation in borderline personality disorder. *American Journal of Psychiatry*, **151**, 1305–1311.

Eells, T.D. (1997). Psychotherapy case formulation: History and current status. In T.D. Eells (Ed.), *Handbook of psychotherapy case formulation* (pp. 1–25). New York: Guilford Press.

Erikson, E. (1950). *Childhood and society*. New York: Norton.

Eubanks-Carter, C., Muran, J.C., & Safran, J.D. (2010). Alliance ruptures and resolution. In J.C. Muran & J.P. Barber (Ed.), *The therapeutic alliance: An evidence-based guide to practice* (pp. 74–94). New York, NY, US: Guilford Press.

Evans, K., Tyrer, P., Catalan, J., Schmidt, U., Davidson, K., Tata, P., et al. (1999). Manual-Assisted Cognitive-behavioral Therapy (MACT): A randomized controlled trial of a brief intervention with bibliotherapy in the treatment of recurrent deliberate self-harm. *Psychological Medicine*, **29**, 19–25.

Ezriel, H. (1952). Notes on psychoanalytic group therapy: II. Interpretation. *Research Psychiatry*, **15**, 119.

Fernandez-Alvarez, H., Clarkin, J.F., Sagueiro, M., & Critchfield, K.L. (2006). Participant factors in treating personality disorders. In L.G. Castonguay & L.E. Beutler (Eds.), *Principles of therapeutic change that work* (pp. 203–218). New York: Oxford University Press.

Foa, E.B., Keane, T.M., Friedman, M.J., & Cohen, J.A. (2009). *Effective treatments for PTSD: Practice guidelines from the*

International Society for Traumatic Stress Studies (2nd ed.). New York: Guildford Press.

Fonagy, P., & Luyten P. (in press). Attachment, mentalization, and the self. In W.J. Livesley & R.L. Larstone (Eds.), *Handbook of personality disorders* (2nd ed.). New York: Guilford.

Frances, A.J. (1992). Foreword. In L.H. Rockland (Ed.), *Supportive therapy for borderline patients* (pp. vii–viii). New York: Guildford Press.

Frank, A.F. (1992). The therapeutic alliances of borderline patients. In J.F. Clarkin, E. Marziali, & H. Munroe-Blum (Eds.), *Borderline personality disorder: Clinical and empirical perspectives* (pp. 220–247). New York: Guilford Press.

Frank, J. (1963). *Persuasion and healing: A comparative study of psychotherapy.* Baltimore: Johns Hopkins University Press.

Friedman, R.C., Aronoff, M.S., Clarkin, J.F., Corn, R., & Hurt, S.W. (1983). History of suicidal behavior in depressed borderline inpatients. *American Journal of Psychiatry*, **140**, 1023–1026.

Fyer, M.R., Frances, A.J., Sullivan, T., Hurt, S.W., & Clarkin, J.F. (1988). Suicide attempts in patients with borderline personality disorder. *American Journal of Psychiatry*, **145**, 737–739.

Gaston, L. (1990). The concept of the alliance and its role in psychotherapy: Theoretical and empirical considerations. *Psychotherapy*, **27**, 143–153.

Giesen-Bloo, J., van Dyck, R., Spinhoven, P., van Tilberg, W., Dirksen, C., van Asselt, T., et al. (2006). Outpatient psychotherapy for borderline personality disorder: Randomized trial of schema-focused therapy vs. transference-focused therapy. *Archives of General Psychiatry*, **63**, 649–658.

Gold, J.R. (1996). *Key concepts in psychotherapy integration.* New York: Plenum Press.

Goldberg, L.R. (1993). The structure of phenotypic personality traits. *American Psychologist*, **48**, 26–34.

Gray, J.A. (1978). Myers lecture: The neuropsychology of anxiety. *British Journal of Psychiatry*, **69**, 417–434.

Gray, J.A. (1987). *The psychology of fear and stress.* Cambridge: Cambridge University Press.

Greenberg, L.S., & Paivio, S.C., (1997). *Working with emotions in psychotherapy.* New York: Guilford.

Gross, J.J., & Thompson, R.A. (2007). Emotional regulation: Conceptual foundations. In J.J. Gross (Ed.), *Handbook of emotion regulation* (pp. 3–24). New York: Guilford Press.

Gunderson, J.G. (1984). *Borderline personality disorder.* Washington, DC: American Psychiatric Association.

Gunderson, J.G. (Ed.), (1989). Personality disorders. In American Psychiatric Association, et al. (Eds.), *Treatments of psychiatric disorders: A task force report of the American Psychiatric Association* (Vol. **1–3** & Index Vol. pp. 2633–2813). Washington, DC: American Psychiatric Press, Inc.

Gunderson, J.G., Frank, A.F., Ronningstam, E.F., et al. (1989). Early discontinuance of borderline patients from psychotherapy. *Journal of Nervous and Mental Disease*, **177**, 38–42.

Gunderson, J.G., & Links, P.S. (2008). *Borderline personality disorder. A clinical guide* (2nd ed.). Washington, DC: American Psychiatric Publishing Inc.

Habermas, T., & Bluck, S. (2000). Getting a life: The emergence of the life story in adolescence. *Psychological Bulletin*, **126**, 748–769.

Hamackek, D.E. (1971). *Encounters with the self.* New York: Holt, Rinehart, & Winston.

Harned, M.S., Korslund, K.E., & Linehan, M.M. (2014). A pilot randomized controlled trial of dialectical behavior therapy with and without the dialectical behavior therapy prolonged exposure protocol for suicidal and self-injuring women with borderline personality disorder and PTSD. *Behaviour Research and Therapy*, **55**, 7–17.

Harper, H. (1989). *Coding guide I: Identification of confrontation challenges in exploratory therapy.* Unpublished manuscript, University of Sheffield, Sheffield, England (Cited by Tufekcioglu, S., Muran, J.C., 2015).

Hartley, D.E. (1985). Research on the therapeutic alliance in psychotherapy. In R. Hales & A. Frances (Eds.), *Psychiatric update: American Psychiatric Press annual review of psychiatry* (Vol. **4**, pp. 532–549). Washington, DC: American Psychiatric Association Press.

Hatcher, R.L. (2010). Alliance theory and measurement. In J.C. Muran and J.P. Barber (Eds.), *The therapeutic alliance: An evidence-based guide to practice* (pp. 7–28). New York: Guilford Press.

Hatcher, R.L., & Barends, A.W. (1996). Patients' view of the alliance in psychotherapy: Explanatory factor analysis of three alliance measures. *Journal of Consulting and Clinical Psychology*, **64**, 1326–1336.

Hayes, S.C., Strosahl, K.D., & Wilson, K.G. (1999). *Acceptance and commitment therapy: An experiential approach to behavioral change*. New York: Guilford Press.

Heatherton, T.F., & Nichols, P.A. (1994). Conceptual issues in assessing whether personality can change. In T.F. Heatherton, J.L. Weinberger, et al. (Eds.), *Can personality change?* (pp. 3–18). Washington, DC: American Psychological Association.

Heckhausen, J., & Schulz, R. (1995). A life-span theory of control. *Psychological Review*, **102**, 284–304.

Helegeland, M.I., & Torgersen, S. (2004). Developmental antecedents of borderline personality disorder. *Comprehensive Psychiatry*, **45**, 138–147.

Hilsenroth, M.J., & Cromer, T.D. (2007). Clinical interventions related to alliance during the initial interview and psychological assessment. *Psychotherapy: Research, Theory, and Practice*, **44**, 205–208.

Hirsh, J.B., Quilty, L.C., Bagby, M., & McMain, D.F. (2012). The relationship between agreeableness and the development of the working alliance in patients with borderline personality disorder. *Journal of Personality Disorders*, **26**, 616–627.

Hoglend, P., Sortie, T., Heyerdahl, O., Sorbye, O., & Amlo, S. (1993). Brief dynamic psychotherapy: Patient suitability, treatment length, and outcome. *Journal of Psychotherapy Practice and Research*, **2**, 230–241.

Hollin, C.R. (1995). The meaning and implications of "programme integrity." In J. McGuire (Ed.), *What works: Reducing reoffending: Guidelines from research and practice* (pp. 195–208). Oxford, England: John Wiley & Sons.

Hopwood, C.J., Malone, J.C., Ansell, E.B., Sanislow, C.A., Grilo, C.M., McGlashan, T.H., et al. (2011). Personality assessment in DSM-5: Empirical support for rating severity, style, and traits. *Journal of Personality Disorders*, **25**, 305–320.

Horowitz, L.M. (2004). *Interpersonal foundations of psychopathology*. Washington, DC: American Psychological Association.

Horowitz, L.M., Wilson, K.R., Turan, B., Zolotsev, P., Constantino, M.J., & Henderson, L. (2006). How interpersonal motives clarify the meaning of interpersonal behavior: A revised circumplex model. *Personality and Social Psychology Review*, **10**, 67–86.

Horowitz, M.J. (1998). *Cognitive psychodynamics: From conflict to character*. New York: Wiley.

Horvath, A.O., & Greenberg, L.S. (1994a). Introduction. In A. Horvath, & L.S. Greenberg (Eds.), *The working alliance* (pp. 1–9). New York: John Wiley & Sons.

Horvath, A.O., & Greenberg, L.S. (Eds.). (1994b). *The working alliance*. New York: John Wiley & Sons.

Ingenhoven, T., Lafay, P., Rinne, T., Passchier, J., & Duivenvoorden, H. (2010). Effectiveness of pharmacotherapy for severe personality disorders: Meta-analyses of randomized controlled trials. *Journal of Clinical Psychiatry*, **71**, 14–25.

James, W. (1890). *The principles of psychology*. New York: Holt.

Jang, K.L., Livesley, W.J., Vernon, P.A., & Jackson, D.N. (1996). Heritability of personality disorder traits: A twin study. *Acta Psychiatrica Scandinavica*, **94**, 438–444.

Jorgensen, C.R. (2006a). Disturbed sense of identity in borderline personality disorder. *Journal of Personality Disorders*, **20**, 618–644.

Jorgensen, C.R. (2006b). Identity and borderline personality disorder. *Journal of Personality Disorders*, **19**, 344–364.

Jorgensen, C.R. (2009). Identity style in patients with borderline personality disorder and normal controls. *Journal of Personality Disorders*, **23**, 101–112.

Jørgensen, C.R. (2010). Invited essay: Identity and borderline personality disorder. *Journal of Personality Disorders*, **24**, 344–364.

Jorgensen, C.R. (in press). Identity. In W.J. Livesley & R. Larstone (Eds.), *The handbook of personality disorders* (2nd ed.). New York: Guilford Press.

Jorgensen, C.R., Freund, C., Boye, R., Jordet, H., Andersen, D., & Kjolbye, M. (2013). Mentalizing-based therapy versus psychodynamic supportive therapy. *Acta Psychiatrica Scandinavica*, **127**, 305–317.

Joseph, B. (1983). On understanding and not understanding: Some technical issues.

International Journal of Psychoanalysis, **64**, 291–298.

Jovev, M., & Jackson, H.J. (2004). Early maladaptive schemas in personality disordered individuals. *Journal of Personality Disorders*, **18**, 467–478.

Kabat-Zinn, J. (2005a). *Coming to our senses: Healing ourselves and the world through mindfulness*. New York: Hyperion.

Kabat-Zinn, Jon. (2005b). *Full catastrophe living: Using the wisdom of your body and mind to face stress, pain, and illness* (15th anniversary ed., pp. xxxiii, 471). New York, NY, US: Delta Trade Paperback/Bantam Dell.

Kahneman, D. (2011). *Thinking, fast and slow*. Toronto: Doubleday Canada.

Kemperman, I., Russ, M.J., & Shearin, E. (1997). Self-injurious behavior and mood regulation in borderline patients. *Journal of Personality Disorders*, **11**, 146–157.

Kernberg, O.F. (1984). *Severe personality disorders*. New Haven, CT: Yale University Press.

Kiesler, D.J. (1996). *Contemporary interpersonal theory and research: Personality, psychopathology, and psychotherapy*. Hoboken, NJ: John Wiley & Sons.

Kjelsberg, E., Eikeseth, P.H., & Dahl, A.A. (1991). Suicide in borderline patients – predictive factors. *Acta Psychiatrica Scandinavica*, **94**, 283–287.

Klonsky, E.D. (2007). The functions of deliberate self-injury: A review of the evidence. *Clinical Psychology Review*, **27**, 226–239.

Knox, J. (2011). *Self-agency in psychotherapy*. New York: Norton.

Kohut, H. (1971). *The analysis of the self*. New York: International Universities Press.

Kohut, H. (1977). *The restoration of the self*. New York: International Universities Press.

Kroll, J. (1988). *The challenge of the borderline patient*. New York: Basic Books.

Kroll, J. (2000). Use of no-suicide contracts by psychiatrists in Minnesota. *American Journal of Psychiatry*, **157**, 1684–1686.

Kruglanski, A.W., & Webster, D.M. (1996). Motivated closing of the mind: "Seizing" and "freezing." *Psychological Review*, **103**, 263–283.

Layden, M.A., Newman, C.F., Freeman, A., & Morse, S.B. (1993). *Cognitive therapy of borderline personality disorder*. Needham Heights, MS: Allyn & Bacon.

Leahy, R.L. (2015). Emotional schemas. In W.J. Livesley, G. Dimaggio, & J.F. Clarkin (Eds.), *Integrated treatment for personality disorder* (pp. 258–281). New York: Guilford Press.

Leary, M.R., & Tangney, J.P. (2012). The self as an organizing construct in the behavioral and social sciences. In M.R. Leary & J.P. Tangney (Eds.), *Handbook of self and identity* (pp. 1–18). New York: Guilford Press.

Leichsenring, F., & Leibing, E. (2003). The effectiveness of psychodynamic therapy and cognitive behavioural therapy in the treatment of personality disorders: A meta-analysis. *American Journal of Psychiatry*, **160**, 1223–1232.

Leichsenring, F., Leibing, E., Kruse, J., New, A.S., & Lewke, F. (2011). Borderline personality disorder. *Lancet*, **377**, 74–84.

Levy, K.N., Meehan, K.B., Kelly, K.M., Reynoso, J.S., Weber, M., Clarkin, J.F., & Kernberg, O.F. (2006). Change in attachment patterns and reflective function in a randomized control trial of transference-focused psychotherapy for borderline personality disorder. *Journal of Consulting and Clinical Psychology*, **74**, 1027–1040.

Lieb, K., Völlm, B., Rücker, G., Timmer, A., & Stoffers, J.M. (2010). Pharmacotherapy for borderline personality disorder: Cochrane systematic review of randomised trials. *British Journal of Psychiatry*, **196**, 4–12.

Linehan, M.M. (1993). *Cognitive-behavioural treatment of borderline personality disorder*. New York: Guilford Press.

Linehan, M.M., Armstrong, H.E., Suarez, A., Allmon, D., & Heard, H. (1991). Cognitive-behavioural treatment of chronically parasuicidal borderline patients. *Archives of General Psychiatry*, **48**, 1060–1064.

Linehan, M.M., Heard, H.L., & Armstrong, H.E. (1993). Naturalistic follow-up of a behavioral treatment for chronically parasuicidal borderline patients. *Archives of General Psychiatry*, **50**, 971–974.

Links, P.S., & Bergmans, Y. (2015). Managing suicidal and other crises. In W.J. Livesley, G. Dimaggio, & J.F. Clarkin (Eds.), *Integrated treatment for personality disorder: A modular approach* (pp. 197–210). New York: Guilford Press.

Links, P.S., & Kolla, N. (2005). Assessing and managing suicide risk. In J. Oldham, A. Skodal, & D. Bender (Eds.), *Textbook of personality disorders* (pp. 449–462).

Washington, DC: American Psychiatric Press.

Links, P.S., Mercer, D., & Novicks, J. (2015). Establishing a treatment framework and therapeutic alliance. In W.J. Livesley, G. Dimaggio, & J.F. Clarkin (Eds.), *Integrated treatment for personality disorder: A modular approach* (pp. 101–111). New York: Guilford Press.

Liotti, G. (2004). Trauma, dissociation and disorganized attachment: Three strands of a single braid. *Psychotherapy: Theory, Research, Practice, Training*, **41**, 472–486.

Liotti, G. (2009). Attachment and dissociation. In P. Dell & J.A. O'Neil (Eds.), *Dissociation and the dissociative disorders: DSM-V and beyond* (pp. 53–66). New York: Routledge.

Liotti, G. (2011). Attachment disorganization and the clinical dialogue: Theme and variations. In J. Solomon & C. George (Eds.), *Disorganization of attachment and caregiving* (pp. 383–413). New York: Guilford Press.

Lipsey, M.W. (1995). What do we learn from 400 research studies on the effectiveness of treatment with juvenile delinquents? In J. McGuire (Ed.), *What works: Reducing reoffending: Guidelines from research and practice* (pp. 63–78). Oxford, England: John Wiley & Sons.

Lipsey, M.W. (2009).The primary factors that characterize effective interventions with juvenile offenders: A meta-analytic overview. *Victims and Offenders*, **4**, 124–147.

Livesley, W.J. (1998). Suggestions for a framework for an empirically based classification of personality disorder. *Canadian Journal of Psychiatry*, **43**, 137–147.

Livesley, W.J. (2003a). Diagnostic dilemmas in the classification of personality disorder. In K. Phillips, M. First, & H.A. Pincus (Eds.), *Advancing DSM: Dilemmas in psychiatric diagnosis* (pp. 153–189). Arlington, VA: American Psychiatric Association Press.

Livesley, W.J. (2003b). *Practical management of personality disorder*. New York: Guilford Press.

Livesley, W.J. (2007). Integrated therapy for complex cases of personality disorder. *Journal of Clinical Psychology: In Session*, **64**, 207–221.

Livesley, W.J. (2008). Toward a genetically informed model of borderline personality disorder. *Journal of Personality Disorders*, **22**, 42–71.

Livesley, W.J. (2011). Suggestions for a framework for an empirically based classification of personality disorder. *Journal of Personality Disorders*, **25**, 397–420.

Livesley, W.J. (2012). Moving beyond specialized therapies for borderline personality disorder: The importance of integrated domain-focused treatment. *Psychodynamic Psychiatry*, **40**(1), 47–74.

Livesley, W.J. (2015). A modular strategy for treating emotional dysregulation. In W.J. Livesley, G. Dimaggio, & J.F. Clarkin (Eds.), *Integrated treatment for personality disorder: A modular approach* (pp. 232–257). New York: Guilford Press.

Livesley, W.J., & Clarkin, J.F. (2015a). A general framework for integrated modular treatment. In W.J. Livesley, G. Diaggio, & J.F. Clarkin (Eds.), *Integrated treatment for personality disorder: A modular approach* (pp. 19–47). New York: Guilford Press.

Livesley, W.J., & Clarkin, J.F. (2015b). Diagnosis and assessment. In W.J. Livesley, G. Diaggio, & J.F. Clarkin (eds.), *Integrated treatment for personality disorder: A modular approach* (pp. 51–79). New York: Guilford Press.

Livesley, W.J., & Clarkin, J.F. (2015c). Formulation and treatment planning. In W.J. Livesley, G. Dimaggio, & J.F. Clarkin (Eds.), *Integrated treatment for personality disorder: A modular approach* (pp. 80–100). New York: Guilford Press.

Livesley, W.J., & Jackson, D.N. (2009). *Dimensional assessment of personality pathology – Basic questionnaire technical manual*. Port Huron, MI: Sigma Press.

Livesley, W.J., Jackson, D.N., & Schroeder, M.L. (1989). A study of the factorial structure of personality pathology. *Journal of Personality Disorders*, **3**, 292–306.

Livesley, W.J., Jackson, D.N., & Schroeder, M.L. (1992). Factorial structure of personality disorders in clinical and general population samples. *Journal of Abnormal Psychology*, **101**, 432–440.

Livesley, W.J., & Jang, K.L. (2005). Diffentiating normal, abnormal, and disordered personality. *European Journal of Personality*, **19**(4), 257–268.

Livesley, W.J., Jang, K.L., Jackson, D.N., & Vernon, P.A. (1993). Genetic and environmental contributions to dimensions of personality disorder. *American Journal of Psychiatry*, **150**, 1826–1831.

Livesley, W.J., Jang, K.L., & Vernon, P.A. (1998). The phenotypic and genetic architecture of traits delineating personality disorder. *Archives of General Psychiatry*, **55**, 941–948.

Livesley, W.J., Schroeder, M.L., Jackson, D.N., & Jang, K.L. (1994). Categorical distinctions in the study of personality disorder: Implications for classification. *Journal of Abnormal Psychology*, **103**, 6–17.

Luborsky, L. (1976). Helping alliance in psychotherapy. In J. L. Claghorn (Ed.), *Successful psychotherapy*. New York: Brunne/Mazel.

Luborsky, L. (1984). *Principles of psychoanalytic psychotherapy*. New York: Basic Books.

Luborsky, L. (1994). Therapeutic alliances as predictors of psychotherapy outcomes: Factors explaining the predictive success. In A.O. Horvath & L.S. Greenberg (Eds.), *The working alliance* (pp. 38–50). New York: John Wiley & Sons.

Luborsky, L., Crits-Christoph, P., Mintz, J., & Auerbach, A. (1988). *Who will benefit from psychotherapy? Predicting therapeutic conditions*. New York: Basic Books.

Luborsky, L., McLellan, A.T., Woody, G.E., O'Brien, C.P., & Auerbach, A. (1985). Therapist success and its determinants. *Archives of General Psychiatry*, **42**, 602–611.

Malan, D.H. (1979). *Individual psychotherapy and the science of psychodynamics*. London: Butterworth's.

Markovitz, P. (in press). Psychopharmacology. In W.J. Livesley & R. Larstone (Eds.), *Handbook of personality disorders*. New York: Guilford Press.

Mayer, J.D. (2005). A tale of two visions: Can a new view of personality help to integrate psychology? *American Psychologist*, **60**, 294–307.

McAdams, D.P., & Janis, L. (2004). Narrative identity and narrative therapy. In L.E. Angus & J. McLeod (Eds.), *The handbook of narrative and psychotherapy* (pp. 159–173). Thousand Oaks, CA: Sage Publications.

McAdams, D.P., & Pals, J.L. (2006). A new big five: Fundamental principles for an integrative science of personality. *American Psychologist*, **61**, 204–217.

McCallum, M., & Piper, W.E. (1997). The psychological mindedness assessment procedure. In M. McCallum & W.E. Piper (Eds.), *Psychological mindedness* (pp. 27–58). MahWah, NJ: Lawrence Erlbaum Associates.

McCullough-Vaillant, L. (1997). *Changing character*. New York: Basic Books.

McGlashan, T.H. (1986). The Chestnut Lodge follow up study III: Long-term outcome of borderline personalities. *Archives of General Psychiatry*, **43**, 2–30.

McMain, S.F., Links, P.S., Gnam, W.H., Guimond, T., Cardish, R.J., Korman, L., & Streiner, D.L. (2009). A randomized controlled trial of dialectical behavior therapy versus general psychiatry management for borderline personality disorder. *American Journal of Psychiatry*, **166**, 1365–1374.

Mehlum, L., Vaglum, P., & Karterud, S. (1994). The longitudinal pattern of suicidal behavior in borderline personality disorder: A prospective follow-up study. *Acta Psychiatric Scandinavica*, **90**, 124–130.

Mehlum, L., Vaglum, P., & Karterud, S. (1994). The longitudinal pattern of suicidal behavior in borderline personality disorder: A prospective follow-up study. *Acta Psychiatric Scandinavica*, **90**, 124–130.

Meichenbaum, D., & Turk, D.C. (1987). *Facilitating treatment adherence: A practitioners' guidebook*. New York: Plenum Press.

Meissner, W.W. (1984). *The borderline spectrum: Differential diagnosis and developmental issues*. Northvale, NJ: Jason Aronson. CH 3

Meyer, B., Ajchenbrenner, M., & Bowles, D.P. (2005). Sensory sensitivity, attachment experiences, and rejection responses among adults with borderline and avoidant features. *Journal of Personality Disorders*, **19**, 641–658.

Mikulincer, M. (1997). Adult attachment style and information processing: Individual differences in curiosity and cognitive closure. *Journal of Personality and Social Psychology*, **72**, 1217–1230.

Miller, W.R., Moyers, T.B., Amrhein, P., & Rollnick, S. (2006). A consensus statement on defining change talk. *MINT Bulletin*, **13**, 6–7.

Miller, W.R., & Rollnick, S. (1991). *Motivational interviewing: Preparing people to change addictive behavior*. New York: Guilford Press.

Miller, W.R., & Rollnick, S. (2002). *Motivational interviewing: Preparing people for change* (2nd ed.). New York: Guilford Press.

Miller, W.R., & Rollnick, S. (2013). *Motivational interviewing: Helping people change* (3rd ed.). New York: Guilford Press.

Mitchell, S.A. (1993). *Hope and dread in psychoanalysis.* New York, NY: Basic Books.

Morgan, T.A., & Zimmerman, M. (in press). Epidemiology. In W.J. Livesley & R.L. Larstone (Eds.), *Handbook of personality disorder* (2nd ed.). New York: Guilford.

Moritz, S., Schilling, L., Wingenfeld, K., Köther, U., Wittekind, C., Terfehr, K., & Spitzer, C. (2011). Psychotic-like cognitive biases in borderline personality disorder. *Journal of Behavior Therapy and Experimental Psychiatry*, **42**, 349–354.

Mulder, R.T., Newton-Howes, G., Crawford, M.J., & Tyrer, P. (2011). The central domains of personality pathology in psychiatric patients. *Journal of Personality Disorders*, **25**, 364–377.

Muran, J.C., Segal, Z.V., Samstag, L.W., & Crawford, C. (1994). Patient pretreatment interpersonal problems and therapeutic alliance in short-term cognitive therapy. *Journal of Consulting and Clinical Psychology*, **62**, 185–190.

Muraven, M., & Baumeister, R.F. (2000). Self-regulation and depletion of limited resources: Does self-control resemble a muscle? *Psychological Bulletin*, **126**, 247–259.

Napolitano, L., & McKay, D. (2007). Dichotomous thinking in borderline personality disorder. *Cognitive Therapy and Research*, **31**, 717–726.

Newman, M. (2000). Recommendations for a cost-offset model of psychotherapy allocation using generalized anxiety disorder as an example. *Journal of Consulting and Clinical Psychology*, **68**, 549–555.

Nolen-Hoeksema, S. (2012). Emotion regulation and psychopathology: The role of gender. *Annual Review of Clinical Psychology*, **6**, 161–187.

Ofrat, S., Krueger, R.F., & Clark, L.A. (in press). Dimensional approaches to personality disorder classification. In W.J. Livesley & R. Larstone (Eds.), *The handbook of personality disorders* (2nd ed.). New York: Guilford Press.

Olson, E.T. (1999). There is no problem of the self. In S. Gallagher & J. Shear (Eds.), *Models of the self* (pp. 49–61). Exeter: Imprint Academic.

Orlinsky, D.E., Grawe, K., & Parks, B.K. (1994). Process and outcome in psychotherapy – Noch einmel. In A.E. Begin & S.L. Garfield (Eds.), *Handbook of psychotherapy and behavioral change* (3rd ed. pp. 270–376). New York: John Wiley & Sons.

Orlinsky, D.E., & Howard, K.I. (1986). Process and outcome in psychotherapy. In A.E. Begin & S.L. Garfield (Eds.), *Handbook of psychotherapy and behavioral change* (3rd ed. pp. 311–381). New York: John Wiley & Sons.

Osatuke, K., Glick, M.J., Gray, M.A., Reynolds, D.J., Humphreys, C.L., Salvi, L.M., & Stiles, W.B. (2004). Assimilation and narrative: Stories as meaning bridges. In L.E. Angus & J. McLeod (Eds.), *The handbook of narrative and psychotherapy* (pp. 193–210). Thousand Oaks, CA: Sage Publications.

Ottavi, P., Passarella, T., Pasinetti, M., Salvatore, G., & Dimaggio, G. (2015). Adapting mindfulness for treating personality disorder. In W.J. Livesley, G. Dimaggio, & J.F. Clarkin (Eds.), *Integrated treatment for personality disorder: A modular approach* (pp. 282–302). New York: Guilford Press.

Paris, J. (2001). Psychosocial adversity. In W.J. Livesley (Ed.), *Handbook of personality disorders* (pp. 231–241). New York: Guilford Press.

Paris, J. (2003). *Personality disorders over time.* Washington, DC: American Psychiatric Publishing.

Paris, J. (in press). Childhood adversities and personality disorders. In W.J. Livesley & R.L. Larstone (Eds.), *Handbook of personality disorders* (2nd ed., pp.). New York: Guilford Press.

Paris J., Brown, R., & Nowlis, D. (1987). Long-term follow-up of borderline patients in a general hospital. *Comprehensive Psychiatry*, **28**, 530–535.

Paris J., Nowlis, D., & Brown, R. (1989). Predictors of suicide in borderline personality disorder. *Canadian Journal of Psychiatry*, **34**, 8–9.

Paris J., & Zweig-Frank H. (2001). A 27-year follow-up of borderline patients. *Comprehensive Psychiatry*, **42**, 482–487.

Perry, S., Cooper, A.R., & Michels, R. (1987). The psychodynamic formulation: Its purpose, structure, and clinical application. *American Journal of Psychiatry*, **144**, 543–550.

Perry, C. J., Fowler, J. C., Bailey, A., Clemence, A. J., Plakun, E. M., Zheutlin, B., et al. (2009). Improvement and recovery from suicidal and self-destructive phenomena in treatment-refractory disorders. *The Journal of Nervous and Mental Disease*, **197**, 28–34.

Pierro, A., & Kruglanski, A.W. (2008). "Seizing and freezing" on a significant-person schema: Need for closure and the transference effect in social judgment. *Personality and Social Psychology Bulletin*, **34**, 1492–1503.

Pincus, A.L., & Ansell, E.B. (2012). Interpersonal theory of personality. In J. Suls & H. Tennen (Eds.), *Handbook of Psychology Vol. 5: Personality and social psycyhology* (2nd ed., pp. 141–159). Hoboken, NJ: Wiley.

Piper, W.E., Azim, H.F.A., Joyce, A.S., McCallum, M., Nixon, G.W.H., & Segal, P.S. (1991). Quality of object relations versus interpersonal functioning as predictors of therapeutic alliance and psychotherapy outcome. *Journal of Nervous and Mental Disease*, **179**, 432–438.

Piper, W.E., & Joyce, A.S. (2001). Psychosocial treatment outcome. In W.J. Livesley (Ed.), *Handbook of personality disorders: Theory, research, and treatment* (pp. 323–343). New York: Guilford Press.

Piper, W.E., Rosie, J.S., Azim, H.F.A., & Joyce, A.S. (1993). A randomized trial of psychiatric day treatment for patients with affective and personality disorders. *Hospital and Community Psychiatry*, **44**, 757–763.

Piper, W.E., Rosie, J.S., Joyce, A.S., & Azim, H.F.A. (1996). *Time-limited day treatment for personality disorders: Integration of research and practice in a group program*. Washington, DC: American Psychological Association Press.

Pretzer, J. (1990). Borderline personality disorder. In T.A. Beck, A. Freeman, & Associates (Eds.), *Cognitive therapy of personality disorders* (pp. 176–207). New York: The Guilford Press.

Prochaska, J.O., & DiClemente, C.C. (1992). The transtheoretical approach. In J.C. Norcross & M.R. Goldfried (Eds.), *Handbook of psychotherapy integration*. New York: Basic Books.

Prochaska, J.O., DiClemente, C.C., & Norcross, J.C. (1992). In search of how people change. *American Psychologist*, **47**, 1102–1114.

Prochaska, J.O., Norcross, J.C., & DiClemente, C.C. (1994). *Changing for good: The revolutionary program that explains the six stages of change and teaches you how to free yourself from bad habits*. New York: William Morrow.

Rafaeli, E., Bernstein, D.P., & Young, J. (2011). *Schema therapy: Distinctive features*. New York: Routledge.

Ricoeur, P. (1981). The narrative function. In P. Ricoeur, *Hermeneutics and the human sciences* (J.B. Thompson Ed. & Trans., pp. 165–181). Cambridge, UK: Cambridge University Press.

Ridolfi, M.E., & Gunderson, J.G. (in press). Psychoeducation for patients with borderline personality disorder. In W.J. Livesley & R. Larstone (Eds.), *Handbook of personality disorder* (2nd ed.). New York: Guilford.

Robins, C.J., Ivanoff, A.M., & Linehan, M.M. (2001). Dialectic behavior therapy. In W.J. Livesley (Ed.), *Handbook of personality disorders* (pp. 437–459). New York: Guilford Press.

Robins, C.J., Zerubavel, N., Ivanoff, A.M., & Linehan, M.M. (in press). Dialectic behavior therapy. In W.J. Livesley & R. Laarsone (Eds.), *Handbook of personality disorders*. New York: Guilford Press.

Rockland, L.H. (1992). *Supportive therapy for borderline patients*. New York: Guilford Press.

Roemer, L., & Orsillo, S.M. (2009). *Mindfulness- and acceptance-based behavioral therapies in practice*. New York: Guilford Press.

Rogers, C.R. (1951). *Client centered therapy: Its current practice, implications, and theory*. Boston: Houghton.

Rogers, C.R. (1957). The necessary and sufficient conditions of therapeutic personality change. *Journal of Counselling Psychology*, **21**, 95–103.

Romero-Canyas, R., Downey, G., Berenson, K., Ayduk, O., & Kang, N.L., (2010). Rejection sensitivity and the rejection–hostility link in romantic relationships. *Journal of Personality*, **78**, 119–145.

Rosengren, D.B. (2009). *Building motivational interviewing skills: A practitioner workbook*. New York: Guilford Press.

Roth, A., & Fonagy, P. (2005). *What works for whom?* (2nd ed.). New York: Guilford Press.

Ruiz-Sancho, A.M., Smith, G.W., & Gunderson, J.E. (2001). Psychoeducational approaches. In W.J. Livesley (Ed.), *Handbook of personality disorders: Theory, research, and treatment* (pp. 460–474). New York: Guilford Press.

Ryan, R.M., Deci, E.L., & Grolnick, W.S. (1995). Autonomy, relatedness, and the self: Their relation to development and psychopathology. In D. Cicchetti & D.J. Cohen (Eds.), *Developmental psychopathology: Vol. I. Theory and methods* (pp. 618–655). New York: Wiley.

Ryle, A. (1975). *Frames and cages.* London: Sussex University Press.

Ryle, A. (1997). *Cognitive analytic therapy and borderline personality disorder.* Chichester, UK: Wiley.

Sadikaj, G., Russell, J.J., Moskowitz, D.S., & Paris, J. (2010). Affect dysregulation in individuals with borderline personality disorder: Persistence and interpersonal triggers. *Journal of Personality Assessment,* **92** (6), 490–500.

Safran, J.D., Crocker, P., McMain, S., & Murray, P. (1990). Therapeutic alliance rupture as a therapy event for empirical investigation. *Psychotherapy,* 27, 154–165.

Safran, J.D., & Muran, J.C. (2000). *Negotiating the therapeutic alliance: A relational treatment guide.* New York, NY, US: Guilford Press.

Safran, J.D., Muran, J.C., Demaria, A., Boutwell, C., Eubank-Carter, C., & Winston, A. (2014). The impact of alliance-focused training on interpersonal process in a cognitive-behavioral therapy for personality disorders. *Psychotherapy Research,* **24,** 269–285.

Safran, J.D., Muran, J.C., & Samstag, L.N. (1994). Resolving therapeutic alliance ruptures: A task analytic investigation. In A.O. Horvath, L.S. Greenberg, et al. (Eds.), *The working alliance: Theory, research, and practice* (pp. 225–255). New York: John Wiley & Sons.

Safran, J.D., Muran, J.C., Samstag, L.W., & Stevens, C. (2002). Repairing alliance ruptures. In J.C. Norcross (Ed.), *Psychotherapy relationships that work: Therapist contributions and responsiveness to patients* (pp. 235–254). New York: Oxford University Press.

Salvatore, G., Popolo, R., & Dimaggio, G. (2015). Promoting integration between different self-stages through ongoing reformulation. In W.J. Livesley, G. Dimaggio, & J.F. Clarkin (Eds.), *Integrated treatment for personality disorder* (pp. 419–435). New York: Guilford Press.

Samstag, L.W., Batchelder, S., Muran, J.C., Safran, J.D., & Winston, A. (1998). Predicting treatment failure from in-session interpersonal variables. *Journal of Psychotherapy Practice & Research,* 5, 126–143.

Sanderson, C., & Clarkin, J.F. (2013). Further use of the NEO-PI-R personality dimensions in differential treatment planning. In T.A. Widiger & P.T. Costa (Eds.), *Personality disorders and the five factor model of personality* (3rd ed., pp. 325–348). Washington, DC: American Psychological Association.

Sansome, R.A. (2004). Chronic suicidality and borderline personality. *Journal of Personality Disorders,* 18, 215–225.

Saunders, E.F., & Silk, K.R. (2009). Personality trait dimensions and the pharmacological treatment of borderline personality disorder. *Journal of Clinical Psychopharmacology,* **29,** 461–467.

Schmideberg, M. (1947). The treatment of psychopathic and borderline patients. *American Journal of Psychotherapy,* **1,** 45–71.

Schoeneman, T.J., & Curry, S. (1990). Attributions for successful and unsuccessful health behavior change. *Basic and Applied Social Psychology,* 11, 421–431.

Sexton, H., Littauer, H., Sexton, A., & Tommeras, E. (2005). Building the alliance: Early therapeutic process and the client-therapist connection. *Psychotherapy Research,* 15, 103–116.

Shapiro, D. (1965). *Neurotic styles.* New York: Basic Books.

Shapiro, D. (1981). *Autonomy and rigid character.* New York: Basic Books.

Shearer, S.L., Peter, C.P., Quaytman, M.S., & Wadman, B.E. (1988). Intent and lethality of suicide attempts among female borderline patients. *American Journal of Psychiatry,* **145,** 1424–1427.

Sheldon, K.M., & Elliot, A.J. (1999). Goal striving, need satisfaction, and longitudinal well-being: The self-concordance model. *Journal of Personality and Social Psychology*, **76**, 482–497.

Sheldon, K.M., Ryan, R.M., Rawsthorne, L.J., & Ilardi, B. (1997). Trait self and true self: Cross-role variation in the big-five personality traits and its relations with psychological authenticity and subjective well-being. *Journal of Personality and Social Psychology*, **73**, 1380–1393.

Shenk, C.E., & Fruzzetti, A.E. (2011). The impact of validating and invalidating responses on emotional reactivity. *Journal of Social and Clinical Psychology*, **30**, 163–183.

Sieswerda, S., Barnow, S., Verheul, R., & Arntz, A. (2013). Neither dichotomous nor split, but schema-related negative interpersonal evaluations characterize borderline patients. *Journal of Personality Disorders*, **27**, 36–52.

Silk, K.R., & Friedel, R.O. (2015). Psychopharmacological considerations in the integrated treatment of personality disorder. In W.J. Livesley, G. Dimaggio, & J.F. Clarkin (Eds.), *Integrated treatment for personality disorder* (pp. 211–231). New York: Guilford Press.

Singer, J.A. (2004). Narrative-identity and meaning-making across the lifespan: An introduction. *Journal of Personality*, **72**, 437–459.

Skinner, E.A. (1996). A guide to constructs of control. *Journal of Personality and Social Psychology*, **71**, 549–570.

Soloff, P.H. (2000). Psychopharmacology of borderline personality disorder. *Psychiatric Clinics of North America*, **23**, 169–190.

Soloff, P.H., Lis, J.A., Kelly, T., Cornelius, J., & Ulrich, R. (1994). Self-mutilation and suicidal behavior in borderline personality disorder. *Journal of Personality Disorders*, **8**, 257–267.

Sommerfeld, E., Orbach, I., Zim, S., & Mikulincer, M. (2008). An in-session exploration of ruptures in working alliance and their associations with clients' core conflictual relationship themes, alliance-related discourse, and clients' post-session evaluations. *Psychotherapy Research*, **18**(4), 377–388.

Sonne, J.L., & Janoff, D.S. (1979). The effect of treatment attributions on the maintenance of weight reduction: A replication and extension. *Cognitive Therapy and Research*, **3**, 389–387.

Staebler, K., Renneberg, B., Stopsack, M., Fiedler, P., Weiler, M., & Roepke, S. (2011). Facial emotional expression in reaction to social exclusion in borderline personality disorder. *Psychological Medicine*, **41**, 1929–1938.

Stanford, E., Goetz, R.R., & Bloom, J.D. (1994). The no harm contract in the emergency assessment of suicidal risk. *Journal of Clinical Psychiatry*, **55**, 344–348.

Stanghellini, G., & Rosfort, R. (2013). *Emotions and personhood*. Oxford, UK: Oxford University Press.

Steiner, J. (1994). Patient-centered and analyst-centered interpretations: Some implications of containment and countertransference. *Psychoanalytic Quarterly*, **14**, 406–422.

Stepp, S.D., Pilkonis, P.A., Yaggi, K.E., Morse, J.Q., & Feske, U. (2009). Interpersonal and emotional experiences of social interactions in borderline personality disorder. *Journal of Nervous and Mental Disease*, **197**, 484–491.

Stiles, W.B. (2011). Coming to terms. *Psychotherapy Research*, **21**, 367–384.

Stone, M.H. (1989). The course of borderline personality disorder. In A. Tasman, R.E. Hales, & A.J. Frances (Eds.), *American Psychiatric Press review of psychiatry* (vol. **8**, pp. 103–122). Washington, DC: American Psychiatric Press.

Stone, M.H. (1990). *The fate of borderline patients*. New York: Guilford Press.

Stone, M.H. (1993). Long-term outcome in personality disorders. *British Journal of Psychiatry*, **162**, 299–353.

Stone, M.H. (2001). Natural history and long-term outcome. In W.J. Livesley (Ed.), *Handbook of personality disorder* (pp. 259–273). New York: Guilford Press.

Strupp, H.H., Fox, R.E., & Lessler, K. (1969). *Patients view their psychotherapy*. Baltimore, MD: Johns Hopkins Press.

Sullivan, H.S. (1953). *The interpersonal theory of psychiatry*. New York, NY: Norton.

Suyemoto, K.L. (1998). The functions of self-mutilation. *Clinical Psychology Review*, **18**, 531–554.

Swenson, C. (1989). Kernberg and Linehan: Two approaches to the borderline patient. *Journal of Personality Disorders*, **3**, 26–35.

Taylor, S.E. (1983). Adjustment to threatening events: A theory of cognitive adaptation. *American Psychologist*, **38**, 1161–1173.

Teasdale, J.D., Segal, Z., & Williams, J.M.G. (1995). How does cognitive therapy prevent depressive relapse and why should attentional control (mindfulness) training help? *Behavior Therapy and Research*, **33**, 25–39.

Thompson, S.C., & Spacaman, S. (1991). Perceptions of control in vulnerable populations. *Journal of Social Issues*, **47**, 1–21.

Tickle, J.J., Heatherton, T.F., & Wittenberg, L.G. (2001). Can personality change? In W.J. Livesley (Ed.), *Handbook of personality disorders: Theory, research, and treatment* (pp. 242–258). New York: Guilford Press.

Torgensen, S. (2012). Epidemiology. In T.A. Widiger (Ed.), *Handbook of personality disorders* (pp. 186–205). New York: Oxford University Press.

Torgersen, S., Lygren, S., Oien, P.A., Skre, I., Onstad, S., Edvardsen, J., Tambs, K., & Kringlen, E. (2000). A twin study of personality disorders. *Comprehensive Psychiatry*, **41**, 416–425.

Toulmin. S. (1978). Self-knowledge and knowledge of the "self." In T. Mischel (Ed.), *The self: Psychological and philosophical issues* (pp. 291–317). Oxford: Oxford University Press.

Tufekcioglu, S., & Muran, J.C. (2015). A relational approach to personality disorder and alliance rupture. In W.J. Livesley, G. Dimaggio, & J.F. Clarkin (Eds.), *Integrated treatment for personality disorder: A modular approach* (pp. 123–147). New York: Guilford Press.

Tyrer, P., & Johnson, T. (1996). Establishing the severity of personality disorder. *American Journal of Psychiatry*, **153**, 1593–1597.

Tyron, G.S. (1988). Session depth and smoothness in relation to the concept of engagement in counseling. *Psychotherapy*, **26**, 54–61.

Tyron, G.S., & Kane, A.S. (1990). The helping alliance and premature termination. *Counseling Psychology Quarterly*, **3**, 233–238.

Tyron, G.S., & Kane, A.S. (1993). Relationship of working alliance to mutual and unilateral termination. *Journal of Counseling Psychology*, **40**, 33–36.

Tyron, G.S., & Kane, A.S. (1995). Client involvement, working alliance and type of therapy termination. *Psychotherapy Research*, **5**(3), 189–198.

Vaillant, G.E. (1992). The beginning of wisdom is never calling a patient a borderline. *Journal of Psychotherapy Practice and Research*, **1**, 117–134.

Veen, G., & Arntz, A. (2000). Multidimensional dichotomous thinking characterizes borderline personality disorder. *Cognitive Therapy and Research*, **24**(1), 23–45.

Verheul, R., Andrea, H., Berghout, C.C., Dolan, C., Busschbach, J.J.V., van der Kroft, P.J.A., & Fonagy, P. (2008). Severity Indices of Personality Problems (SIPP-118): Development, factor structure, reliability, and validity. *Psychological Assessment*, **20**, 23–34.

Vernon, P.E. (1964). *Personality assessment: A critical survey*. London: Methuen.

Wagner, A.W., & Linehan, M.M. (1999). Facial expression recognition among women with borderline personality disorder: Implications for emotion regulation? *Journal of Personality Disorders*, **13**, 329–344.

Wagner, D.D., & Heatherton, T.F. (2011). Giving in to temptation: The emerging cognitive-neuroscience of self-regulatory failure. In K.D. Vohs & R.F. Baumeister (Eds.), *Handbook of self-regulation: Research, theory, and applications* (2nd ed., pp. 41–63). New York: Guilford Press.

Waldinger, R.J. (1987). Intensive psychodynamic therapy with borderline patients: An overview. *American Journal of Psychiatry*, **144**, 267–274.

Waldinger, R.T., & Gunderson, J.G. (1989). *Effective psychotherapy with borderline patients*. Washington, DC: American Psychiatric Association.

Walton, G.M., Paunesku, D., & Dweck, C.S. (2012). Expandable selves. In M.R. Leary & J.P. Tangney (Eds.), *Handbook of self and identity* (2nd ed., pp. 141–154). New York: Guilford Press.

Weiner, B. (1985). An attributional model of achievement motivation and emotion. *Psychological Review*, **92**, 548–573.

Wicklund, R.A. (1975). Objective self-awareness. In L. Berkowitz (Ed.), *Advances in experimental social psychology* (Vol. **8**, pp. 233–275). New York: Academic Press.

Wicklund, R.A., & Duval, S. (1971). Opinion change and performance facilitation as a result of objective self-awareness. *Journal of Experimental Social Psychology, 7,* 319–342.

Widiger, T.A., Costa, P.T., Jr., & McCrea, R.R. (2002). A proposal for Axis II: Diagnosing personality disorders using the five-factor model. In P.T. Costa, Jr., & T.A. Widiger (Eds.), *Personality disorders and the five-factor model of personality* (2nd ed., pp. 431–456). Washington, DC: American Psychological Association.

Wild, J. (1965). Authentic existence: A new approach to "value theory." In J.M. Edie (Ed.), *An invitation to phenomenology: Studies in the philosophy of experience* (pp. 59–78). Chicago: Quadrangle Books.

Willi, J. (1999). *Ecological psychotherapy.* Seattle: Hogrefe & Huber.

Wise, M.J., & Rinn, R.C. (1983). Premature client termination from psychotherapy as a function of continuity of care. *Journal of Psychiatric Treatment and Evaluation, 5,* 63–65.

Wolpe, J. (1958). *Psychotherapy by reciprocal inhibition.* Stanford, CA: Stanford University Press.

Yalom, I.D. (1985). *The theory and practice of group psychotherapy* (3rd ed.). New York: Basic Books.

Yeomans, F. (2007). Questions concerning the randomized trial of schema-focused therapy vs. transference-focused psychotherapy. *Archives of General Psychiatry, 64,* 609–610.

Young, J.E. (1994). *Cognitive therapy for personality disorders: A schema-focused approach.* Sarasota, FL, US: Professional Resource Press.

Young, J.E., Klosko, J.S., & Weishaar, M.E. (2003). *Schema therapy: A practitioner's guide.* New York: Guilford Press.

Zaheer, J., Links, P.S., & Liu, E. (2008). Assessment and emergency management of suicidality in personality disorders. *Psychiatric Clinics of North America, 31,* 527–543.

Zanarini, M.C., Frankenburg, F.R., Hennen, J., Reich, D.B., & Silk, K.R. (2006). Prediction of the 10-year course of borderline personality disorder. *American Journal of Psychiatry, 16,* 827–832.

Zanarini, M.C., Frankenburg, F.R., Hennen, J., & Silk, K.R. (2004). Mental health service utilization by borderline personality disorder patients and Axis II comparison subjects followed prospectively for 6 years. *Journal of Clinical Psychiatry, 65,* 28–36.

Zweig-Frank, H., Paris, J., & Guzder, J. (1994). Psychological risk factors for dissociation and self-mutilation in female patients with borderline personality disorder. *Canadian Journal of Psychiatry, 39,* 259–264.

Index